Ethnic Factors in Pain Management:
Is Anyone Listening?

William Edward Ackerman III, MD

Ethnic Factors In Pain Management: Is Anyone Listening?

Copyright © 2016 by William Edward Ackerman III, MD

LCCN: 2016906097

Publisher: Create Space: **City:** Charleston, South Carolina

This book is dedicated to my significant other whom I love and cherish.

Acknowledgments

I wish to acknowledge my patients and staff. Patient populations in most clinical settings are diverse. Therefore, one would not expect a "one size fits all" medical management approach to be successful. My patients and staff are diverse. My success as a pain management physician is due to the fact that I recognize that no patients are biologically the same and that gender, ethnicity, age and diversity must be taken into consideration when treating any pain patient.

Thanks to President Obama and the Surgeon General of the United States, Vivek Murthy MD for their support and implementation of the National Precision Medicine Initiative. Dr. Murthy was the president of Doctors for America, a non-profit organization comprised of more than 16,000 physicians and medical students in all 50 states who work with patients and policymakers to build a high quality, affordable healthcare system for all.

This goal can be accomplished if physicians understand the importance of these goals and help to implement these goals in their individual practices. Recognition that physicians need to take individual patient variability into account is driving huge interest in 'precision' medicine. In President Barack Obama announced a US $215-million National Precision Medicine Initiative.

Discovering that an intervention works well in certain groups happens rarely and frequently by chance. Researchers typically get disappointing results with a drug in large, population-based trials. This leads them to conduct ad hoc post trial analyses, to try to identify the factors that cause some of the people in the trial to seem to be responsive.

Data from future observations will lead to more specific care for individual patients and should end the "one size fits all" attitude noted in pain management practices that are prevalent today.

Foreword

Considerable evidence demonstrates substantial disparities in the prevalence, treatment, progression and outcomes of pain-related conditions. Elucidating the mechanisms underlying these group differences is of crucial importance in reducing and eliminating disparities in the pain experience. Over recent years, accumulating confirmation has identified a variety of processes, from neurophysiological factors to structural elements of the healthcare system, which may contribute to shaping individual differences in pain.

Ethnicity refers to cultural factors, including nationality, regional culture, ancestry, and language. An example of race is brown, white, or black skin (all from various parts of the world), while an example of ethnicity is German or Spanish ancestry (regardless of race).

Diversity refers to human characteristics that are different from your own and from those of groups to which you belong. Diversity may be visible or invisible. Visible diversity is external and includes age, race, ethnicity, gender, and physical attributes. Invisible diversity includes those attributes that are not readily seen, such as work experience, marital status, educational background, parental status, income, religious beliefs and affiliations, geographic location, or socioeconomic status.

Patient populations in most clinical settings are demographically diverse. The diversity of approaches for lumbar spine pain for example suggests perhaps that the ideal technique has not been determined for the treatment of low back pain. Multidisciplinary approaches to the management of low back pain for example may be expected to be most beneficial in diverse populations as opposed to only one single therapy. The nature of the particular patient population being treated enhances our understanding of potential differences in the definition of symptom issues, variation of clinical practice, and cultural and psychosocial influences. It is unfortunate that many academic pain text books do not address diversity in pain treatments and only present a "one size fits all approach".

Every day, millions of people are taking medications that will not help them. Human characteristics imply diversity and therefore, medical treatments must address ethnicity and diversity to be effective. However, the question that remains to be answered: is anyone listening?

Table of Contents

1. What is Ethnicity?

The specialty of pain management is a challenging practice of medicine. Pain affects all ages, both genders and all ethnic groups. The most prevalent consensus on pain management addresses only the pathology and physiology of a painful disease and subsequently recommends certain generic medications, injections and/or surgical procedures for pain relief without consideration of the important demographics previously mentioned.

Ethnicity refers to ethnic groups and actually the terms can be used interchangeably. Ethnicity pertains to a group of people who share a common heritage, language, culture, religion, and ideologies.

Diversity refers to human characteristics that are different from your own and from those of groups to which you belong. Diversity may be visible or invisible. Visible diversity is external and includes age, race, ethnicity, gender, and physical attributes. Invisible diversity includes those attributes that are not readily seen, such as work experience, marital status, educational background, parental status, income, religious beliefs and affiliations, geographic location, or socioeconomic status. A pain patient population in general is usually demographically diverse.

Patient populations in most clinical settings are diverse. Therefore, one would not expect a "one size fits all" approach to be successful. Once you take a medication, it is transformed in your body by complex chemical reactions. The sum of all chemical reactions within a living body is known as metabolism. Drug metabolism is the body's way of transforming drugs, from the original chemical substance to another chemical so that they can be excreted from your body. Many drugs are converted to active metabolites, which are capable of exerting their own pharmacologic action. Hydrocodone, for example, is converted to hydromorphone, which helps to decrease your pain. The metabolic rate can vary significantly from person to person, and drug dosages that work quickly and effectively in one individual may not work well for another.

Factors such as genetics, environment, nutrition, and age influence drug metabolism. Genetic variation among people can greatly affect the metabolism of some drugs as well. You need to be aware that individuals who metabolize a drug poorly may be prone to overdose even when taking a low dose of the drug. On the other hand, extensive metabolizers of a drug may need a higher dosage of the drug to obtain a therapeutic effect and consequently, your drug may not work for you. Your physician can do genetic testing in many instances to determine what type of drug metabolizer that you are. You will then be prescribed the appropriate medication.

Multidisciplinary approaches to the management of pain may be expected to be most beneficial in diverse populations as opposed to only one single therapy. The exact nature of the particular patient population being treated enhances our understanding of potential differences in the definition of symptom issues, variation of clinical practice, and cultural and psychosocial influences. It is unfortunate that many academic pain text books do not address diversity in pain treatments and only present a "one size fits all approach".

Human characteristics imply diversity and therefore, medical treatments must address this diversity to be effective. It is now well documented that substantial disparities exist in the quality and quantity of medical care received by minority Americans, especially those of African, Asian and Hispanic heritage. Research on disparities in the treatment of pain has shown that minorities receive less aggressive pain management than non-minorities.[1] In addition; the special needs and responses to pharmaceutical treatment of these groups have been undervalued or ignored. Age, gender and ethnicity must be given consideration to each patient before a rational treatment plan can be formulated. Unfortunately, this is not always the case. Patients are currently treated in many occasions with a "cookbook" approach.

In most instances, ethnicity or effects on race are not included in many of the studies originally done by pharmaceutical companies with respect to each company's specific medication. Racial and ethnic minorities unfortunately tend to receive a lower quality of healthcare than non-minorities. Patients can benefit from culturally appropriate education programs to improve their knowledge of how to access care and their ability to participate in clinical-decision making.

A therapeutic goal should be to inform patients, pharmacists, care givers and families that a "one size fits all" approach is not relevant for effective pain management. It is anticipated that someday a patient will be able to discuss applicable pain management modalities with his or her medical provider in order to outline potential appropriate treatment options. In other words, why is a particular drug any better than its competitor drug? It is unreasonable for one to believe that a specific arthritis drug, for example, will be generally effective in all ages, both genders and all ethnic groups.

In some instances however, age, gender, and race/ethnicity have no clinically relevant effects on the steady-state pharmacokinetics of some drugs in healthy adults. Therefore, dosage adjustments based on these covariates are unnecessary. A patient must understand that a particular drug that helps one patient may not help another. The best overall pain-management treatment is one that is tailored to all patients as individuals with attention to age, gender and ethnicity. A flexible combination of pharmacological agents and physical therapy and/or manipulative therapy must be individually designed for each patient.

The basic principles underlying personalized medicine require a treating physician take into account not only empirically based guidelines, but also the individual characteristics of the person needing therapy. Bias, stereotyping, prejudice, and clinical uncertainty on the part of healthcare providers may contribute to racial and ethnic disparities in healthcare. It must not be forgotten that one's environment, diet, age, lifestyle, and state of health all influence a person's response to a medicine.

The healthcare workforce and its ability to deliver quality care for racial and ethnic minorities can be improved substantially by increasing the proportion of underrepresented racial and ethnic minorities among health care professionals. Racial and ethnic minorities are more likely than whites to be enrolled in lower-end health plans, which are characterized by higher per capita resource constraints and strict limits on covered medical services. Equalizing access to high-quality plans can limit such fragmentation. Public healthcare payers such as Medicaid should strive to help beneficiaries access the same health products as privately-insured patients.

It is with great hope that racial and ethnic disparities in healthcare exist and are recognized and that positive actions must be undertaken by all individuals involved in health care to end these inequalities. Given that ethnic groups may differ in the outcomes of specific treatments, ethnicity should be one factor that clinicians consider when selecting and recommending treatments. There is no reason for certain diverse groups to receive suboptimal treatment, and greater efforts should be made to offer consistent treatment to all patients. There is also a need for improved training for health care providers and educational interventions for patients.

Ethnic differences in the perception, experience, and impact of pain have received growing attention in recent years.[2] Race and ethnicity influence the presentation and treatment of chronic pain. A significant proportion of this research has been carried out in the USA, and reveals that African–Americans, compared to non-Hispanic whites, suffer a greater burden of pain and pain-related suffering. Pain was reported to be highly prevalent across ethnic groups, and there are racial and ethnic differences in pain experience and treatment preferences.[3] Revealing the mechanisms underlying these inequalities are of crucial importance in reducing and eliminating disparities in the pain experience. Physicians in general sometimes treat women and minorities less aggressively for their pain.[4]

An example of inequality in care is that Black patients with heart failure have a poorer prognosis than white patients, a difference that has not been adequately explained.[5] Whether racial differences in the response to drug treatment contribute to differences in this outcome is unclear. The mortality rate of Black Americans with heart failure is at least 30% higher than that of White Americans.[6] When treated in a conventional manner, available data have been inconsistent, and reliable drug efficacy has not been demonstrated.

It is anticipated that an enhanced understanding of genetic contributions to pain responses will ultimately improve diagnosis and treatment of clinical pain conditions. Increasing evidence suggests that genetic factors contribute significantly to individual differences in responses to both clinical and experimental pain.[7] When treating pain, gender and racial differences were evident only when the role of physician gender was examined, suggesting that male and female physicians may react differently to gender and/or racial cues.8

Approximately 20 per cent of new drugs approved in the past six years demonstrated differences in exposure and/or response across racial/ethnic groups, translating to population-specific prescribing recommendations in a few cases.[9] Most patients were willing to undergo molecular testing and minimally invasive procedures to guide approved or experimental therapy. There were significant differences in attitudes toward molecular testing between racial groups; nonwhites were less willing to undergo testing even if the results would guide their own therapy.[10]

Is anyone listening? Yes, evidence demonstrates that individuals in medical science are beginning to listen and are attempting to promote action which will ultimately improve the diagnosis and treatment of not only clinical pain conditions but also in most other medical specialties as well.

References

1.   Weisse CS, Foster KK, Fisher EA. The influence of experimenter gender and race on pain reporting: does racial or gender concordance matter? Pain Med. 2005;6(1):80-87.

2.   Edwards RR, Moric M, Husfeldt B, Buvanendran A, Ivankovich O. Ethnic similarities and differences in the chronic pain experience: a comparison of african american, Hispanic, and white patients. Pain Med. 2005;6(1):88-98.

3.   Portenoy RK, Ugarte C, Fuller I, Haas G. Population-based survey of pain in the United States: differences among white, African American, and Hispanic subjects. J Pain. 2004;5(6):317-328.

4.   Weisse CS, Sorum PC, Dominguez RE. The influence of gender and race on physicians' pain management decisions. J Pain. 2003;4(9):505-510.

5.   Exner DV, Dries DL, Domanski MJ, Cohn JN. Lesser response to angiotensin-converting-enzyme inhibitor therapy in black as compared with white patients with left ventricular dysfunction. N Engl J Med. 2001;344(18):1351-1357.

6.   . Yancy CW. Heart failure in blacks: etiologic and epidemiologic differences. Curr Cardiol Rep. 2001;3(3):191-197.

7.   Fillingim RB, Wallace MR, Herbstman DM, Ribeiro-Dasilva M, Staud R. Genetic contributions to pain: a review of findings in humans. Oral Dis. 2008;14(8):673-682.

8.   Weisse CS, Sorum PC, Sanders KN, Syat BL. Do gender and race affect decisions about pain management? J Gen Intern Med. 2001;16(4):211-217.

9.   Ramamoorthy A, Pacanowski MA, Bull J, Zhang L. Racial/ethnic differences in drug disposition and response: review of recently approved drugs. Clin Pharmacol Ther. 2015;97(3):263-273.

10.   Yusuf RA, Rogith D, Hovick SR, et al. Attitudes toward molecular testing for personalized cancer therapy. Cancer. 2015;121(2):243-250.

2. Disparities in Pain Treatments

US Census reports show that 1 in 4 Americans are of a race other than White; 1 in 3 children are African American, Hispanic, or Asian; and 1 in 10 people are foreign-born. Racial and gender disparities in health are well documented in health science literature. Racial minorities and women are known to receive disproportionately poorer quality of health care when compared to non-Hispanic Whites. It is unknown why women and particular racial and ethnic minorities are more susceptible to experience disparities in patient care. However, it's unwise, even false and prejudicial, to assume that everyone from a certain culture will respond the same way.

Moreover, with pain being the most common complaint for those entering the healthcare system, gaps in understanding the potential relationship between the nurse provider's gender and/or race and ethnicity and pain management deserve exploration. When illness or injury strikes, White patients are typically intolerant to pain, unlike many other cultures, where pain is seen as part of life. White patients also have a high expectation that their disease will be cured, or at least well managed, through technology and powerful drugs.

Each ethnic group brings its own perspectives and values to the health care system, and many health care beliefs and health practices differ from those of the traditional American health care culture. Unfortunately, the expectation of many health care professionals has been that patients will conform to mainstream values. Such expectations have frequently created barriers to care that have been compounded by differences in language and education between patients and providers from different backgrounds

Race refers to a person's physical characteristics, such as bone structure and skin, hair, or eyes. Ethnicity, however, refers to cultural factors, including nationality, regional culture, ancestry, and language.[1] Some genetic disorders are more likely to occur among people who trace their ancestry to a particular geographic area. People in an ethnic group often share certain versions of their genes, which have been passed down from common ancestors. If one of these shared genes contains a disease-causing mutation, a particular genetic disorder may be more frequently seen in the group.

Examples of genetic conditions that are more common in particular ethnic groups are sickle cell anemia, which is more common in people of African, African American, or Mediterranean heritage; and Tay-Sachs disease, which is more likely to occur among people of Ashkenazi (eastern and central European) Jewish or French Canadian ancestry. It is important to note, however, that these disorders can occur in any ethnic group. African Americans and Native Americans often doubt the need for medications when symptoms ease, and may discontinue drugs like antibiotics and antidepressants.

A patient's race or ethnic background influences how medications are metabolized. Common genetic polymorphisms (multiple forms of enzymes used for drug metabolism) affect the metabolism of many important medications. For some polymorphisms, the proportion of rapid metabolizers and slow metabolizers varies based on ethnicity. For example, only 3% to 5% of Whites are poor metabolizers of drugs affected by mephenytoin polymorphism (e.g., diazepam, imipramine), but 15% to 20% of Chinese and Japanese are poor metabolizes of mephenytoin and related drugs. Ethnic differences in the metabolism of specific drugs may differ within a class.

There are some diseases that have very limited distributions around the world due to the fact that they are caused by unique combinations of environmental circumstances and cultural practices. Kuru is a specific disease of the brain and nervous system. Death almost always occurs within 6-12 months of the onset of symptoms. Dr. Carleton Gajdusek came to Papua, New Guinea to try to study the disease. Through the microscopic examination of tissue from people who died of Kuru, he discovered that the disease organism was carried in the blood and was concentrated in brain tissue. The means of transmission was cannibalism.

The South Foré ate their dead relatives as part of their funerary practices. Kuru is closely related to two other well-known fatal diseases that affect the brain and nervous system. The disease has been connected to eating beef from cattle that had acquired the disease as a result of eating food supplements made from ground up dead sheep and perhaps other farm animals.

Racial prejudice remains a continuing problem throughout the world. It is known that the causes and treatment of pain are different for men and women of different ethnic groups. The study of the differences between how men and women feel pain and are treated for it is a relatively new branch of medicine. Your age, physical design, hormones, psychological issues, and social issues all play a part in why you feel pain. These things also determine how your doctor will treat your pain. In the future, doctors will be able to design treatments that are specific to men and women.

Pharmacogenomics is the study of how an individual's genome influences his or her response to a specific drug. Pharmacogenetics is the study of individual genetic differences in drug absorption, metabolism, distribution, and excretion. Pharmacogenetics is a field that seeks to unravel the genetic underpinnings of variable drug responses. Some polymorphisms that raise variability in drug metabolism occur at higher frequencies in the genomes of particular races. The P-glycoprotein (PGP) is a transporter that distributes many types of drugs, including those used in chemotherapy. Globally, there is an immense genetic variation in the gene encoding PGP. What is interesting in the case of PGP is that different races have been characterized as having higher frequencies of certain PGP polymorphisms. Studies have shown that African people have about an 80% chance of having one specific version while Asian and European peoples have half that chance. [2]

The advent of BiDil marks the first drug in America to be marketed exclusively for African Americans. Data from the trial that studied the effects of BiDil on congestive heart failure among African American patients showed a 43% improvement in survival rate.[3] The following diseases are examples of cases where consideration of race has been played a strong role in directing advances in healthcare and the applicability of pharmacogenomics. BRCA1 and BRCA2, two of the genes associated with the onset of breast cancer, have several polymorphisms identified .[4] In particular, three polymorphisms in these two genes are approximately ten times more prevalent in Ashkenazi Jewish women than in American women.

In Type-2 diabetes mellitus, the primary defect responsible for this disease is varied among populations, especially in Japanese and Caucasians. As the development of type-2 diabetes can arise from two different paths (i.e., impaired insulin secretion or impaired insulin sensitivity), recent studies have shown that diabetes in Japanese people arise primarily through problems in secretion whereas Caucasian diabetics primarily have problems with sensitivity. [5]

Phenylketonuria (PKU). PKU is an autosomal recessive metabolic condition that has been used as a classic model for teaching hereditary diseases in biology. The occurrence of PKU varies among different races (1/10,000 in Caucasians, 1/120,000 in Japanese, and 1/41,000 in Koreans). [6] Colorectal cancer Greater drug efficacy was found in tumor cells with particular mutations, confirming the effectiveness of treatment options based on genetic information.[7]

With regard to the health disparities associated with race, it has been noted that more than 29 drugs have been claimed by various literatures to have different levels of efficacy among different racial groups.[8] These differences may be attributable to intrinsic factors, extrinsic factors, or interactions between these factors. For example, in the United States, Whites are more likely than persons of Asian and African heritage to have abnormally low levels of an important enzyme (CYP2D6) that metabolizes drugs belonging to a variety of therapeutic areas, such as antidepressants, antipsychotics, and beta blockers.[9][10]

Other studies have shown that Blacks respond poorly to several classes of antihypertensive agents (beta blockers and angiotensin converting enzyme (ACE) inhibitors)[9] Although the FDA has long requested race and ethnicity data on subjects in certain clinical trials, the Agency has not previously made explicit recommendations on the categories to use when collecting and reporting the data. The race categories can be modified to reflect the following, as appropriate: American Indian or Alaska Native, Asian, Black, Native Hawaiian or Other Pacific Islander or White.

Ethnicity is one factor that may account for the observed differences in both pharmacokinetics (PK) and pharmacodynamics (PD) of drugs, resulting in variability in response to drug therapy. Given that the applicability of clinical study results to the treatment of an individual patient is a critical consideration in a physician's choice of drug therapy, drug development should seek to ensure that a clinical pharmacologic evaluation includes a population that is representative of the target therapeutic population.

Ethnic diversity in drug response with respect to safety and efficacy and the resulting differences in recommended doses have been well described for some drugs. Some of these differential responses may be related to the pharmacogenomics of a particular drug. In the early 1980s, clinical differences in response to the blood pressure lowering effects of β-blockers and, to a lesser extent, diuretics were noted between ethnic groups.

Pain is a very individual and personal experience. Things that cause pain in you may not cause pain in someone else. Without a psychological component to your type of pain, the repeated experience of the same type of pain would not be considered to be as painful as the first episode. This is the reason why a professional football player continues to play in a big game in spite of a broken bone. The psychology of the game distracts the broken-bone pain. Pain perception varies between person to person based on gender and age. When you feel pain, your response is to stay away from everything that would cause you to feel more pain. This is the response that aids your body in tissue healing.

Examining within-race-group variability suggests that chronic pain differentially affects the quality of life and health status of black Americans and white Americans across age groups. Intra race differences exist among black and white Americans presenting for chronic pain management. Ethnic differences in the metabolism of specific drugs may differ within a class. Previous studies indicated that patients from Black, Asian and minority ethnic groups tend to receive less analgesics compared to Caucasian (White) patients after similar surgical procedures.[11]

Differences between men and women exist with physical characteristics, hormones, and social expectations, just to name a few. One of the reasons men and women feel pain differently has to do with hormones. Sex differences affect the absorption, metabolism (breakdown of drugs), and excretion (elimination of drugs) of many medications.

Women respond more favorably to a class of antidepressant medications called serotonin-specific reuptake inhibitors, or SSRIs (Prozac), than to other antidepressants known as tricyclics (Elavil). Sexual differences between men and women are important with respect to drug action. A medication that works well for one person with schizophrenia often doesn't work well for another. Genetic variations are thought to play a key role in this difference in response. While patients search for the right medications, their illnesses may worsen.

The way receptors respond to drugs and hormones effects the body's response to both drugs and hormones. For example, giving estrogen to a man does not affect his brain like it does a woman. In the same way, giving androgens (male hormones) to a female brain does not cause the same response as in a male. Researchers have therefore concluded that hormone and hormonal receptor differences between men and women also influence the regulation and transmission of the nervous impulses that transmit pain. Estrogen (the female hormone) affects the central nervous system levels of dopamine and serotonin, which are involved with mood disorders.

Women experience more depression than males. Men may have more serotonin receptors, which may be a reason why they suffer from a lower incidence of depression. As a result, a woman's greater sensitivity to pain may be dependent on the fact that she has less serotonin in the brain and spinal cord. Studies show that sex hormones modulate neural function and affect the central nervous system with respect to the perception of pain. In rats hormone receptors for male and female hormones are also present and modulate the function of the peripheral nerves (nerves outside the brain and spinal cord).[12]

Neurons are not in direct contact with each other; in order to communicate with each other, they rely on highly specialized chemicals called neurotransmitters. Neurotransmitters are chemical messengers that coordinate the transmission of signals from one nerve cell (neuron) to the next. These all important brain chemicals interact with target sites called receptors located throughout the brain and body to regulate a wide variety of processes including emotions, fear, pleasure, joy, anger, mood, memory, cognition, attention, concentration, alertness, energy, appetite, cravings, sleep, and the perception of pain. Furthermore, neurotransmitters chemically link the brain and spinal cord with the rest of your body: muscles, organs, and glands. The four major neurotransmitters that regulate mood are Serotonin, Dopamine, GABA and Norepinephrine. The Inhibitory System comprises mainly GABA and serotonin. There are no good studies that have shown neurotransmitter ethnic differences but there are gender differences.

When you are reading this book, you may be struck by the diversity of factors that affect your pain diagnosis and pain management whether these factors are genetic, hormonal, psychological, physiological, or pharmacological or all combined. You should now be aware that women and men really are different and that ethnicity can affect pain treatment.[13]

Ultimately, a better understanding of these differences is necessary to enhance your doctor's ability to diagnose and treat all types of pain. Studies into how and why men and women feel pain differently have begun in the past few years. These studies are important and must cross the life cycle of men and women, because age can also affect hormones and physical characteristics. In the future, your doctor will be able to use such research to design treatments that will work just for you.

Pain perception will vary from person to person. While, men and women report the same number of negative (or adverse) reactions during and following treatment with therapeutic medications, negative effects of medicines are higher and more serious in women than in men. This disparity may be influenced by the fact that women use medications more often than men and in different doses, and also because the different ways the drugs are absorbed, metabolized (broken down), and removed from the body by men and women.

Women often report more migraine headaches and arthritic pain than men. Women also have a greater discomfort for the same type of pain than men and are more likely to develop long-term pain after an injury. Women also use more over-the-counter pain medications and have more doctor visits than men. Because of these differences, research is being done on why women are more likely to suffer from painful conditions than men and which medications work better for men and women.

Reviews of major medical journals show clinical drug studies rarely test to determine how medication will affect different ethnic and men and women differently. Women are excluded from many clinical drug study trials. Because of the potential for pregnancy and the potential harmful effects of a new drug on a developing baby, most researchers have been hesitant to include women in their studies. Early studies primarily consisted of male prisoners.

In 1993, Congress made it mandatory that women, as well as minorities, be included in clinical drug trials. Also in 1993, the FDA began allowing women of child-bearing age to take part in clinical drug trials. In 1994, the National Institutes of Health issued guidelines to grant applications to confirm that researchers complied with the inclusion of women of child-bearing age in their studies. Recent studies in 1997 showed that women exceeded 50 percent of the study participants. (U.S. Food and Drug Administration website, www.fda.gov).

Published clinical trial results today often include data analyzing how the studied drug affected men and women. Data submitted to the FDA for drug approval must include the gender, age, height, and weight of each participant. It also has been recommended that the data include whether any participating women are pre- or postmenopausal, because levels of hormones can affect how pain much pain is felt. However, ethnicity differences in drug efficacy needs to be addressed as well. Only few laboratory studies have examined race differences in pain perception.

The anatomic differences between men and women also influence their reactions to medications. In general, women have lower body weights and organ sizes and a higher percentage of body fat, factors that need to be taken into account when discussing the way the body handles drugs and their use in men and women. For example, the muscle relaxant Valium (diazepam) causes more impairment of voluntary muscle control in women than in men, probably because of lower body weight of women as compared to men.

There are no good generalized studies to date with reference to ethnicity and drug absorption. It is known however, that Asians and Eskimos need lower doses of anxiolytics than white patients. Asians, Indians, and Pakistanis require lower doses of lithium and antipsychotic drugs. African Americans' symptoms generally improve faster after taking neuroleptics and anxiolytics. Hispanics may require lower doses of antidepressants than Whites. Since various drugs within the same class are often cleared by different metabolic pathways, ethnic differences in the metabolism of specific drugs may differ within a class and further studies are certainly necessary to confirm this hypothesis.[14-16]

Differences in drug reactions are caused by differences in the way men and women process drugs.[17] The transport of drugs within the bloodstream and the chemicals that break down drugs differ in men and women. Enzymes in the liver help break down drugs. One of these enzymes is the CYP 3A4 liver enzyme. This enzyme breaks down more than 50 percent of all therapeutic drugs. In women, drugs that have been metabolized in the liver are delivered more slowly to the bloodstream, where they are then sent to the kidneys for excretion from the body. Because more of the pain medications are not taken out of the liver, a higher concentration of these drugs in the liver requires processing. The liver enzymes in women have to process higher concentrations of the drugs than males. Liver enzymes in women may also not metabolize the antidepressants of the selective serotonin-specific reuptake inhibitor class.

Women have a lower stomach acid secretion than men. This can increase the absorption of more basic drugs such as Elavil or Valium, and decrease the absorption of acidic drugs such as Dilantin and barbiturates. Women weigh less than men and have a lower total blood value than men. Body fat is 11 percent higher in women between the ages of 25 and 35. After a drug is absorbed from either the stomach or the small intestine, the drug is distributed throughout the tissues in the body.

Drugs that have a high affinity for fat and are called fat-soluble drugs. If an individual has a high body fat content, some drugs may rapidly enter the fatty tissue. This action will decrease the level of medication in the blood and make it less effective. However, if repetitive administration of a drug causes a high concentration of that drug in body fat, it will eventually be released back into the bloodstream, which can cause a significantly higher blood level of the drug at that time.

The liver breaks down and eliminates most drugs. Biologic systems, including the liver, may be more efficient in men than in women. Drugs may be eliminated from the body more effectively by the kidneys in men when compared to women. As a result, equal doses of medication could result in a higher blood level of that particular drug in a woman than in a man. [18] This in turn could cause serious side effects in the woman but not in the man.

The effects of hormones on neurotransmitters in the brain during the premenstrual cycle can affect the sensitivity of neurotransmitters or nervous system receptors. A doctor may have to increase the total dosage of a specific medication throughout the entire menstrual cycle and may have to decrease the medication two to three days after the cycle has been completed.

Oral contraceptives used by some women can decrease the effect of anti-anxiety drugs such as the Valium. Studies are currently investigating whether estrogen can be effective in treating depression in women. The effects of estrogen on certain drugs in postmenopausal women is also currently under study.

Men and women respond differently to antidepressant medications. In women, pre- and postmenopausal effects must be taken into account when prescribing an antidepressant medication. Age also influences the effects of drugs. Because older people break down drugs more slowly in their livers, older individuals typically need a smaller dose of a drug. However, age effects are less prevalent in women than in men.

Older men have a decreased ability to excrete drugs than women. Age can also influence how sensitive you may be to pain. The intensity of pain felt by children lessens as they grow older. As puberty approaches, girls will notice and report more pain than boys do. To date there are no good studies with reference to age/ethnicity drug dosing effects.

Gender bias can occur in a doctor's management of pain. Men and women are treated differently by some doctors because of a gender-stereotyped attitude. Both men and women doctors contribute to the gender-disparate treatment.[19] Patient–physician communication during medical visits differs among African American versus White patients. Interventions that increase physicians' patient-centeredness and awareness of affective cues with African Americans patients and that activate African American patients to participate in their health care are important strategies for addressing racial/ethnic disparities in health care.

Ethnic minorities are poorly represented among physicians and other health professionals.[20] In what is called "race-discordant" relationships, patients from ethnic groups frequently are treated by professionals from a different ethnic background. While Hispanics, African Americans, and Native Americans represent more than 25 percent of the U.S. population, they comprise fewer than 6 percent of doctors and 9 percent of nurses. [21] Black and Hispanic Americans sought care from physicians of their own race because of personal preference and language, not solely because of geographic accessibility.

In summary, there is reasonable evidence that patient–provider race concordance is associated with better patient ratings of care among adult primary care patients. The need for concerted quality-improvement efforts to ensure that all patients, regardless of race/ethnicity, receive optimal access to pain relief.[22] There is no reason for certain groups to receive suboptimal treatment, and greater efforts should be made to offer consistent treatment to all patients.

References

1.   Tan AK, Duman I, Taskaynatan MA, Hazneci B, Kalyon TA. The effect of gabapentin in earlier stage of reflex sympathetic dystrophy. Clinical rheumatology. 2007;26(4):561-565.

2.   Kim SH, Ye YM, Palikhe NS, Kim JE, Park HS. Genetic and ethnic risk factors associated with drug hypersensitivity. Curr Opin Allergy Clin Immunol. 2010;10(4):280-290.

3.   Taylor PR, Bell RE. Combined carotid and coronary artery disease. Acta Chir Belg. 2004;104(6):622-625.

4.   McClain MR, Nathanson KL, Palomaki GE, Haddow JE. An evaluation of BRCA1 and BRCA2 founder mutations penetrance estimates for breast cancer among Ashkenazi Jewish women. Genet Med. 2005;7(1):34-39.

5.   Martin BC, Warram JH, Krolewski AS, Bergman RN, Soeldner JS, Kahn CR. Role of glucose and insulin resistance in development of type 2 diabetes mellitus: results of a 25-year follow-up study. Lancet. 1992;340(8825):925-929.

6.   Aoki H, Akao M, Ito A, Nakamura S. [Crystal chemistry of hydroxyapatite]. Kokubyo Gakkai Zasshi. 1988;55(3):451-459.

7.   Etienne MC, Ilc K, Formento JL, et al. Thymidylate synthase and methylenetetrahydrofolate reductase gene polymorphisms: relationships with 5-fluorouracil sensitivity. Br J Cancer. 2004;90(2):526-534.

8.   Goldstein DB, Hirschhorn JN. In genetic control of disease, does 'race' matter? Nat Genet. 2004;36(12):1243-1244.

9.	Exner DV, Dries DL, Domanski MJ, Cohn JN. Lesser response to angiotensin-converting-enzyme inhibitor therapy in black as compared with white patients with left ventricular dysfunction. N Engl J Med. 2001;344(18):1351-1357.

10.	Xie HG, Kim RB, Wood AJ, Stein CM. Molecular basis of ethnic differences in drug disposition and response. Annu Rev Pharmacol Toxicol. 2001;41:815-850.

11.	Al-Hashimi M, Scott S, Griffin-Teall N, Thompson J. Influence of ethnicity on the perception and treatment of early post-operative pain. Br J Pain. 2015;9(3):167-172.

12.	Gleiter CH, Gundert-Remy U. Gender differences in pharmacokinetics. Eur J Drug Metab Pharmacokinet. 1996;21(2):123-128.

13.	Lin MY, Kressin NR. Race/ethnicity and Americans' experiences with treatment decision making. Patient Educ Couns. 2015.

14.	Li J, Lao X, Zhang C, Tian L, Lu D, Xu S. Increased genetic diversity of ADME genes in African Americans compared with their putative ancestral source populations and implications for pharmacogenomics. BMC Genet. 2014;15:52.

15.	El Desoky ES, Sabarinath SN, Hamdi MM, Bewernitz M, Derendorf H. Population pharmacokinetics of steady-state carbamazepine in Egyptian epilepsy patients. J Clin Pharm Ther. 2012;37(3):352-355.

16.	Musshoff F, Stamer UM, Madea B. Pharmacogenetics and forensic toxicology. Forensic Sci Int. 2010;203(1-3):53-62.

17.	Ohana S, Mash R. Physician and patient perceptions of cultural competency and medical compliance. Health Educ Res. 2015;30(6):923-934.

18.	Burt J, Lloyd C, Campbell J, Roland M, Abel G. Variations in GP-patient communication by ethnicity, age, and gender: evidence from a national primary care patient survey. Br J Gen Pract. 2016;66(642):e47-52.

19.	Maldonado ME, Fried ED, DuBose TD, Nelson C, Breida M. The role that graduate medical education must play in ensuring health equity and eliminating health care disparities. Ann Am Thorac Soc. 2014;11(4):603-607.

20.	Simon AE, Marsteller JA, Lin SX. Physician-patient race concordance from the physician perspective. Journal of the National Medical Association. 2013;105(2):150-156.

21.	Vina ER, Utset TO, Hannon MJ, Masi CM, Roberts N, Kwoh CK. Racial differences in treatment preferences among lupus patients: a two-site study. Clin Exp Rheumatol. 2014;32(5):680-688.

22.　　Shah AA, Zogg CK, Zafar SN, et al. Analgesic Access for Acute Abdominal Pain in the Emergency Department Among Racial/Ethnic Minority Patients: A Nationwide Examination. Medical care. 2015;53(12):1000-1009.

3. Pain Intensity Reporting in Diverse Groups

Pain costs almost $100 billion a year in the United States. Each year, more than 500 million work days are lost, and 40 million doctor visits are made for the treatment of painful conditions. According to the Wall Street Journal in 2001, until the past decade, no new pain treatments had been developed for more than 30 years. With the beginning of the pain medicine specialty, new methods for the treatment of pain are becoming more available. And as research is developed, new methods that have fewer side effects and are more effective are being developed. You do not need to fear a lifetime of agony as a result of your pain. Research into the processes that cause pain has resulted in the development of more drugs to block nervous system pathways that transmit pain in your body.

Sex, gender, and ethnic differences exist in the pathophysiology, diagnosis, and provision of care for patients with pain. In other words sex, gender, and ethnic differences exist in the pathophysiology, diagnosis, and provision of care for patients with pain. Sex, gender, ethnicity, and religion are powerful factors that affect a patient's pain experience.[1] Recently, gender role expectations of pain were suggested to account for some of the differences in pain perception between men and women.[2]

Some researchers have implied that gender and ethnic differences with respect to the treatment and management of your pain are relatively minor. However, other researchers have reported that gender and ethnic differences significantly influence responses to pain. Which of these opinions is correct? Both may be correct. Be aware that pain research can be influenced by whether the study is in an experimental situation or an acute or chronic pain situation.[3] Pain treatment should be based on science because there is not "a one size fits all" treatment approach.

During laboratory experiments and clinical trials, gender differences are well documented with respect to pain responses. The problem that exists among doctors who treat pain in their day to day practices is that many do not identify gender or ethnic differences, which can influence your pain diagnosis and treatment. As discussed in Chapter 1, studies of large numbers of people (epidemiological data) clearly show that women are at greater risk for developing certain pain syndromes than men and that these is a result of hormonal factors and other differences between the sexes but are not significantly related to ethnic differences.

Women have more frequent/intense heartburn and extra-esophageal symptoms and more discomfort from abdominal pain, indigestion and constipation than men. Comorbid anxiety and depression may contribute to the increased symptom burden in women.[4] With respect to post-surgical pain, women have more pain and slower recovery of shoulder motion than men during the first 3 months after rotator cuff repair.[5] Women have higher initial pain levels in the acute whiplash injury. Age and ethnicity have less impact on those pain levels.[6] Pain is common among older adults and there are significant differences between the sexes. With women reporting higher pain intensity the men.[7]

Hormonal differences between men and women may account for the fact that predominantly those seeking pain management treatment are women. Whether a woman is experiencing her menstrual cycle also significantly influences her response to pain and medication. In other words, a female with a pain syndrome may respond differently from one day to the next depending on where she is in her menstrual cycle. At one time it was thought that the menstrual cycles in animals were obstacles to experimental research.

However, with the advancement of gender-specific medicine, it is thought that the menstrual cycles in laboratory animals are opportunities. The problem in doing gender-specific pain medicine studies arises from the emphasis on the equality of the sexes that became dominant in the 1980s. This factor may have delayed the onset of gender-specific medical research. It has been reported and demonstrated that sex differentiates the reaction to chronic pain with females reporting more pain than males.[8]

Many factors determine how well a particular medicine will work on your body. Pain is your body's way of telling you that something is harming your body. For example, chest pain tells you that you may be having a heart attack. Pain will cause your body to become restricted or immobile so that healing can occur. When your pain becomes severe, it tells you to seek medical attention. The problem exists when your body's pain alarm system fails to quit working and the pain continues. When pain becomes uncontrolled, depression, anxiety, and loss of sleep can result, making your perception of the pain worse. The onset of depression or anxiety happens when your pain reduces certain levels of chemicals in your brain and spinal cord.

Pain is an individual experience that is difficult to study. The International Association for the Study of Pain defines pain as an unpleasant emotional and sensory experience that results from tissue injury or the threat of tissue injury. The sensation of pain in different places on your body usually begins with the peripheral nervous system. The peripheral nervous system includes all nerves located outside of your spinal cord and brain, such as in your arms and legs. The spinal cord and brain together are called the central nervous system. Nerve fibers in the peripheral nervous system send painful impulses from nerve endings in your body directly to your spinal cord and brain.

There are two main classes of nerve fibers that transmit pain in your body. The first class of pain fibers is called Alpha delta fibers. These fibers are able to send sharp pain and transmit pain impulses rapidly. The second class of pain fibers is called C fibers. These are smaller fibers and send burning types of pain more slowly than the Alpha delta fibers. If you were to hit your finger with a hammer, you would experience two components of pain. First, you would feel a fast, sharp pain (Alpha delta fiber), followed by a second slow, throbbing or burning (C fiber) pain. The throbbing or burning types pain last longer than sharp pain.

Specific pathways exist that transmit pain information from the damaged part, or tissue, through your spinal cord to a center of pain perception in your brain. When you are hurt, chemicals called neurotransmitters are released by the injured tissue that stimulates your nerve endings to feel pain. As a result, the pain you feel comes from the place of your tissue injury. The effects of several of these neurotransmitters have been studied well. Some of these chemical substances make your nerve endings more sensitive to pain. This process is called transduction.

If a type of neurotransmitter called prostaglandin is in the hurt area of tissue, the size of your blood vessels will grow and increase your blood circulation to that area. This will cause you to have swelling, redness and warmth in the injured area. The pain impulse travels along the length of your nerve to a junction where the nerve enters the spinal cord. This junction between the nerve and the spinal cord is the command center for many pain syndromes. Transmission occurs when the pain impulse from the injured tissue flows to the junction at your spinal cord. From this area, the sensation of pain is transmitted to the back of your spinal cord. When the pain impulse reaches your spinal cord, it can lessen your sensation of pain. This process is called modulation.

Nerves communicate with each another when neurotransmitter chemicals are released, causing other nerves around the injured area to transmit painful impulses. Another chemical released from injured tissue is bradykinin. Bradykinin causes C fibers to transmit pain, and also causes another type of neurotransmitter called prostaglandins to be produced.

Prostaglandins decrease the level of pain tolerance that C fibers can withstand, which causes an increased sensitivity to feelings of pain. There are some medications available that can block these prostaglandins from casing pain. A common prostaglandin blocker is Ibuprofen.

When the pain fibers enter the spinal cord, they terminate in different parts of the spinal cord. Nerve cells in the spinal cord receive and respond to pain impulses from both the large and small fibers. Activation of receptors by the continual bombardment by pain impulses can result in a significant increase in your pain. The spinal cord is "upregulated" to magnify pain impulses and result in excruciating disabling pain.

Another type of pain fiber exists that transmits impulses from the peripheral nervous system to the spinal cord. The third fiber that is important in understanding the transmission of pain are large nerve fibers called A beta fibers. These fibers respond to non-pain-producing stimuli such as touch, pressure or movement of joints. These fibers also end at the spinal cord. They are important because these nerves can either activate or inhibit pain impulses.

The convergence of different types of nerves including pain-producing nerves as well as touch and pressure producing nerves can be a source of an unusual experience referred to as referred pain. Referred pain occurs when an individual feels pain, for example, in the shoulder when the actual pain producing tissue is the heart as is noted when an individual suffers a heart attack. This referred pain from the heart travels to the shoulder because some of the receptors in the spinal cord also receive nervous impulses from both the peripheral nervous system and arms and legs as well as within the organs within the body. In this case, the brain misinterprets the location of the injured tissue stimulus.

When a hammer strikes your finger, rubbing the injured finger can result in considerable pain relief. This phenomenon was explained in 1965 by two pain researchers who published the gate-control theory of pain. Their studies revealed that only a limited amount of sensory information can be processed by the brain and spinal cord at any given moment. When pain fibers from the periphery such as the arms or legs, activate pain transmission cells in the spinal cord, signals from the non-pain-producing large fibers can inhibit or increase activation of these the pain impulses from these pain transmitting nerves.

As a result, pain impulses appear to be dependent on a balance of activity in both the large and small fibers. This is the basis of the gate-control theory of pain. When the balance of nerve activity is directed toward the pain transmission fibers, the gate is open which allows transmission of painful signals to go from the spinal cord to the brain. On the other hand, when the large non-pain fibers predominate electrical impulses, the gate is closed and the pain signals are decreased. In some instances they may be completely blocked.

Once the pain impulses have reached the spinal cord, the pathways for pain are crossed. Pain originating from peripheral nerves on the left side of the body is transmitted to the spinal cord on the right side of the body. Pain transmission then reaches the brain by two main pathways, called tracts. Chronic pain can make pain nerve endings more sensitive which results in more pain that continues to worsen over time. After a while the pain from the pain transmitting fibers can "cross wires" with the large nerves that transmit touch and movement sensation so that even a slight change in movement or light touch can cause severe agony to a patient.

Gender differences in body structure and brain function develop when a fetus is still in the mother's womb. These differences show themselves in childhood. These factors combine with family lifestyles and school and socio-cultural sex roles to act uniquely on the individual. All of these events factor into gender-specific patterns of pain perception. During adolescence, gender differences in pain syndromes emerge, such as dysmenorrhea in women and cluster headaches in men. Smoking and other dangerous activities can influence the onset of these chronic pain syndromes in both men and women.

When acute pain becomes chronic, a self-perpetuating cycle of maladies can occur, resulting in changes in your body as well as behavior that make your pain worse. For example, after an injury, changes can occur in the regrowth of damaged nerve endings and where pain nerves connect with other nerves. This can result in muscle tension, making muscles extra sensitive because they are tense rather than relaxed. The increased stress from chronic pain can increase the release of a naturally occurring chemical in the brain called norepinephrine, eventually leading to its depletion and resulting depression and exhaustion. The depression can magnify the physical pain, which in turn depletes serotonin in both the spinal cord and brain.

Persistent pain can decrease an individual's sleep. This depletes the body's supply of endorphins, chemicals that decrease pain. With the depletion of endorphins, pain can become worse. As a result of the increase in pain, people often place themselves into guarded positions to avoid pain. However, these unnatural positions can strain other muscles, which in turn spread more pain to other parts of the body. Other, unused muscles shrink, or atrophy, with a resulting loss of strength causing more discomfort. The goal and purpose of pain medicine is to interrupt this vicious cycle.

Some pain syndromes are affected by changes in sex hormones. For example, migraine headaches resolve during pregnancy as a result of elevated blood levels of progesterone. Experimental animal pain responses are reduced during lactation as a result of increased progesterone. When estrogen decreases (following menopause, for instance), joint pains increase in females. In men, a decrease in testosterone will increase the frequency of angina. With an increase in testosterone, cluster headaches are more prevalent in men. With an increase in progesterone, testosterone, and estrogen, both men and women experience an equal increase in temporomandibular jaw (TMJ) pain.

Positron Emission Tomography (PET) scanning has shown areas in the brain where sex steroid hormones can affect gender differences in pain control. A PET scan is a nuclear medicine device which enables a physician to assess functional activity of tissue. PET scan imaging has determined that pain can vary from person to person. Furthermore, studies have shown that pain within each person is based on life experiences.

Endorphins, mentioned previously, can shut the gate to pain. Endorphins are natural morphine like drugs (chemically related to opium) that switch off the pain alarm. Several types have been identified that modulate pain at the spinal cord and the brain. Because pain can affect breathing, blood flow, heart rate, and digestion, the body naturally releases endorphins to deal with pain. Moreover, pain can affect the limbic system, which is a complex area of nerve pathways in the brain that controls emotions such as mood, self-preservation, rage, fear, and pleasure. Certain areas of the spinal cord contain high concentrations of endorphin receptors. The body also produces enkephalins and dynorphins, two neurochemicals also involved in pain modulation. Another important neurochemical is gamma aminobutyric acid (GABA), an inhibitory pain mediator. GABA inhibits pain transmission in the spinal cord.

Genetics also produce gender-related pain differences. Gender-linked genetic disorders affect both males and females. Chromosome differences in two strains of mice have revealed different perception to opioid therapy in male mice. Stress can influence an animal's response to pain. There is a difference in stress-induced analgesia between male and female rodents, with the females having a greater pain response to stress. The reason for this observation is unknown and is believed not to be a result of the effect of hormones. On the other hand, estrogen, a female hormone, regulates the formation of the pain transmitter chemical substance P as well as some of the other chemicals in the nervous system that do cause pain.

Women go through a 5 to 10 year period of menopause. During this time, changes occur in hormones, most notably a decrease in the hormones in the female bloodstream. In men hormone changes occur over approximately 20 years. Body structure changes occur in both males and females. Lifestyle changes also occur during this time. Increases in the incidence of disease occur during this time in both men and women. There also is an alteration of drug metabolism in both men and women.

During adulthood, social roles and lifestyles become entrenched. Be aware that health-care providers also have ideas that have become entrenched with respect to gender specificity in pain management. Not only does lifestyle affect one's perception of pain, this in combination with nutrition and hormone status combine to affect one's perception of pain.

Nicotine can have a gender-specific effect on pain as well. [9] Doctors usually ask their patients about recent nicotine use. When conducting research, however, many researchers fail to ask their subjects about nicotine consumption. It has been shown that nicotine increases the amount of stimulus needed to cause pain in men but not in women. Smokers had more severe postoperative pain and required a higher quantity of postoperative opioid than nonsmokers. With increasing nicotine dependence, postoperative pain severity and postoperative opioid requirement increased.[10]

In human patients, the effects of pain-relieving drugs are greater in men than in women. Men report greater pain relief than women when morphine or morphine like drugs are used for pain control. In contrast, drugs that stimulate other receptors than the morphine receptors, such as butorphanol (Stadol), provide greater pain relief in women than men in a clinical setting.

According to physiologic cardiovascular parameters, male rodents exhibit greater levels of analgesia following stressful laboratory manipulations than female rodents. This may be a result of the effects of stress on the pain systems in these animals. It is known that significant differences exist between men and women as to sensitivity to painful stimuli. Laboratory studies show that sex hormones do affect pain perception. When sex hormones are at their peak in the female, pain sensitivity is decreased.

Women have a higher incidence of migraine headaches, with an aura that precedes the headaches. An aura is a sensation which forewarns of an attack of a neurological condition, such as migraine.

Men can have migraine headaches, but do not usually experience an aura. Females suffer more from chronic tension headaches related to an increase in muscle tone, whereas men suffer more from something called cluster headaches. Women often suffer spinal headaches after epidural needle placement from childbirth. They often suffer spinal headaches as a result of epidural needle placement for surgery or for myelograms as opposed to men. Women experience a higher incidence of headaches that begin in the neck and go to the rear ridges of the skull or to the top of the head. These different types of headaches are discussed later in this book. Women have a greater vulnerability to increased pain awareness in the brain and spinal cord than men, which is believed to be related to estrogen. Women experience a higher incidence of tic douloureux, a severe form of pain in the facial area. Women also experience a higher incidence of carpal tunnel syndrome as well as Raynaud's disease, a condition that causes some areas of your body to feel numb and cool in response to cold temperatures or stress. Reflex sympathetic dystrophy (a chronic condition that usually affects the arms or legs and causes intense aching and burning pain along with swelling, skin discoloration and temperature changes) is more prevalent in females as is a piriformis muscle syndrome (a spasm of the gluteal [buttocks] muscles).

Men experience a higher incidence of nerve disorders in the arms and legs than females. Women experience a higher incidence of irritable bowel syndrome as well as interstitial cystitis than males. Males experience a higher incidence of pancreatic disease, which can cause significant pain. Fibromyalgia and rheumatoid arthritis are more prevalent in females. Post-herpetic neuralgia, on the other hand, is more prevalent in males. This is a painful condition that affects your nerve fibers and skin and is a result of shingles.

Cold pressor tests were done in black and white African subjects. The cold pressor test elicited significant blood pressure elevations with higher relative increases in the black Africans. The higher blood pressure reactivity in black Africans was accompanied by a substantially greater cardiac response and lower parasympathetic outflow as compared with white Africans. Black Africans also reported higher chronic stress levels and rated the stimulus as more painful than their white counterparts.. A higher cognitive appraisal of pain may contribute to the exaggerated blood pressure reactivity in black Africans.

There are potentially important ethnic/racial group differences in experimental pain perception. Elucidating ethnic group differences has translational merit for culturally competent clinical care and for addressing and reducing pain treatment disparities among ethnically/racially diverse groups. Interestingly, verbal pain ratings at NFR threshold were not significantly different between ethnic groups, suggesting that the lower stimulation intensities required to elicit a reflex in African-American versus non-Hispanic white participants were perceived as similar.

It appears that men and women have different referred pain patterns. Referred pain from your organs can go to other structures such as your arms or legs. This is noted when a person has a heart attack. The pain in men can go to the upper-left extremity. With respect to a heart attack, there is gender specificity: Women may not experience pain in the upper-left extremity but only pressure in the area about the heart. Pain in the neck related to a disc or degeneration of the bones and joints can give an area of referred pain to the face. Referred pain is a difficult entity for a neurological scientist to completely find. You feel the pain in an area that is not essentially involved with tissue trauma or destruction.

The sympathetic nervous system and its release of pain neuro-stimulating chemicals can increase a woman's susceptibility to reflex sympathetic dystrophy (RSD) or causalgia. Reflex sympathetic dystrophy and causalgia are usually caused by trauma to a nerve. These entities are more common in women.

Differences in the mechanisms of pain inhibition in the brain and spinal cord are presently being studied. This is important because preliminary studies have noted that equivalent doses of pain-relieving drugs differ for males and females and between some ethnic groups. It is obvious that men and women differ with respect to pain. This is also true with regard to the treatment of pain. Doctors are beginning to realize that men and women respond differently to different pain therapies. As stated earlier, the effects of the absorption and metabolism of drugs differ in men and women. It also has been mentioned that different types of drugs such as opioids and antidepressants may work differently in men and women.

The menstrual cycle results in women being affected more than men with respect to the absorption of drugs through their stomach and intestine. Women experience a decreased absorption of drugs in the mid cycle of the menstrual period. When women are using hormones, there is a decreased attachment of drugs to proteins in their bloodstream after the drug has been absorbed through the intestine. Removal of drugs from the bloodstream by the kidneys appears to be equal in males and females, and this "clearance" appears to decrease as both men and women age.

With respect to race and ethnicity, a study was done to determine whether there were systematic differences in Emergency Severity Index (ESI) scores, which are intended to determine priority of treatment and anticipate resource needs, across categories of race and ethnicity, after accounting for patient-presenting vital signs and examiner characteristics. Medical records of emergency department (ED) patients from twenty-two U.S. Department of Veterans Affairs ED stations were analyzed to determine whether ESI assignments differ systematically by race or ethnicity. Black patients were assigned less urgent ESI scores than White patients, and this effect was more prominent for Black males compared with Black females. A similar interaction was found for Hispanic males. A pain management protocol might reduce bias in pain management in the acute whiplash injury in the ED.[11]

Minority race/ethnicity was not consistently associated with worse processes or outcomes in some managed care settings, and not all differences favored Whites.[12] Regular aspirin use, particularly as secondary prevention, reduces morbidity from heart disease and stroke. African Americans and Hispanics are less likely to take aspirin than their White counterparts. Differences in sociodemographic characteristics and cardiovascular disease risk factors do not account for lower aspirin use among racial/ethnic minorities.[13] Researchers studying disparities in pain care face a number of ethical and methodological challenges that must be addressed to advance the field towards eliminating disparities.[14] Racial discrimination may influence the clinical pain severity of African Americans via the nociceptive processing of painful stimuli.[15] There is important racial and age-related variability in the symptom severity of patients with chronic pain presenting with similar physical, emotional, and pain characteristics to some a pain centers.[16]

Ethnicity disparities have been reported to occur in workman's compensation settlements when compared to white injured workers. Race differences in diagnostic specificity and rates of surgery may mediate documented differences in workers' compensation case management outcomes and settlement awards between African Americans and whites with low back injuries. Whites were 40% more likely than African Americans to receive a herniated disc diagnosis. Of claimants with the latter diagnosis and whites were 110% more likely than African Americans to undergo surgery. Race differences in diagnostic specificity and rates of surgery may mediate documented differences in workers' compensation case management outcomes and settlement awards between African Americans and whites with low back injuries.[17]

References

1.   Kamath AF, O'Connor MI. Breakout session: Gender and ethnic disparities in pain management. Clinical orthopaedics and related research. 2011;469(7):1962-1966.

2.   Defrin R, Eli I, Pud D. Interactions among sex, ethnicity, religion, and gender role expectations of pain. Gend Med. 2011;8(3):172-183.

3.   Campbell CM, France CR, Robinson ME, Logan HL, Geffken GR, Fillingim RB. Ethnic differences in the nociceptive flexion reflex (NFR). Pain. 2008;134(1-2):91-96.

4.   Vakil N, Niklasson A, Denison H, Ryden A. Gender differences in symptoms in partial responders to proton pump inhibitors for gastro-oesophageal reflux disease. United European Gastroenterol J. 2015;3(5):443-452.

5.   Cho CH, Ye HU, Jung JW, Lee YK. Gender Affects Early Postoperative Outcomes of Rotator Cuff Repair. Clin Orthop Surg. 2015;7(2):234-240.

6.   Koren L, Peled E, Trogan R, Norman D, Berkovich Y, Israelit S. Gender, age and ethnicity influence on pain levels and analgesic use in the acute whiplash injury. Eur J Trauma Emerg Surg. 2015;41(3):287-291.

7.   Wranker LS, Rennemark M, Berglund J. Pain among older adults from a gender perspective: findings from the Swedish National Study on Aging and Care (SNAC-Blekinge). Scand J Public Health. 2015.

8.   Rzeszutek M, Oniszczenko W, Schier K, Biernat-Kaluza E, Gasik R. Sex differences in trauma symptoms, body image and intensity of pain in a Polish sample of patients suffering from chronic pain. Psychol Health Med. 2015.1-9.

9.   Hawkins JL, Denson JE, Miley DR, Durham PL. Nicotine stimulates expression of proteins implicated in peripheral and central sensitization. Neuroscience. 2015;290:115-125.

10.   Yu A, Cai X, Zhang Z, et al. Effect of nicotine dependence on opioid requirements of patients after thoracic surgery. Acta Anaesthesiol Scand. 2015;59(1):115-122.

11. Boissoneault J, Bunch JR, Robinson M. The roles of ethnicity, sex, and parental pain modeling in rating of experienced and imagined pain events. J Behav Med. 2015;38(5):809-816.

12. Brown AF, Gregg EW, Stevens MR, et al. Race, ethnicity, socioeconomic position, and quality of care for adults with diabetes enrolled in managed care: the Translating Research Into Action for Diabetes (TRIAD) study. Diabetes Care. 2005;28(12):2864-2870.

13. Brown DW, Shepard D, Giles WH, Greenlund KJ, Croft JB. Racial differences in the use of aspirin: an important tool for preventing heart disease and stroke. Ethn Dis. 2005;15(4):620-626.

14. Campbell LC, Robinson K, Meghani SH, Vallerand A, Schatman M, Sonty N. Challenges and opportunities in pain management disparities research: implications for clinical practice, advocacy, and policy. J Pain. 2012;13(7):611-619.

15. Goodin BR, Pham QT, Glover TL, et al. Perceived racial discrimination, but not mistrust of medical researchers, predicts the heat pain tolerance of African Americans with symptomatic knee osteoarthritis. Health Psychol. 2013;32(11):1117-1126.

16. Green CR, Ndao-Brumblay SK, Nagrant AM, Baker TA, Rothman E. Race, age, and gender influences among clusters of African American and white patients with chronic pain. J Pain. 2004;5(3):171-182.

17. Chibnall JT, Tait RC, Andresen EM, Hadler NM. Race differences in diagnosis and surgery for occupational low back injuries. Spine (Phila Pa 1976). 2006;31(11):1272-1275.

4. Genetic Testing

When you take a pain pill by mouth, it goes to your stomach and/or small intestine and the molecules in the pill go to receptors in throughout your body by means of your blood flow and will attach to receptors in your body specific for that medication. For example, codeine will go to mu receptors throughout your body. The majority of mu receptors are in your brain and spinal cord. Before the codeine attaches to these receptors the codeine will be converted to morphine by enzymes in your body. You will then begin to experience pain relief because of the morphine's effects on your receptors. In some individuals, a genetic abnormality is present which prevents conversion of codeine into morphine. If this happens you will have no pain relief.

Codeine is one example of a drug whose metabolism is greatly influenced by genetics. In order for codeine to exert an effect, it first has to be converted into morphine by the body's enzymes. This chemical reaction occurs in the liver and is catalyzed by the cytochrome P450 enzyme, CYP2D6. However, up to 10% of individuals have a mutation in the CYP2D6 gene that abolishes enzyme activity. Thus, codeine may have very little or no impact on these patients. People with this mutation cannot convert codeine to morphine and thereby cannot benefit from the analgesic effects of the drug. Identification of the CYP2D6 mutation before therapy would allow physicians to prescribe a different pain control regimen, instead of resorting to trial and error.

In most individuals, codeine is converted to morphine and you experience pain relief. In another subset of patients the morphine is not broken down into its component chemical molecules after it relieves your pain. Your body should break the morphine down (called metabolism) into its chemical components so that your body can rid itself of these component chemicals. If this does not happen subsequent doses of codeine could cause you to experience a possible drug overdose because the previous morphine dose has not been eliminated. In another group of individuals, the morphine is promptly broken down into its basic chemicals causing you to only experience a rapid pain relief causing your pain to quickly return. This overall process is called pharmacogenetics. Age, gender and ethnicity can all affect pharmacogenetics.

Patients vary widely in their response to drugs. Genetic factors can account for 20 to 95 percent of patient variability. A gene is the basic physical and functional unit of heredity. Genes are made up of DNA. DNA contains the instructions for our genes. Our body contains much DNA and the DNA is tightly packaged into small structures called chromosomes. Genes are located within our DNA and one strand of DNA can contain many genes. The genes direct our bodies to create certain proteins in order for our bodies to function. Inside of each cell are long and complex molecules called DNA. DNA tells your body's cells how to create new cells. Your genes code your body's instructions for making proteins. Proteins do the work within our cells throughout your body.

In humans, most genes are arranged on chromosomes. The whole set of genes is called the genotype, and the total effect of genes on the body is called the phenotype (e.g. what you look like). During the process of DNA replication, errors sometimes occur which cause mutations that may have an effect on the phenotype of an organism. Random changes (mutations) in the DNA can result in slight changes in organisms. As these mutations accumulate, there can be changes in organisms, resulting in evolution. Beneficial mutations tend to be preserved and as these mutations accumulate, the species can gradually adapt to its environment.

The pharmaceutical industry has been focused on the drug that can yield billions of dollars in revenue. The industry is concerned that it will not be able to maximize the patient base able to use a certain drug, and thereby revenue and profits, if it adopts genetic testing. Studies showing how the body metabolizes a drug in African Americans, Asian Americans and other minorities in the United States, are rare. Precision medicine is an emerging approach for disease treatment and prevention that takes into account individual variability in genes, environment, and lifestyle for each person. This approach will allow doctors and researchers to predict more accurately which treatment and prevention strategies for a particular disease will work in which groups of people.

Drug therapy is ineffective in patients in from 38% to 75% of therapeutic areas because of genetic influences which could be remedied with genetic testing. Alleles are alternative forms of the same gene. Alleles for a trait are located at corresponding positions on homologous chromosomes. Since a living thing has two copies of each gene, it can have two different alleles of it at the same time. Often, one allele will be dominant, meaning that the living thing looks and acts as if it had only that one allele. The unexpressed allele is called recessive. In other cases, you end up with something in between the two possibilities.

Research shows that genetic factors account for a substantial proportion of all elements contributing to a patient's response to drugs in addition to age, sex, weight and liver function. Genes provide your body with instructions for making enzymes, which help break down drugs in your system, allowing your body to benefit from the medicine that you take. Differences in your enzymes can affect how your body metabolizes a drug and how long the drug stays your body.

People of different racial and/or ethnic origin may respond to drugs differently. Genes in your cells provide your body with instructions for making enzymes. These enzymes are responsible for affecting how your medications work within your body. The study of genetic variations in drug response is called pharmacogenetics when studying an individual gene, or pharmacogenetics when studying all genes. People of Asian descent metabolize some antidepressants and antipsychotic drugs more slowly than Caucasians. People of African and Asian descent may respond differently to psychotropic drugs.

Drug studies fall generally under two categories: pharmacokinetics (how the body affects the drugs, i.e., how the drug is metabolized); and pharmacodynamics (how the drug affects the body, i.e., efficacy and safety). Pharmacogenetics is the study of the role of genetics in a drug response. A person's genotype is his or her genetic makeup. The term can pertain to all genes or to a specific gene. The phenotype is a person's outward physical appearance or function resulting from the interaction between the genotype and the environment.

Genetic polymorphisms are naturally-occurring variants in gene structure that occur in more than 1 percent of the population. Common variations (polymorphisms) in cytochrome P450 genes can affect the function of the enzymes. The effects of polymorphisms are most prominently seen in the breakdown of medications. Depending on the gene and the polymorphism, drugs can be metabolized quickly or slowly. If a cytochrome P450 enzyme metabolizes a drug slowly, the drug stays active longer and less is needed to get the desired effect.

The clinical consequence of the CYP2D6 polymorphism can be either occurrence of adverse drug reactions or altered drug response. Drugs that are most affected by CYP2D6 polymorphisms are commonly those in which CYP2D6 represents a substantial metabolic pathway either in the activation to form active metabolites or clearance of the agent.[1] The CYP2D6 activity ranges considerably within a population and includes ultra-rapid metabolizers, extensive metabolizers , intermediate metabolizers and poor metabolizers . Be aware that many pain medications are metabolized to the active drug that relieves your pain.

There is a considerable variability in the CYP2D6 allele distribution among different ethnic groups, resulting in variable percentages of the different metabolizer types in a given population. As a consequence, drug adverse effects or lack of drug effect may occur if standard doses are applied. For example a poor metabolizer drug may not convert to the active pain relieving chemical and you therefore will not experience pain relief.

A drug that is quickly metabolized is broken down sooner, and a higher dose might be needed to be effective. Cytochrome P450 enzymes account for 70 percent to 80 percent of enzymes involved in drug metabolism. An allele is one of a number of alternative forms of the same gene. Subjects possessing certain allelic variants will show normal, decreased, or no CYP2D6 function, depending on the allele. Ethnicity is a factor in the occurrence of CYP2D6 variability. The prevalence of CYP2D6 poor metabolizers is approximately 6–10% in White populations, but is lower in most other ethnic groups such as Asians (2%).

In African-Americans, the frequency of poor metabolizers is greater than for whites, while the occurrence of CYP2D6 ultrarapid metabolizers is greater among Middle Easterners and North Africans. As a consequence, drug adverse effects or lack of drug effect may occur if standard doses are applied. The alleles *10, *17, *36 and *41 give rise to substrate-dependent decreased activity. Concordant genotype-phenotype correlation provides a basis for predicting the phenotype based on genetic testing, which has the potential to achieve optimal pharmacotherapy. However, genotype testing for CYP2D6 is not routinely performed in clinical practice.

The most prevalent drug-metabolizing enzymes are the Cytochrome P450 enzymes. The human Cytochrome P450 family consists of 57 genes, with 18 families and 44 subfamilies. In the nucleus of each cell, the DNA molecule is packaged into thread-like structures called chromosomes. Cytochrome P450 proteins are conveniently arranged into these families and subfamilies based on similarities identified between amino acid sequences. Enzymes that share 35-40% identity are assigned to the same family by an Arabic numeral, and those that share 55-70% make up a particular subfamily with a designated letter. For example, CYP2D6 refers to family 2, subfamily D, and gene number 6.

From a clinical perspective, the most commonly tested Cytochrome P450 enzymes include: CYP2D6, CYP2C19, CYP2C9,

CYP3A4 and CYP3A5. These genes account for the metabolism of approximately 80-90% of current prescription drugs. Each cytochrome P450 gene is named with CYP, indicating that it is part of the cytochrome P450 gene family. The gene is also given a number associated with a specific group within the gene family, a letter representing the gene's subfamily, and a number assigned to the exact gene within the subfamily. For example, the cytochrome P450 gene that is in group 26, subfamily B, gene 2 is written as CYP26B2. Individuals presenting these variations may have an altered level of MOR expression. A possible association of these genomic variants on efficacy and side effects of opioid treatment in different ethnic groups.[2]

Polymorphism is the condition of one of two or more variants of a particular DNA sequence occurring in several different forms. Polymorphisms may influence a drug's action by changing its pharmacokinetics or its pharmacodynamics. Enzymes are needed for your body to break down drugs so your body can get the benefit from the medicine. Differences in genes can affect the speed of action of different enzymes you have in your body. This affects how well your body can use medicines and how well drugs work in your body. Differences in your enzymes can affect how your body can break down a drug and how long the drug stays your body. Based on what type of genes you carry, you may be: a poor drug metabolizer, an extensive or "normal" drug metabolizer.

For many drugs, there exist patients that are poor metabolizers (PM), intermediate metabolizers (IM), and ultra-rapid metabolizers (UM). The risk of toxicity may increase for poor and intermediate metabolizers whereas for ultrapid metabolizers, these patients may require higher than normal doses for a therapeutic effect. If you are a "poor metabolizer", you do not break down drugs well. This may result in too many drugs or too much drug mass in your body which may lead to a dangerous side effect or even death. In some cases, your body may not be able to break down certain drugs to their working form and therefore, the drugs will not work properly.

You metabolize drugs at the normal rate if you are an extensive or "normal" drug metabolizer. In other words, you metabolize drugs at a normal rate. If you are an "ultra-rapid" metabolizer, this means you break down drugs too fast, causing them to be of no use in the body. If medications do not work properly, conditions such as high blood pressure, blood disorders, and cancer will be left untreated and may even lead to death. Your doctor will adjust the dose of your medication so that it is the correct right dose for you. Poor metabolizers might need to take a lower dose of drug than normal metabolizers because they break down drugs slowly. Ultra-rapid metabolizers might need a higher dose because they break down drugs too fast.

Enzymes produced from the cytochrome P450 genes are involved in the formation and breakdown of various molecules and chemicals within cells. Cytochrome P450 enzymes play a role in the synthesis of many molecules, including steroid hormones, cholesterol and other fatty acids, and acids used to digest fats. Additional cytochrome P450 enzymes metabolize external substances, such as medications that are ingested and internal substances, such as toxins that are formed within cells. There are approximately 60 cytochrome P450 genes in humans.

Cytochrome P450 enzymes are primarily found in liver cells but are also located in cells throughout the body. Within cells, cytochrome P450 enzymes are located in a structure involved in protein processing and transport and the energy-producing centers of cells. The enzymes found in the inner aspects of cells (mitochondria) are generally involved in the synthesis and metabolism of internal substances, while enzymes in the outer part of the cell (endoplasmic reticulum) usually metabolize external substances, primarily medications and environmental pollutants.

Diseases caused by mutations in cytochrome P450 genes typically involve the buildup of substances in the body that are harmful in large amounts or that prevent other necessary molecules from being produced. Common pain medications require activation by an enzyme called CYP2D6 to become effective. Approximately half of patients have genes that alter the function of CYP2D6. Testing for these gene alterations allows for changes to dosage regimens in order to compensate for altered metabolisms and can optimize the efficacy of your pain medication. Ultra-rapid metabolizers break down medications rapidly. Individuals who frequently need more doses of medication in order to relieve pain may be ultra-rapid metabolizers. Poor metabolizers, on the other hand, tend to have severe side effects at low doses.

Some patients being treated with pain medication, for example, may not experience expected pain relief if they are ultra-rapid or poor metabolizers. Cytochrome P450 may also be inhibited or induced by drugs, resulting in drug-drug interactions and leading to unanticipated, adverse drug reactions. Most drugs in common clinical use are metabolized in the liver by the family of enzymes. Patients can exhibit inconsistent responses to drug therapies, which are influenced by variations in DNA coding of the Cytochrome P450 enzyme family. These enzymes affect the extent of drug metabolism, and understanding patient metabolism rate can help physicians determine accurate dosage of proper pain management medication. Identifying CYP450 polymorphisms in 2D6, 2C19, 3A4 and 3A5 will indicate the rate at which patients can be expected to metabolize a drug. These tests can classify a patient as an ultra-rapid metabolizer, extensive metabolizer, intermediate metabolizer or poor metabolizer.

Differences in drug metabolism can lead to potential drug interactions, overdosing, or under dosing. More than 85% of patients have significant genetic variations in the most important cytochromes: CYP2D6, CYP2C9, CYP2C19, CYP3A4 and CYP3A5. For example, CYP3A4 and CYP3A5 affect the metabolism of one-half of the drugs in clinical use. In terms of CYP-related drug metabolism, there are nine CYP enzymes of known clinical importance and they are referred to as CYP1A2, CYP2B6, CYP2C9, CYP2C18, CYP2C19, CYP-D6, CYP2E1, and CYP3A4.3

DNA in a cell determines the rate of metabolic activity. If the enzymes are fully functional, the person is an extensive (normal) metabolizer. Changes in the DNA can alter the rate of metabolism. There are at least three categories for this: (1) If a person had duplications of this genetic material, he or she would metabolize the drug so quickly that therapeutic levels of the drug could never be reached. This is called ultrarapid metabolism. (2) On the other hand, someone can inherit genetic material which produces none of the desired enzyme, so that person will not be able to metabolize a drug at all; this person would be a poor metabolizers. (3) If a person carried genetic material that codes for less CYP2D6 enzyme activity than normal, he would be an intermediate metabolizer, and metabolize the drug very slowly. People who are intermediate and poor metabolizers often have more severe side effects.

Many of the pioneer pharmacogentic studies were conducted in Sweden, where a large population of Chinese immigrants lived near the university and forward thinking researchers conducted a comparative pharmacogenetic study. They observed that the Chinese population metabolized drugs involving the CYP2D6 enzymes considerably slower than did Caucasians. Meanwhile, pharmacogenetic studies in African also showed unique genetic variations. For example, studies conducted in Zimbabwe identified another "reduced function" genetic variation (CYP2D6*17), which occurs frequently in people of African descent, and is responsible for slower metabolic rate.

Studies using drugs metabolized by CYP2D6 show that many people of African descent metabolize these drugs more slowly than Caucasians. Therefore, it is predicted that when prescribed the same doses as Caucasians, about 40% of people of African descent will have higher blood levels of drugs metabolized by CYP2D6. It has been shown that up to 10% of Whites, 2% of Blacks, and 1% of Asians exhibit CYP-2D6 polymorphism.

An individual's genetic material can also influence how effective a drug will be in reducing the symptoms of an illness, and determine the occurrence and/or severity of side effects. The examples above show that a person's unique genetic make-up can determine how quickly or slowly a drug will be metabolized. Recently, industry began offering genomic testing for enzymes of drug metabolism. Genetic testing can be a vital component of personalized medicine, assisting clinicians in choosing medications based on patient genetics to increase benefit and decreased risks.

Patients who are poor metabolizers may have an increased risk of drug-induced side effects, or may experience inadequate pain relief. Patients characterized as poor metabolizers or ultra-rapid metabolizers may need adjustments in dosage depending on the drug. Cytochrome P450 test results may help develop a treatment strategy for patients using some medications. If your medicine does not work, ask your physician if genetic testing is appropriate for you to help determine why your medication does not work.

Pharmacogenetic testing may enable physicians to understand why patients react differently to various drugs and to make better decisions about therapy. Pharmacogenetics is a field that deals with the relationship between genetic variations and the effects and side-effects of drugs. Genetic variations in drug-metabolizing enzymes, transporters, receptors, and other drug targets have been linked to individual differences in the efficacy and safety of many drugs.

Variation in responses to pain medication may be explained or predicted by a patient's genetics. How a patient handles a drug often depends on genetic differences that affect pharmacokinetics or pharmacodynamics (i.e. the response of the body to the drug, whether positive or negative). Those individuals who express poor or a complete lack of enzyme function (non-metabolizers) are predisposed to the accumulation of the parent drug and will possibly achieve excessive serum levels and prolonged half-lives of some of these drugs. These individuals have a tendency to become toxic on the "usual" doses of a medication.

Genes may affect pain in a race or ethnicity specific manner. Research in a genetically mixed population evaluating the role of several candidate genes in human pain sensitivity revealed that gender, ethnicity, and temperament contributed to individual variation in thermal and cold sensitivity. In opioid abuse and addiction, twin studies have shown that heritability estimates of addictions range from 0.39 (hallucinogens) to 0.72 (cocaine), and heritability estimates for addiction are usually higher than for substance use. Similar to pain genes, opioid addiction-related genes also have ethnicity- and sex-specific effects. Functional alleles may independently contribute to heroin dependence in female patients, while a polymorphism was associated with heroin dependency risk in males only.

Drug metabolism is controlled by a number of specific enzymes, and the action of these enzymes varies among individuals. For example, most individuals show normal activity of the IID6 isoenzyme that is responsible for the metabolism of many tricyclic antidepressant medications and most antipsychotic drugs. However, studies have found that one-third of Asian Americans and one-third of African Americans have a genetic alteration that decreases the metabolic rate of the IID6 isoenzyme, leading to a greater risk of side effects and toxicity. The CYP2D6 enzyme is important for the way in which the liver clears many drugs from the body and varies greatly between individuals in ways that can be ethnically specific. Though enzyme activity is genetically influenced, it can also be altered by cultural and environmental factors such as diet, the use of other medications, alcohol and disease states.

It is clear from the past decade of study that we are making progress in determining that genetic variations in individuals can and do impact drug response. In order to truly offer personalized medicine advantages for all Americans, more emphasis needs to be placed on determining genetic variations not only of people of European Caucasian descent, but also in people of African and Asian descent.

The appeal of pharmacogenetics lies in the possibility of personalized medicine. This sort of care has always been the goal of the doctor-patient relationship, with physicians considering a patient's family history and lifestyle when prescribing treatment. Access to information about an individual's genetic makeup would provide yet another source of personalized data and would therefore enable doctors to better define the nature of a disease and find the most effective treatment for a particular patient. With the help of pharmacogenetic studies, physicians will be able to administer treatment regimens that are personalized and adapted to each person's genetic makeup. Two people with the same diagnosis might receive different therapies or drug dosages. This might in turn reduce health care costs, because physicians would be able to prescribe more targeted drugs and pharmaceutical companies would be able to develop and market drugs to specific groups of patients.

African Americans have been treated as a representative population for African ancestry for many purposes, including pharmacogenomic studies. The contribution of European ancestry is expected to result in considerable differences in the genetic architecture of African American individuals compared with an African genome. As a result, drug responses in admixed populations such as African Americans may be altered from those individuals with only African ancestry. The different genetic diversity between African Americans and Africans indicated that ethnic differences in pharmacologic studies exist despite that African ancestry is dominant in Africans Americans.[3]

Approximately 50 years ago, pharmacogenetics was described as a new field of medicine that may explain human drug action.4 Genetic variations that may provide a molecular basis for ethnic differences in drug metabolizing enzymes (CYP 2C9, 2C19, 2D6, and 3A4), drug transporter (P-glycoprotein), drug receptors (adrenoceptors), and other functionally important proteins (eNOS and G proteins) are discussed. A better understanding of the molecular basis underlying ethnic differences in drug metabolism, transport, and response will contribute to improved individualization of drug therapy.[5]

Genomic variations influencing basal pain sensitivity, the likelihood of developing chronic pain diseases as well as the response to pharmacotherapy of pain. Polymorphisms of the cytochrome P450 enzymes influence the analgesic efficacy of codeine, tramadol, tricyclic antidepressants and nonsteroidal anti-inflammatory drugs.[6] A genetic test helps a physician when prescribing medications . Genetic variations affect a patient's ability to metabolize drugs. Drugs that metabolize in the liver account for approximately 80% of all medications. Unfortunately medications are developed with the assumption that patients are normal metabolizers. Pharmacogenetics is a way to know if a patient will respond to a medication. And will decrease a chance of an adverse drug reaction.

Inability to predict the therapeutic effect of a drug in individual pain patients prolongs the process of drug and dose finding until satisfactory pharmacotherapy can be achieved. Many chronic pain conditions are associated with hypersensitivity of the nervous system or impaired endogenous pain modulation.[7] Genomic testing for enzymes of drug metabolism has significant potential for improving the efficacy of drug treatment and reducing adverse drug reactions.[8]

Drug half-life calculations can be used as functional markers of the cumulative effect of pharmacogenetics and drug-drug interactions.[9] Assessment of half-life and therapeutic effects may be more useful than genetic testing in preventing adverse drug reactions to pain medications, while ensuring effective analgesia. Definitive, mass spectrometry-based methods, capable of measuring parent drug and metabolite levels, are the most useful assays for this purpose. Pain-perception regulation and modulation are still not fully understood, and thus more knowledge of the genetic background for pain relief will be needed.[10]

Physicians should evaluate the extent to which their communication with patients varies by patient race/ethnicity, and make efforts to ensure that they share equally with all patients regarding the rationale for treatment recommendations. There is an increased recognition regarding the complexity of pain research, acknowledging the additional role of epigenetic, transcriptomic, proteomic, and metabolic factors in the development, experience, and treatment of pain.[11]

References

1.   Zhou SF. Polymorphism of human cytochrome P450 2D6 and its clinical significance: Part I. Clin Pharmacokinet. 2009;48(11):689-723.

2.   Bayerer B, Stamer U, Hoeft A, Stuber F. Genomic variations and transcriptional regulation of the human mu-opioid receptor gene. Eur J Pain. 2007;11(4):421-427.

3.   Li J, Lao X, Zhang C, Tian L, Lu D, Xu S. Increased genetic diversity of ADME genes in African Americans compared with their putative ancestral source populations and implications for pharmacogenomics. BMC Genet. 2014;15:52.

4.   Landau R, Bollag LA, Kraft JC. Pharmacogenetics and anaesthesia: the value of genetic profiling. Anaesthesia. 2012;67(2):165-179.

5.   Xie HG, Kim RB, Wood AJ, Stein CM. Molecular basis of ethnic differences in drug disposition and response. Annu Rev Pharmacol Toxicol. 2001;41:815-850.

6.   Stamer UM, Stuber F. Genetic factors in pain and its treatment. Curr Opin Anaesthesiol. 2007;20(5):478-484.

7.   Siegenthaler A, Schliessbach J, Vuilleumier PH, et al. Linking altered central pain processing and genetic polymorphism to drug efficacy in chronic low back pain. BMC Pharmacol Toxicol. 2015;16:23.

8.   Fishbain DA, Fishbain D, Lewis J, et al. Genetic testing for enzymes of drug metabolism: does it have clinical utility for pain medicine at the present time? A structured review. Pain Med. 2004;5(1):81-93.

9.   Kapur BM, Lala PK, Shaw JL. Pharmacogenetics of chronic pain management. Clin Biochem. 2014;47(13-14):1169-1187.

10.   Svetlik S, Hronova K, Bakhouche H, Matouskova O, Slanar O. Pharmacogenetics of chronic pain and its treatment. Mediators Inflamm. 2013;2013:864319.

11.   Jimenez N, Galinkin JL. Personalizing pediatric pain medicine: using population-specific pharmacogenetics, genomics, and other -omics approaches to predict response. Anesth Analg. 2015;121(1):183-187.

5. Physician Diversity Influence on Treatment

There is growing evidence that disparities in the treatment of pain occur by medical providers because of differences in race. Considerable evidence demonstrates substantial ethnic disparities in the prevalence, treatment, progression and outcomes of pain-related conditions. These disparities extend to the prevalence, treatment, progression and outcomes of pain-related conditions.

Equal treatment by race for example, occurs in nonopioid related therapies, but White patients are more likely than Black patients to be treated with opioids. For persistent back pain, female physicians prescribed lower doses of hydrocodone, especially to male patients. For renal colic, lower doses were prescribed to Black versus White patients when the patient was female, whereas the reverse was true when patients were male.[1]

There is a need for better understanding of the way a complex interplay of non-clinical characteristics affects physician and other health care provider behaviors in order to improve quality of pain management and other clinical decision-making. Patient characteristics including race, age, chronic pain, and trauma influence prescription of emergency department opioids. Fewer opioids were prescribed for Black patients than for White patients. Younger patients, those with trauma, and those with chronic pain received more opioids and discharge analgesics compared with older patients and those without trauma or chronic pain.[2]

Race is a term often used, but may be ill defined. It can incorporate biological, social, and cultural characteristics of patients and can refer to both genetic and behavioral traits. Various investigators have reported differences between racial and ethnic groups in health status, disease manifestation and outcome, resource utilization, and health care access, often specifying neither a definition of race.

When treating pain, gender and racial differences were evident only when the role of physician gender was examined, suggesting that male and female physicians may react differently to gender and/or racial cues. Male patients reported higher pain scores to male practitioners when experiencing relatively low pain levels, and both male and female patients reported higher pain scores to female practitioners when experiencing relatively high pain levels.[3]

It is unclear why treatment approaches varied according to the gender of the physician. The reasons for these differences can only be speculative. Physicians may sympathize or identify with patients of the same gender or race, or with patients of disadvantaged groups in the case of female physicians. It is also unclear why physician gender interacted with patient race when treating acute kidney stone pain but with patient gender when treating persistent lower back pain.

Physicians have under recognized the influence of their own demographically based predispositions in medical practice, and the medical literature evidences the presumption that clinicians are neutral operators governed by objective science and are unaffected by personal variables. There is sufficient evidence for the hypothesis that provider behavior contributes to race/ethnicity disparities in medical care.[4]

Physicians are believed to be demographically homogeneous, and that any heterogeneity is not clinically relevant. In fact, the physician workforce is not homogeneous as more than 20% of North American physicians come from ethnic minorities, and more than 25% are women. Studies on pain management have suggested that physicians are more likely to withhold or under prescribe opioid analgesics to minority patients compared with white ones.[5] Physicians' preferences for their own treatment influence their estimates of their patients' preferences for their treatments. Physicians' religious affinities also affect practice. For example, Catholic or Jewish physicians may be less willing to withdraw life support from their patients than physicians with other religious beliefs.[6]

An overriding health care objective is to improve the consistency and quality of care rendered by diverse health professionals to even more dissimilar populations of patients. Various psychological mechanisms may lead to unintentional provider bias in decisions about pain treatment.[7]

Patients presenting to an outpatient cardiology clinic with a new complaint of angina were prospectively followed to determine if there was a gender bias in the management of suspected coronary artery disease when physicians trained in cardiology managed their care. Overall, there were no differences in the percentage of women who underwent noninvasive evaluation, invasive evaluation, and treatment of suspected coronary artery disease compared with men.[8] A gender-based clinical hierarchy operates in the clinical management of angina pectoris in primary care. Women with angina have been shown to receive less intensive clinical care than similar men.[9]

Strong bias clinicians reserve for reported pain may lead them to overrate pathology, treat patients inappropriately, prescribe unnecessary imaging tests, and generate unfounded medical opinions that are responsible for many disputes.[10] Proposals of nonspecific somatic diagnoses, psychosocial questions, drug prescriptions, and the expressed need of diagnostic support from a physiotherapist and an orthopedist were more common with females. Laboratory tests were requested more often in males. Both male and female physicians contributed to the gender differences. When assessing the impact of the patient-doctor relationship for health outcome, male physicians underlined the importance of patient compliance foremost in female patients, and female physicians did the opposite.[11]

Prior studies suggest a gender-based difference in the management of myocardial ischemia in nonacute settings. In patients chest pain, women were evaluated and managed less aggressively than men.[12] The interaction effects between health care need and gender to explain variations in use of health care services indicates that users of services varied in ways that suggest a bias or barrier of their own or of service providers to access services.[13] Provider gender, as well as patient gender, may affect the clinical assessment and treatment of pain. With respect to anesthesia, pain treatment strategies were indistinguishable between male and female anesthetists, as well as between male and female patients.[14]

Findings indicate that the interdisciplinary teams in specialist healthcare may discriminate against women with chronic pain when physiotherapy and radiological investigation are recommended.[15] Age bias has been reported to result in under treatment of elderly patients with various medical conditions.[16] However, research has detected no bias in the use of arthritis treatment compared with younger patients. Clinical arthritis studies also showed that the elderly patients with arthritis were faring at least as well as the younger arthritic patients.

It is hoped that medical practitioners can become aware of any bias that may exist toward their patients and that treatment can instead be based on Evidence Based Medicine Principles.

References

1.   Weisse CS, Sorum PC, Dominguez RE. The influence of gender and race on physicians' pain management decisions. J Pain. 2003;4(9):505-510.

2.   Heins JK, Heins A, Grammas M, Costello M, Huang K, Mishra S. Disparities in analgesia and opioid prescribing practices for patients with musculoskeletal pain in the emergency department. J Emerg Nurs. 2006;32(3):219-224.

3.   Vigil JM, Alcock J. Tough guys or sensitive guys? Disentangling the role of examiner sex on patient pain reports. Pain Res Manag. 2014;19(1):e9-e12.

4.   van Ryn M. Research on the provider contribution to race/ethnicity disparities in medical care. Medical care. 2002;40(1 Suppl):I140-151.

5.   Tamayo-Sarver JH, Hinze SW, Cydulka RK, Baker DW. Racial and ethnic disparities in emergency department analgesic prescription. Am J Public Health. 2003;93(12):2067-2073.

6.   Christakis NA, Asch DA. Physician characteristics associated with decisions to withdraw life support. Am J Public Health. 1995;85(3):367-372.

7.   Burgess DJ, van Ryn M, Crowley-Matoka M, Malat J. Understanding the provider contribution to race/ethnicity disparities in pain treatment: insights from dual process models of stereotyping. Pain Med. 2006;7(2):119-134.

8.   Blum M, Slade M, Boden D, Cabin H, Caulin-Glaser T. Examination of gender bias in the evaluation and treatment of angina pectoris by cardiologists. Am J Cardiol. 2004;93(6):765-767.

9.   Crilly MA, Bundred PE, Leckey LC, Johnstone FC. Gender bias in the clinical management of women with angina: another look at the Yentl syndrome. J Womens Health (Larchmt). 2008;17(3):331-342.

10.   Gracovetsky SA, Marriott A, Richards MP, Newman NM, Asselin S. The impact of inefficient clinical diagnosis on the cost of managing low back pain. J Healthc Risk Manag. 1997;17(3):21-31.

11.   Hamberg K, Risberg G, Johansson EE, Westman G. Gender bias in physicians' management of neck pain: a study of the answers in a Swedish national examination. J Womens Health Gend Based Med. 2002;11(7):653-666.

12.   Heston TF, Lewis LM. Gender bias in the evaluation and management of acute nontraumatic chest pain. The St. Louis Emergency Physicians' Association Research Group. Fam Pract Res J. 1992;12(4):383-389.

13.   Weir R, Browne G, Tunks E, Gafni A, Roberts J. Gender differences in psychosocial adjustment to chronic pain and expenditures for health care services used. Clin J Pain. 1996;12(4):277-290.

14.   Criste A. Do nurse anesthetists demonstrate gender bias in treating pain? A national survey using a standardized pain model. AANA J. 2003;71(3):206-209.

15.   Stalnacke BM, Haukenes I, Lehti A, Wiklund AF, Wiklund M, Hammarstrom A. Is there a gender bias in recommendations for further rehabilitation in primary care of patients with chronic pain after an interdisciplinary team assessment? J Rehabil Med. 2015;47(4):365-371.

16.   Harrison MJ, Kim CA, Silverberg M, Paget SA. Does age bias the aggressive treatment of elderly patients with rheumatoid arthritis? J Rheumatol. 2005;32(7):1243-1248.

6. Psychologic Aspects of Pain

Men and women perceive and respond to painful experiences in different ways. Debate that has spanned many generations continues over who can stand more pain, men or women.[1] Chronic pain may be perceived differently according to gender and race, which may affect physical health and psychological wellbeing. In this chapter you will also learn how your own psychology affects how you perceive your pain and how pain is perceived differently by men and women and by different ethnic groups. Anxiety, pain thresholds, and pain tolerance will be discussed. It is important for you to keep the psychology of your pain in mind as you begin to take control of your total pain treatment.

The International Association for the Study of Pain (IASP) defines pain as an unpleasant sensory and emotion experience associated with tissue injury as a result of trauma (for instance, bone fracture) or disease (for instance, cancer or shingles). Pain is psychological in that it is a mental processing of sensation impulses that reach the pain center in the brain, whereas pain "intensity" depends on how an individual reacts to pain. Injury or illness experienced when you were young may influence the way you relates to pain.

When pain becomes chronic, it becomes a personal problem. However, pain can also become a social problem, perhaps disrupting the family and resulting in loss of self-esteem. Lower individualized pain intensity and unpleasantness ratings were associated with higher levels of ambulatory blood pressure. African Americans and women reported higher levels of pain intensity when using the standard verbal rating scale but not when using the individually ordered rating scale.[2] Collectively, these results support previous research relating reduced pain sensitivity with increased blood pressure among men and women.

The following findings relate to how an individual's psychological state influences his or her perception of and response to pain: Patients who have strongly negative emotions about a situation experience more pain. Women have more negative emotions about situations in general than men and, therefore, have a higher incidence of pain. However, women cope better with pain than men. In general, women have a lower tolerance to pain than men. Even though the tissue trauma can be the same for multiple individuals, the response to pain is individualized based on education, psychological makeup, gender, and cultural influences.

"Pain medicine" as a specialty has evolved in a short time to realize that pain is a multidimensional entity influenced by psychological, neurological, social, ethnic, and cultural factors. Before the advent of this specialty, many doctors looked only at tissue injury and not at the patient as a whole. Pain cannot be observed or objectively measured. Instead, a pain "diagnosis" is based on verbal and nonverbal communication from the individual suffering pain. Doctors should diagnose pain based on both physical and psychological data. Physical data may include a physical examination and interpretation of x-rays, CT scans, and MRI) images. Doctors use this information to tailor therapies to the individual patient.

In summary, ethnic differences in pain responses and pain management have been observed persistently in a broad array of settings. Despite advances in pain care, minorities remain at risk for inadequate pain control. As society grows more and more ethnically diverse, the examination of disparities between wide varieties of ethnic groups should increasingly be requested of research studies in a variety of settings disparities and not only between African Americans and non-Hispanic whites. Previous research rarely examines and reports interactions between ethnic group membership and other important variables, such as gender and age, which are both recognized as factors that influence pain perception.

Because emotional factors can affect pain perception and intensity, a pain specialist's complete assessment of pain should include not only a physical examination but also analysis of the psychological, emotional, and behavioral aspects of pain. Personality greatly influences an individual's response to pain and his or her chosen coping strategies. In general, people who have underlying anxiety are more likely to seek higher doses of pain medications. Pain is a subjective complaint and is affected by a patient's emotions.

Unfortunately, persistent pain can change a patient's behavior. Persistent pain can increase patient anxiety and depression. As a result, it is difficult for a doctor to ascertain whether the pain came first or the psychological dysfunction. Most pain patients can benefit from behavioral treatments designed to improve their ability to cope with pain.

Both the patient and the doctor need to identify situations that reinforce pain behavior. Patients can use a pain diary to help identify what behavior signals pain. Most people with pain respond to routine treatments, such as oral medication and nerve injections of anti-inflammatory drugs (corticosteroids, for instance) as well as physical or manipulative therapy. When an individual fails to respond to these methods, psychological intervention is necessary. Many chronic pain patients have suffered emotionally traumatic childhoods; a history of this trauma should be sought by the doctors caring for these patients. Emotional disorders can also be associated with chronic pain. In a somatoform disorder, physical symptoms are compatible with a physical disorder, but there is no evidence of any clear psychiatric or physical problem. These patients overanalyze their bodies and have a tendency to look for abnormal symptoms.

A somatization disorder is a chronic disorder that usually begins before age 30 and primarily affects women. With it, an individual complains of many symptoms but has few physical findings to confirm their complaints. These individuals consult many doctors to validate their symptoms and may even consent to multiple injections by a pain-management doctor or even a surgical procedure for the treatment of pain. A conversion disorder results from an emotional conflict unrelated to bodily disease but resulting in loss of function of a part of the body. An example is losing the use of a hand without an obvious physical problem or injury.

These individuals exaggerate the magnitude of their complaints. Psychogenic pain disorders are complaints of pain without adequate physical findings. Hypochondriasis is a disturbance that involves an unrealistic interpretation of physical disease. These individuals have a preoccupation with the belief that they have a serious disease and are preoccupied with their physical symptoms.

Malingering is uncommon but implies a conscious fabrication of an illness for personal gain and may be seeking narcotic analgesic drugs such as morphine or Dilaudid. The chronic pain-prone patient is often an individual who had a traumatic childhood, perhaps with a history of physical and/or emotional abuse or a history of chronic pain or disability.

Various psychological tests are available to evaluate pain patients. A common test is the Minnesota Multiphase Personality Inventory Test (MMPI), which evaluates multiple dimensions of a pain patient. The Beck Depression Scale can be used to assess depression. The MMPI, consisting of 566 questions, is widely used by psychologists working with pain patients, but cannot consistently distinguish between psychogenic and tissue damage pain. However, people with high hypochondriasis and hysteria scores and lower depression scores may have a physical basis for their pain, rather than a conversion reaction. The MMPI test also proves useful in assessing emotional disorders that occur secondary to a pain experience and personality factors that could affect an individual's response to pain treatment.

Psychological assessments and treatment are now part of the total approach to managing those experiencing chronic pain. Psychologists can teach relaxation techniques and biofeedback and use hypnosis to decrease pain, complementing physical therapy, pharmacological therapy, and injections. Therefore, you should not feel offended if your pain-management doctor wants to send you to a psychologist. A multidisciplinary approach, one that treats the whole patient, is the proper way to manage your pain.

Unfortunately, many pain-relieving methods touted on television and in reputable magazines are not "placebo controlled." To properly assess a drug or a treatment method, read the medical literature. Again, the National Library of Medicine has an excellent website. If you truly believe that you will get better and that you will conquer your pain syndrome, you will.

The effect of prayer also has been documented as a powerful analgesic. If you truly believe that a method will work, in most instances it will. That you are able to control your pain means that you are less dependent on drugs, nerve blocks, and other methods for pain relief. The goal of any pain-management practitioner is to have you control your pain symptoms. Try to take control of your pain and do not let your pain control you.

Some researchers report that the placebo effect is related to your body's release of endorphins, naturally occurring chemicals that we have in our bodies to control pain. A placebo, furthermore, may reduce anxiety. Anxiety can increase the perception of pain. People with positive expectations prior to taking medications generally have more positive results. This finding may be related to endorphin release from the brain and spinal cord. Expectation is a learned trait. This is one reason why a placebo response is not evident in children. Expectation depended on an individual's life experience and personality.

Other methods used by psychologists for the management of pain include relaxation and biofeedback training. These methods are used to treat both acute and chronic pain syndromes. Biofeedback is another method frequently used by psychologists to manage pain. An electromyogram, which measures muscle contractions in different parts of the body, can be used for biofeedback training and pain evaluations.

Other measurements include skin temperature and brainwave forms. When muscles are tense, skin temperature is less than in surrounding tissues because of a decrease in blood flow. Biofeedback techniques can increase blood flow to muscles and skin and increase your temperature. This can be used in combination with relaxation training to manage pain; both techniques are more commonly used by women than by men.

Relaxation treatment has also been shown to be effective for the management of lower back pain. Most back pain is caused by sustained muscle tension. Relaxation training relaxes muscles and increases blood flow and oxygen delivery while removing excessive buildup in muscles of lactic acid. Be aware, however, that muscle relaxation is not effective in all people. Biofeedback and relaxation techniques continue to be studied for the relief of various pain syndromes. If your doctor does not offer you a choice of either of these methods, let your doctor know that you are interested in either or both of these useful analgesics.

Hypnosis is another tool used by psychologists to relieve pain. Hypnosis has a long history of use in various pain syndromes. Hypnosis reduces awareness of painful stimuli by providing suggestions or images that divert attention away from painful stimuli. Hypnosis is a state of consciousness that differs from the normal waking state and is characterized by a significant response to suggestions, although not everyone responds to hypnotic therapy.

A psychologist will teach you relaxation as well as what you can do if you have a relapse of your pain syndrome. Your psychologist will help you take control over any abnormal thoughts or feelings. Your psychologist can train you to change your ways of thinking and alter your feelings and behaviors in a manner that can leave you with positive thoughts and subsequently help you relax and control your chronic pain.

Your psychologist will then assess any levels of psychological abnormalities. Behavioral goals will be explained to you. Your psychologist will discuss with you concerns that you may have with respect to the health-care system and analyze your patterns of medication use. Your psychologist will evaluate the role of family members and how they can help you manage your pain. You will be taught that negative thoughts can occur, and the occurrence of some negative thoughts is normal. However, when they do occur you are to use those thoughts as reminders to initiate coping skills taught to you by your psychologist. Your psychologist will teach you that your pain is a set of multiple problems rather than one single entity.

Occupational, physical, and recreational factors will be assessed and identified as possible etiologies of your pain. Each of these segments will be addressed by both you and your psychologist. This type of pain-relieving therapy is useful in reducing your pain as well as increasing your normal activities of daily living.

Clinicians should make every effort to increase their cultural sensitivity and awareness in order to improve treatment outcomes for minority patients. Given that ethnic groups may differ in the outcomes of specific treatments, ethnicity should be one factor that clinicians consider when selecting and recommending treatments.

Hispanics are more likely to be under treated for pain than Caucasian patients. This may be due to communication barriers, patient being stoic and not asking for pain medicines, patient afraid to take the medicines etc. Patient's ethnicity has a greater impact on the amount of narcotic prescribed by the physician than on the amount of narcotic self-administered by the patient post surgically. Members of different cultures may assume differing attitudes towards these various types of pain. Members of various cultures may react and behave differently to various pain experiences, and this behavior is often dictated by the culture which provides specific norms according to the age, sex and social position of the individual.

In most studies, women report more severe levels of pain, more frequent pain and pain of longer duration than do men. Women are more likely to experience recurrent pain, have moderate and severe pain from menstruation and childbirth and may be at increased risk of disability arising from pain. There is a significant gap between the evaluation and treatment of pain in white people and its evaluation and treatment in African American and Hispanic people.

Differences in pain treatment may be due to differences in needs e.g., resulting from genetic differences or to inequities—unfair differences in access or opportunity. Pharmacokinetic studies of codeine have demonstrated that 10 percent of the White population and 0.5 percent of the African American and Asian populations obtain no pain relief from codeine due to the lack of an enzyme needed for metabolism of codeine to morphine.

In a population-based survey, 27 percent of African Americans and 28 percent of Hispanics over the age of 50 reported having severe pain most of the time; only 17 percent of non-Hispanic whites did. African Americans were found to have lower pain thresholds than whites for cold, heat, pressure, and ischemia. Most studies showed no racial differences in pain intensity ratings, although African Americans described comparable pain intensity as a more unpleasant sensation than did Whites. Racial disparities in reports of pain unpleasantness differed by various condition.

African Americans were more likely than non-Hispanic Whites to underreport pain unpleasantness in the clinical setting, especially in the presence of physicians who were perceived as having "higher social status". African Americans were more likely to attribute pain to personal inadequacies and to use "passive" coping strategies, such as prayer, than were non-Hispanic whites.

African Americans and Hispanics were more afraid than were non-Hispanic whites of opioid addiction. African Americans and Hispanics were less likely than White people to misuse prescription opioids. The overall rate of drug-related deaths was highest among non-Hispanic White people. African Americans and Hispanics were less likely than white patients to receive any pain medication and more likely to receive lower doses of pain medication, despite higher pain scores and they had their pain needs met less frequently in hospice care than did non-Hispanic whites.

Several studies of patients with low back pain found that African Americans reported greater pain and higher levels of disability than whites but were rated by their clinicians as having less severe pain. There is overwhelming evidence that the management of pain in the United States is inequitable. Three mechanisms likely to influence physician judgments across the wide range of clinical encounters with racial/ethnic minorities: (a) prejudice against minorities, (b) greater uncertainty when making judgments regarding minority patients, and (c) stereotypes held by the provider about minorities.

The role of the health care provider is to help patients advocate for what feels appropriate for them within their cultural context. Stoic patients are less expressive of their pain and tend to "grin and bear it." They tend to withdraw socially. Emotive patients are more likely to verbalize their expressions of pain, prefer to have people around and expect others to react to their pain so as to validate their discomfort.

We can make the broad generalization that expressive patients often come from Hispanic, Middle Eastern, and Mediterranean backgrounds, while stoic patients often come from Northern European and Asian backgrounds. Not all cultures describe pain in the same way.

African-American men were more likely to experience particularly severe levels of chronic pain, and were also more likely to exhibit symptoms of depression, than their white counterparts. The findings are reported in the April issue of the Journal of the National Medical

Association and part of a body of work developed by pain medicine physician and anesthesiologist Carmen R. Green, M.D., on racial disparities in the pain experience.[3]

Through previous research Dr. Green has shown that Black women are more severely impacted by chronic pain, and in general minorities have a harder time filling prescriptions for painkillers in their local pharmacies. The latest study shows Black men with chronic pain are in poorer overall health than White men and are at higher risk for not being able to take care of themselves or their families.

For years, physicians never had a course in how to manage pain. That has changed in many places. Many medical schools now have pain management courses, and younger physicians have become more interested in managing it. Pain management is multimodal and multidisciplinary. It includes physical, psychological, social, and even spiritual management. Racial and ethnic disparities in acute pain, chronic cancer pain, and palliative pain care continue to persist. Rigorous research is needed to develop interventions, practices, and policies for eliminating disparities in pain.[4] Differences in pain perception may be associated with different pain mechanisms.[5]African Americans rated the painful stimuli as more unpleasant and showed a tendency to rate it as more intense than whites. Women showed a tendency to rate the stimuli as more unpleasant and more intense than men.

Epidemiological evidence indicates that African Americans in general receive lower quality pain treatment than European Americans.[6] Perceived racial discrimination may influence the clinical pain severity of African Americans via the nociceptive processing of painful stimuli.[7] Different ethnic groups should not be treated as if they were homogeneous.[8] Reactions of Black, White and Puerto Rican patients to pain were studied in a dental emergency room setting.[9] Attitude differences reflected a relative willingness to deny, get rid of or avoid dealing with the pain.

The Puerto Ricans scored highest, Whites lowest, with Blacks in between. Racial/ethnic minority patients with pain need to be empowered to accurately report pain intensity levels, and physicians who treat such patients need to acknowledge their own belief systems regarding pain and develop strategies to overcome unconscious, but potentially harmful, negative stereotyping of minority patients.[10]

It is your choice as to which pain management methods could work best for you with respect to your pain management. As you now know, pain medicine is a relatively new medical specialty. The exact causes of pain and the exact treatments that will cure your pain remain to be studied.

Years ago, Voltaire summarized our current situation. "Doctors pour drugs, of which they know little, for disease, of which they know less, into patients, of which they know nothing." It is your decision whether you want to use the services of a behavioral medicine specialist. Your pain managing specialist should be aware of ethnic, gender and age related causes of pain before attempting behavioral therapy as an adjunct therapy for tour pain management.

References

1.   Brown C, Bachmann GA, Wan J, Foster D. Pain Rating in Women with Provoked Vestibulodynia: Evaluating Influence of Race. J Womens Health (Larchmt). 2016;25(1):57-62.

2.   Campbell TS, Hughes JW, Girdler SS, Maixner W, Sherwood A. Relationship of ethnicity, gender, and ambulatory blood pressure to pain sensitivity: effects of individualized pain rating scales. J Pain. 2004;5(3):183-191.

3.   Green CR, Ndao-Brumblay SK, Nagrant AM, Baker TA, Rothman E. Race, age, and gender influences among clusters of African American and white patients with chronic pain. J Pain. 2004;5(3):171-182.

4.   Anderson KO, Green CR, Payne R. Racial and ethnic disparities in pain: causes and consequences of unequal care. J Pain. 2009;10(12):1187-1204.

5.   Sheffield D, Biles PL, Orom H, Maixner W, Sheps DS. Race and sex differences in cutaneous pain perception. Psychosom Med. 2000;62(4):517-523.

6.   Drwecki BB, Moore CF, Ward SE, Prkachin KM. Reducing racial disparities in pain treatment: the role of empathy and perspective-taking. Pain. 2011;152(5):1001-1006.

7.   Goodin BR, Pham QT, Glover TL, et al. Perceived racial discrimination, but not mistrust of medical researchers, predicts the heat pain tolerance of African Americans with symptomatic knee osteoarthritis. Health Psychol. 2013;32(11):1117-1126.

8.   Ezenwa MO, Ameringer S, Ward SE, Serlin RC. Racial and ethnic disparities in pain management in the United States. J Nurs Scholarsh. 2006;38(3):225-233.

9.   Weisenberg M, Kreindler ML, Schachat R, Werboff J. Pain: anxiety and attitudes in Black, white and Puerto Rican patients. Psychosom Med. 1975;37(2):123-135.

10.   Mossey JM. Defining racial and ethnic disparities in pain management. Clinical orthopaedics and related research. 2011;469(7):1859-1870.

7. Pain Assessments

Ancient tribal concepts of pain were based on beliefs that evil spirits were sent as punishment from their gods to invade one's body and cause severe pain. In the book of Genesis, Eve was condemned to pain during childbirth as a result of her encounter with the devil in the Garden of Eden. It has been reported that a shaman could suck an evil spirit from a wound to decrease one's pain. The ancient Greeks such as Aristotle were the first individuals who believed that pain was derived from various nerves in the body. The exact cause of pain was unknown to them.

Unfortunately, not unlike ancient times, the diagnosis and treatment of many chronic painful conditions today remains mostly guesswork in patients. Pain medicine is for the most part subjectively based, because pain is a subjective symptom while other medical specialties are based upon objective medical evidence. The experience of the sensation of pain in general is not bad. Pain is a protective mechanism that warns you that your body has something wrong at some location.

The sensation of pain tells you to stop activity or to at least slow down your activity. For example if you sprain your ankle, your pain is a warning for you not to put weight on that leg. The International Association for the Study of Pain defines pain as" an unpleasant sensory and emotional experience associated with tissue injury as a result of trauma (e.g. bone fracture) or disease (e.g. cancer, shingles)".

Precise and systematic pain assessment is required to make the correct diagnosis and determine the most efficacious treatment plan for patients presenting with pain. However, in order to do so a treating provider that pain intensity may vary between Pain measures fall into two categories. Single-dimensional scales are those scales which assess a single dimension of pain and, through patient self-reporting, measure only pain intensity. Multidimensional scales are those that measure the intensity, nature, and location of a patient's pain, as well and should include the impact that pain is having on a patient's activity or mood.

Pain assessment can be particularly difficult in elderly patients. The verbal descriptor scale may be the easiest tool for the elderly to use. It allows patients to use common words to describe what they are feeling. Pain can be difficult to assess in cognitively impaired individuals because their reports of pain can be difficult to obtain. Behavioral observation based assessment is optimal in these patients. Frowning, grimacing rigid body postures, tense, guarding, and fidgeting can indicate increased pain.

Pain has psychological effects in some in-stances especially when pain is severe. Pain may cause anxiety and depression. Acute pain is associated with injury, bone fractures, surgery or sprains and strains. Once these entities have healed sometimes, the pain continues. Arthritis is another example of chronic pain. Arthritic pain is caused by continuous joint destruction. However, once the pain becomes chronic, your pain it becomes a problem.

Not only does pain become a personal problem but pain can become a social problem with creation of family problems, loss of self-esteem and lost wages. Fibromyalgia patients have alterations in CNS anatomy, physiology, and chemistry that potentially contribute to the symptoms experienced by these patients.

Assessing various ethnic pain intensity reports is difficult as there is not a valid single test which can assess multi-cultural pain complaints. As a result, there are many pain assessment evaluation forms in existence. There is no consensus as to the most valid test. This chapter addresses some of the different type of pain assessments. One study found important racial and age-related variability in the symptom severity of patients with chronic pain presenting with similar physical, emotional, and pain characteristics to a tertiary care pain center.[1]

A significant proportion of this research has been carried out in the United States, and reveals that African Americans, compared to non-Hispanic Whites, suffer a greater burden of pain and pain related suffering. Several different techniques are available for your doctor to use in determining your level of pain. Elucidating the mechanisms underlying these disparities is of crucial importance in reducing and eliminating disparities in the pain experience.

Ethnic differences in pain perception have been documented in a variety of clinical pain conditions, generally indicating that, for a given condition that is characterized by persistent pain complaints, African Americans report greater pain and suffering when compared with whites. Arthritis-attributable activity, work limitation and severe joint pain were higher for non-Hispanic blacks, Hispanics and multiracial or other participants with arthritis when compared with their non-Hispanic white counterparts. American Indians and Alaska Natives had a higher prevalence of pain symptoms and painful conditions when compared with the general United States population.

Asian patients in one study had similar levels of inflammation and less damage but more pain and disability than the matched European patients with rheumatoid arthritis.[2] Black men have been shown to have higher pain scores, disability, and depression than white men.[1] There are gender related differences on the mechanical pressure pain threshold and not for mechanical pressure sensation threshold.[3] There is an evidence to suggest that the cancer pain experience is different between ethnicities[4] Minority patients face potential barriers for effective pain management due to problems with communication and poor pain assessment

Differences in menstrual pain and found that Australian women rated menstrual pain as more intense, with the duration of pain lasting 36% longer when compared with Chinese women. Italian-born men were more likely to report back pain as frequent, severe and chronic, limiting their behavior and reported having more painful sites when compared with Australian-born men, despite no difference in the prevalence of back pain between the groups. Enhanced physiological pain sensitivity in minority groups has been proposed as a contributing factor that might partially explain the observed ethnic differences in clinical pain report.

Individuals with an ethnic minority background (relative to the country in which they live) demonstrate increased sensitivity to pain relative to groups representing ethnic majorities. Ethnic differences exist in response to multidisciplinary pain treatment. Following a 4-week treatment, African Americans and non-Hispanic whites both improved in depressive symptoms and pain-related interference. However, only non-Hispanic white participants reported reduced pain severity.

The prevalence of persistent pain increases with age. There are increases in joint pain and neuralgias because bones, joints and nerves degenerate. A majority of elderly persons have significant pain problems. Persistent pain interferes with activities of daily living and quality of life in elderly patients. The detection and management of chronic pain remain inadequate in elderly patients. Elderly patients tend to be reluctant to report pain-related symptoms. This reluctance may be due to the belief that pain is a necessary part of older life.

Commonly used techniques to assess pain include verbal, visual, and psychological tests. A pain patient and their doctor are responsible for documenting and recording trends in the intensity and frequency of his or her pain. A pain-experience measurement is extremely valuable to both you and your doctor. It provides a baseline for your doctor to assess any therapy or medications you are currently taking, and it also helps your doctor to prescribe future therapy methods. The current methods doctors have available to measure your pains are imperfect. The perception of pain is based on many things that affect you, and can range from memories of a previous painful event to psychological influences. Pain is not necessarily just a sensory experience, but it is also a result of processes that occur at a higher level in the brain, making pain a psychological experience.

There is no general consensus among pain medicine doctors as to the best test for the measurement of pain. An ideal test for the assessment of pain must bring together experimental as well as clinical knowledge. Right now, there are no adequate tests that can differentiate gender with respect to the assessment of pain. In order to provide adequate pain management, a doctor must combine all of the data given by you concerning your pain complaints.

Hopefully a universally accepted pain assessment test will become available in the near future. In the meantime, you and your doctor must talk not only about pain complaints, but also about your feelings of depression and anxiety during each office visit. You and your doctor must develop a healthy relationship so that the appropriate pain modalities can be rationally prescribed specifically for you.

A short form of the McGill Pain Questionnaire (SF-MPQ) has been developed. The main component of the SF-MPQ consists of 15 descriptors (11 sensory; 4 affective) which are rated on an intensity scale as 0 = none, 1 = mild, 2 = moderate or 3 = severe. Three pain scores are derived from the sum of the intensity rank values of the words chosen for sensory, affective and total descriptors. The SF-MPQ also includes the Present Pain Intensity (PPI) index of the standard MPQ and a visual analogue scale (VAS).[5]

Experiments have shown that White and Black Americans-including registered nurses and nursing students-assume that Black people feel less pain than do White people.[6] This data has important implications for understanding race-related biases and healthcare disparities.

A pain management doctor can use several different pain-assessment forms to monitor a patient's pain-medicine therapy. Which pain assessment form is best for you? There is no definite answer to this question. These assessment scales help you and your doctor plan an individualized pain-management program.

Look over your pain-assessment evaluations carefully. If you are not decreasing your pain, or if your pain is becoming worse, you and your physician must evaluate other treatments for your pain. A functional evaluation, such as reports of your daily activities, must be included in your assessment.

The assessment and measurement of pain has received considerable attention in the past two decades. Progress continues to be made in developing pain-assessment tools. You or your doctor should not oversimplify your pain assessment. Because pain is subjective and can be observed only by you, it is important that the reports of your pain levels come from you. The situations and causes of each person's pain differ, and therefore your doctor may suggest different combinations of methods to help relieve your pain.

A McGill pain questionnaire is a method for assessing pain psychologically. A McGill pain questionnaire gives a multidimensional pain score. You are given 20 word sets that describe a different dimension of your pain. You are asked to select words relevant to your pain from each of these 20 sets. For example, one set includes the words "jumping," "flashing," and "shooting." Another set includes the words "tingling," "itching," "smarting," and "stinging." You circle the word that relates closest to the pain you feel throughout the 20 word sets.

This questionnaire is difficult to administer as well as to interpret. However, it has characteristic response patterns for different pain syndromes such as back pain, arthritis, and cancer. The validity of this questionnaire continues to be studied.

The McGill pain questionnaire consists of four different parts. The first part consists of a human figure drawing on which you are instructed to mark the location of your pain. The second part is the pain-rating index that contains 78 words divided into 20 groups. Each set contains up to six words. Five of these groups describe tension or fear. Each word is assigned a value according to its position within a subclass. The third part of this test asks additional questions about prior pain experiences, as well as the location of the pain and current usage of pain medications. The fourth part consists of a present pain intensity index.

This aspect of the test requests a pain score from 0 to 5 with word descriptors such as no pain, mild pain, discomforting pain, distressing pain, or horrible and excruciating pain. These words also are assigned different values. All the values are added to obtain a total score. All the scores are then evaluated to attempt to assess your total pain experience. The problem with this test is that there is no specific mechanism within the test itself to determine which component truly reflects your pain experience. The value of this test, however, is that it treats pain as a multidimensional experience.

There also is a short form of the McGill pain questionnaire that has been developed. This questionnaire contains fewer words and categories than the long form. This test is sensitive to evaluations of reduction in pain experiences. This test is more useful for rapid evaluation of data following procedures or surgery.

The perception of pain is based on many things that affect you, and can range from memories of a previous painful event to psychological influences. Pain is not necessarily just a sensory experience, but it is also a result of processes that occur at a higher level in the brain, making pain a psychological experience.

There is no general consensus among pain specialists as to the best test for the measurement of pain. An ideal test for the assessment of pain must bring together experimental as well as clinical knowledge. At present, there are no adequate tests that can differentiate gender, age and ethnicity with respect to the assessment of pain. Differences may exist in treatment processes as a function of ethnic group, and will consequently be an important area for future research.[7]

Pain is subjective and does not allow itself to be measured accurately. In other words, it is impossible to visualize "pain." When your doctor interviews you about your pain complaints, he or she will begin by asking the following questions: the time of the onset of your pain, the location of the pain on your body, how long it lasts, and how often it occurs during the day.

Your doctor also will ask you whether your pain is sharp, dull, or cramping. You should tell your doctor whether your pain is mild, moderate, or severe. Women in general are more able to express their pain experiences than men. You must provide your doctor with enough information so that he or she can come up with a reasonable and accurate diagnosis for you.

One way of assessing your pain is to use a numeric scale. This is the simplest method for attempting to measure your pain. During this test, you are asked to rate your pain on a scale of 0 to 5 or to use words such as "none," "slight," "moderate," or "severe." This assessment is also a quick, simple, and reliable way to evaluate the effectiveness of any medications you are taking to manage your pain.

On the numeric scale, 0 equals no pain, 1 equals mild pain, 2 equals moderate pain, 3 equals distressing pain, 4 equals horrible pain, and 5 equals excruciating pain confining you to bed rest. This method is easily understood and may be helpful in guiding the treatment plans your doctor creates for you. Another type of verbal scale asks you to rate your pain on a scale of 1 to 10, with 1 being equivalent to pain that is barely noticeable and 10 relating to excruciating pain.

Pain drawings offer a visual way to evaluate your pain. You will be asked to shade in areas on a human figure outline that correspond to the areas of your pain. The drawing will help your doctor determine where your pain is coming from and how widespread it is on your body. Over time, your pain drawings can be compared to show the changes of your pain and how you are responding to therapy.

Behavioral influences affecting your perception of pain include the amount of medications you use and the number of doctor visits required. Limping and facial grimacing also are appropriate behavioral evaluations of pain. Depression and anxiety are emotional factors that can be measured by tests.

After observing your behavior, your doctor may classify you using the following four-class system: Class 1 consists of patients with low physical injury but high levels of abnormal behavior patterns related to their pain. Class 2 consists of patients with lower physical injury and low behavior pattern abnormalities. Class 3 consists of patients with significant tissue injury in addition to high behavioral pattern abnormalities. Class 4 consists of patients with a high tissue injury and a normal behavioral pattern.

A visual analog scale is another method of assessment that attempts to measure your level of pain. Instead of choosing a number, you are asked to mark a point on a horizontal line that is labeled with "no pain" at one end and "the worst possible pain" at the opposite end.

The line is divided into 10 equal spaces, and you choose number from 1 to 10 based on your level of pain. Some researchers think that the visual analog scale is more accurate than the numeric scale for pain measurements. Another visual scale that is easy to use, especially for children or elderly patients is the face scale. It shows pictures of happy to grimacing faces and patients are asked to circle the face that shows what kind of pain they feel.

Gender and age, are both recognized as factors that influence pain perception. For instance, it may be possible that ethnic differences in pain response fluctuate as a function of age or that ethnic differences are more pronounced among females than males (or vice versa). As a result, a single multi-dimensional standardized test needs to be developed that will assess pain intensity with respect to older individuals, males-females and individuals from different ethnic backgrounds so that any significant statistical differences between groups can be identified.

The SF-MPQ scores obtained from patients in post-surgical and obstetrical wards and physiotherapy and dental departments were compared to the scores obtained with the standard MPQ. The SF-MPQ shows promise as a useful tool in situations in which the standard MPQ takes too long to administer, yet qualitative information is desired and the PPI and VAS are inadequate.

Psychological risk status, depressive symptoms, and pain intensity were predictive of a 6 month recovery status. Furthermore elevated fear-avoidance and depressive symptoms co-occurred with non-recovery at 6 months.[8] Brain imaging can predict the transition to chronic pain but this modality is not practical in a normal clinical setting.[9] in some instances, different ethnic groups and genders may use the same descriptors to report different levels of pain. In the context of clinical pain assessment, it may be important to consider the possibility that descriptions of painful sensations reflect, in part, demographic characteristics.[10]

References

1.   Green CR, Ndao-Brumblay SK, Nagrant AM, Baker TA, Rothman E. Race, age, and gender influences among clusters of African American and white patients with chronic pain. J Pain. 2004;5(3):171-182.

2.   Griffiths B, Situnayake RD, Clark B, Tennant A, Salmon M, Emery P. Racial origin and its effect on disease expression and HLA-DRB1 types in patients with rheumatoid arthritis: a matched cross-sectional study. Rheumatology (Oxford). 2000;39(8):857-864.

3.   Kvachadze I, Tsagareli M, Chichinadze G, Dumbadze Z. Thermal and Mechanical Pain Assessment in Humans: A Preliminary Study. Georgian Med News. 2015(248):57-60.

4.   Kwok W, Bhuvanakrishna T. The relationship between ethnicity and the pain experience of cancer patients: a systematic review. Indian J Palliat Care. 2014;20(3):194-200.

5.   Zinke JL, Lam CS, Harden RN, Fogg L. Examining the cross-cultural validity of the english short-form McGill Pain Questionnaire using the matched moderated regression methodology. Clin J Pain. 2010;26(2):153-162.

6.   Trawalter S, Hoffman KM, Waytz A. Racial bias in perceptions of others' pain. PLoS One. 2012;7(11):e48546.

7.   Merry B, Campbell CM, Buenaver LF, et al. Ethnic Group Differences in the Outcomes of Multidisciplinary Pain Treatment. J Musculoskelet Pain. 2011;19(1):24-30.

8.   George SZ, Beneciuk JM. Psychological predictors of recovery from low back pain: a prospective study. BMC Musculoskelet Disord. 2015;16:49.

9.   Apkarian AV, Baliki MN, Farmer MA. Predicting transition to chronic pain. Curr Opin Neurol. 2013;26(4):360-367.

10.   Campbell TS, Hughes JW, Girdler SS, Maixner W, Sherwood A. Relationship of ethnicity, gender, and ambulatory blood pressure to pain sensitivity: effects of individualized pain rating scales. J Pain. 2004;5(3):183-191.

8. Physical Therapy

Physical therapy is an important modality that can be used to help patients manage their pain. It is important that physical therapy must encompass multiculturalism. Multiculturalism encompasses cultures that differ based on age, color, ethnicity, gender, national origin, political ideology, race, religion, and sexual orientation and includes the presence and participation of people with disabilities and those from different socioeconomic backgrounds.

Older patients need to become aware of physical therapy modalities as well. One study suggested differences by ethnicity in preferred pain interventions for an older adult population.[1] The three racial and ethnic minority groups were more likely to use culturally based treatments (e.g., herbal tea and avocado leaves), home remedies and folk medicine, and/or psychological therapies (e.g., distraction and relaxation) than non-Hispanic whites to manage chronic pain. African-Americans relied on religious coping methods. Non-Hispanic whites were more likely to use physical interventions such as massage and chiropractic treatment. These study findings suggest that there are differences by ethnicity in preferred pain interventions for an older adult population.

There is information about factors related to physical activity among Mexican-Americans with diabetes. Self-efficacy and social support are associated with physical activity. The development of group identity and social cohesion was also a motivator to walk. The belief that the group can improve their lives through collective effort is a viable theoretic construct in the development of physical activity interventions.[2] Ethnic differences in interdisciplinary pain treatment outcome exist.[3] Ethnic minority groups appear to have greater levels of distress compared to Caucasians associated with their pain. Research suggests that racial/ethnic disparities in pain management may operate through limited access to health care and appropriate analgesics.[4]

High-intensity progressive resistance training as an adjunct to standard of care is feasible and effective in improving glycemic control and some of the abnormalities associated with the metabolic syndrome among high-risk older adults with type 2 diabetes.[5] Tai Chi has proven to be effective at improving musculoskeletal fitness by increasing upper and lower body strength, low back flexibility and overall physical health.[6] Tai Chi has the potential of having a beneficial influence on musculoskeletal health-related fitness and self-reported physical health in a mid to older low socioeconomic, ethnically diverse sample.

Most people believe that physical therapy affects only the common musculoskeletal problems such as sore muscles and joints. However, physical therapy addresses a wide variety of difficulties that a patient may have from the common musculoskeletal problems of everyday life to vertigo to chronic and degenerative problems such as Parkinson's and multiple sclerosis. Most patients look for a therapist they can feel comfortable with, who will understand them, and not judge them. For some people, this means finding a therapist who is from their same gender, race, ethnicity, religion, or sexual orientation. For others, it may not matter that their therapist is from the same background, but they at least want a therapist who will be sensitive to their particular experiences. The percentages of African American, Asian/Pacific Islander, and Hispanic/Latino physical therapy graduates have all increased in the past ten years. Furthermore the number of men in physical therapy schools has increased as well.

Older African-Americans have very high rates of hypertension, and they experience one of the highest hypertension-related death rates of all American ethnic groups. They are also one of the most physically inactive groups, which contribute to their hypertension-related health problems. Barriers to physical activity exist among predominantly low-income African-American patients with type 2 diabetes. Interventions are needed to assist them in increasing their exercise activities and thereby gaining better diabetes and hypertension control.[7]

Physical therapists are highly trained individuals who will obtain a medical history from you and perform an examination on you. Your physical therapist will decide what treatment is best for you based on your overall health. Your physical therapist will emphasize to you that you yourself are a major component in your rehabilitation and in the management of your chronic pain. Your physical therapist also will train you to avoid future re-injury and/or a recurrence of your pain problems. An example of how to avoid injury in the work place is by keeping your back straight and bending your knees when lifting.

Not only is a physical therapy evaluation a planned treatment course for your pain, you also will receive an education on future injury prevention using hands-on treatment and verbal education. If you were injured in your workplace, your physical therapist will tell you how to avoid further injury there. You also may be placed in what is called a work-hardening program. This program duplicates your regular work duties and helps increase your muscles' strength and endurance so that you can return safely back to work, hopefully without further injury.

Your physical therapist will emphasize flexibility exercises to you and show you how to do them. You have to be able to move your joints without stiffness and pain. Furthermore, your physical therapist will work with you on your endurance and strength. Most importantly, your pain management treatment will be addressed. Your physical therapist will tell you how to deal with your ongoing pain and emphasize to you that you should try to minimize drug therapy. Your therapist will attempt to get you back to normal daily activity as soon as possible in a safe manner. You do not want to return to activity too soon following the onset of sudden pain because you could re-injure yourself or cause yourself a worse injury. For example, a physical therapist can help you prevent a work re-injury by strengthening both your back and leg muscles.

When you see your physical therapist on your first visit, you should expect the therapist to obtain a detailed medical history from you. To provide you adequate treatment, your therapist will want to know your complete medical history as well as your pain history. For example, if you have a history of angina, your therapist will not overly stress you during exercise-related treatments because this may cause an increase in your heart rate and chest pain. If you have had surgery or have been involved in a motor vehicle accident, it is important that you tell your therapist while he or she is taking your history. Your therapist will become familiar with your pain history as well as your current pain complaints. Your history will give the therapist important information about your pain syndrome, its prognosis, and the appropriate time that you will be under the physical therapist's treatment.

Your therapist also will assess your behavioral response to your pain associated with your injury if you were injured in an accident or at work. Or, if you have arthritis, your therapist will evaluate your pain input and behavior response to the arthritic pain. For example, your therapist will note if you grimace when you move your joints. You should inform your therapist about any previous therapies that you have had for control of your pain, including injection therapies with steroids. Tremendous cultural heterogeneity can exist within one racial group and since even ethnic groups within a single racial category demonstrate variations in the response to pain.[8]

Your therapist may additionally want to ask questions about your social history and family history if they may be relevant to your condition. If you have back pain or neck pain, for example, a family history of rheumatoid arthritis is important for the therapist to know. A family history of some pain causing diseases can increase your chance of developing pain. You should not be reluctant to give your therapist your age.

Many conditions occur within certain age ranges. Osteoarthritis and osteoporosis are known to occur in an older population. Your therapist must know your occupation. If your job involves heavy physical labor, for example, you may be prone to overstress of your back muscles. Tell your therapist when the pain gets worse during the day or notify your therapist if you have increased pain with certain activities. With this information, your therapist can direct an appropriate therapy program for you.

If you have had a similar pain syndrome before your most current pain syndrome, again tell your therapist. If the intensity, duration, and frequency of your pain are increasing during therapy, your therapist may want to send you back to your doctor. This is an indication that you are becoming worse with respect to what is causing your pain.

You should try to remember where your pain was when you first noticed it. Was the pain originally in your back and then later it moved to your leg? This may indicate a disc rupture. If your pain has moved or spread since you first noticed it, be sure to tell your therapist. Tell the therapist what exact movements worsen your pain. Even pain with bowel movements can be an important history fact. A disc rupture can be associated with back pain during the act of defecation. If your pain is worse in the morning and becomes progressively better during the day, this may be an indication that you have arthritis. Your therapist will need to know this information in order to prescribe the proper treatment for you.

Providing a good medical history to your therapist will make it much easier for the therapist to prescribe the proper method of treatment for your pain. You should write down all important information about yourself prior to your first therapy visit. Your therapist will need to know if your pain is in your bones, muscles, nerves, or all of them together. If the pain is in your bones, the pain is usually confined to that particular bone. If your pain is in a nerve, the pain will usually go down your arm or leg from where the therapist is pressing on your spine or neck. If your pain is in your muscles, your physical therapist will note that those muscles will contract more.

Your therapist will examine the range of motion of your joints, including the range of motion of your neck and lower back. If you have a history of dizziness or fainting, tell your therapist before you begin an exercise program. A history of dizziness would alert the therapist to do less vigorous therapy.

Your physical therapist will record how well you move as well as your posture. Your willingness to cooperate with your physical therapist also will be noted. Your therapist will evaluate how you walk. Your muscle size will be observed for unevenness between the right and left sides of your body from your neck down to your feet. This is because muscles can shrink in size from injury and may need more intense physical therapy.

The color of your skin will be noted. Sometimes if you have arthritis, there may be redness about your joints. Your hair pattern in your arms and legs will be evaluated. If you have decreased blood flow, there may be a loss of hair on your skin. Movements of your joints, neck, and lower back will be done to see how flexible you are. Any movements that are painful will be recorded and then will be addressed during your therapy session. Your therapist will decide whether heat or cold could help you with your range of motion or decrease your muscle spasms, which in turn will help decrease your pain.

Your physical therapist's examination will emphasize the joints of your body. The examination by your therapist will probably be more thorough than the examination by your doctor with respect to joint movement. On examination, your therapist will try to determine what movements worsen your pain. As you can see, the examination by your physical therapist can be very extensive. Your physical therapist will examine you for paralysis or a loss of your reflexes in your arms and legs. Any shrinkage of the muscle in your arms and legs will be addressed. For example, if you have decreased muscle size in your thigh, your therapist will target this area to increase strength and muscle mass.

Your therapist will, furthermore, examine you for any loss of sensation in your arms and legs. For example, if you have loss of sensation in your right shoulder, your therapist will be careful not to apply heat on this area for any significant length of time. A heating pad could cause the burning of your skin if you are unable to detect the sensation of heat about your shoulder. After the history and physical examination has been completed, your physical therapist will determine what is causing your pain problem and will design a treatment program for you based on these findings. You will be treated as a complete individual, not just a pain symptom. One goal of physical therapy is to identify the cause of your pain with an attempt to treat the cause of your pain syndrome.

In addition to rehabilitating you following your injury or illness, your physical therapist will attempt to correct any mechanical flaws in your body that could lead to further injury, such as your posture. Your therapist may do a muscle and joint stabilization program to increase your strength and flexibility. For example, if your lower back muscles or stomach muscles have become weak you will need to do vigorous exercises that give your back stabilization, which means that your back (including your discs and joints) will not move when you move. This stabilization will decrease your pain.

Because you will be working closely as a team member with your physical therapist, you must choose a physical therapist that you feel most comfortable with. Your physical therapist will treat you with exercise and strengthening techniques, but also may complement your therapy with whirlpool baths, paraffin baths, or other methods such as using electrical current.

Heat packs can provide you with surface heating, which may reduce the pain in some surface muscles in your back, arms, or legs. Ultrasound is a deep application of heat. This method can relax your deep muscles. Elastic exercise bands and medicine balls may be used to increase your arm and leg strength. The elastic bands can be used to increase your strength, and the medicine balls can be used to increase your range of motion and your flexibility as well as your strength.

Some physical therapists use traction for the management of your pain. Traction on your neck or back can increase blood flow to the injured area of your back. However, if the traction does significantly increase your pain, you must immediately notify your physical therapist. Your physical therapist may instruct you in stretching exercises to be used at home. You must be diligent in doing these exercises provided for you.

Women can have very different fitness and training needs than men. Be aware that the muscle and bone development of adolescent girls is different from that of adolescent boys. A woman's nutritional requirements change with each phase of life. Proper nutrition is crucial to achieve proper hormone balance. For example, be aware that osteoporosis in adult women can be a result of poor nutrition.

Women are more prone to fad dieting and eating disorders. If you have a problem with your diet or have an eating disorder, tell your doctor. A woman's muscle mass in many instances will be less than that of a man, and a woman may have more body fat. Physical therapy is not performed in a cookbook fashion. This is the reason that physical therapy has to be tailored for you as an individual. Because of these gender differences, a physical therapy evaluation is important before initiating an exercise program for you.

Some individuals do not have ready access to physical therapy. Community and academic partners can benefit from funding, structure, and time to create meaningful, trusting, and sustainable relationships committed to improving health. Engaging PT students with community residents provided learning opportunities that promote respect and appreciation of the social, economic, and environmental context of future patients.[9]

However, these individuals can still exercise. Physical therapy students could volunteer to donate time to encourage exercise programs. The individualized and group formats of the Walk With Ease program improved arthritis-related pain, fatigue, and stiffness in African Americans.[10] Culturally appealing arthritis interventions ultimately may increase the use of existing arthritis interventions. One approach to addressing health inequity is community-based participatory research.

Community and academic partners benefitted from funding, structure, and time to create meaningful, trusting, and sustainable relationships committed to improving health. Engaging physical therapy students with community residents provided learning opportunities that promote respect and appreciation of the social, economic, and environmental context of future patients.

Physical therapists are trained to address a woman's health care before and after pregnancy. A therapist can help you with incontinence, vaginal and pelvic pain, pre- and post-delivery muscle and bone pain, and sacroiliac joint pain. The sacroiliac joint is a joint between your back bone and your hip bone. Many times during and after pregnancy, the ligaments in this joint become loose and cause chronic joint pain. Your physical therapist can work on strengthening the muscles around your pelvis and also provide you with a Velcro belt to stabilize your joints until they become stronger again.

Because of the hormones that are released during pregnancy, the joints in your spine and pelvis may become loose. These hormonal effects and the looseness of the ligaments and joints make it easier for you to deliver your baby. These hormonal changes are natural protective mechanisms in your body. Be aware of these hormonal changes and realize that these changes ultimately cause you to have back and joint pain.

Hormonal effects in a woman may be a cause of breast cancer. Women who have had radiation treatment for breast cancer may experience declines in their immune system function. Aerobic exercise programs given to you by your physical therapist can lessen the decline in your immune system function. Moderate-intensity aerobic exercise during radiation treatment for breast cancer is undergoing further study and does appear to be promising. Women undergoing radiation therapy for breast cancer can become tired easily and their mood can become depressed. It has been shown in studies of women undergoing radiation therapy for breast cancer that moderate-intensity aerobic exercise can improve both their mood as well as lessen their tiredness.

Knee injuries are becoming more common in women athletes. As more women participate in sports, more studies are being conducted into the injuries they suffer. The anterior cruciate ligament in a woman's knee has been shown to have a much higher rate of injury as opposed to a man's. It may be related to the looseness of ligaments, depending on the hormone levels of a woman at the time of injury.

Furthermore, a woman's strength may be less than a man's, and other body structure differences can make a woman more prone to this type of injury than a man. Before engaging in sports, women must be preconditioned with muscle-strengthening programs. Physical therapists are a part of this program. Following an anterior cruciate ligament injury, there are no differences between men and women with respect to post-injury rehabilitation.

You must remember that women as opposed to men have a higher percentage of body fat and a smaller muscle mass. The metabolism of a woman can be less than that of a man. These differences in body composition have implications for gender specificity in the muscles and bones of women. These differences affect the way a physical therapist addresses pain syndromes in a man versus a woman. Also remember that men still have more physically demanding occupations and recreational activities. These differences are changing but still exist, which will affect the way in which a physical therapist manages your pain complaints.

Women are more likely to use different methods in physical therapy than men, including relaxation, heat or cold packs, and massage. However, the effects of massage and heat and cold therapies can change for women sensitive during their menstrual cycle. If you consider all the factors mentioned in this chapter, you can see that a physical therapist should use a different approach for both men and women. Therapies should be determined based on gender specificity so that the wide array of methods offered can be selected based on each person's diagnosis, age, and gender rather than at random.

Physical therapists can help you decrease your muscle tension. Your therapist also can educate you on how to decrease muscle tension yourself. Most muscle tension is related to the stress of everyday life. As you know, it is impossible to decrease your discomfort associated with stress when the stress does occur.

While flying on an airplane, you may experience stress when the plane bounces around in turbulent weather. You may experience stress in your job if you have to make a presentation in front of a group. The muscles in your body naturally tense up when you are stressed. When you experience stress, your body has a protective mechanism that increases your muscle tightness. This is an early part of the fight-or-flight response to stressful situations. A generic example of fight-or-flight is perhaps a rattle snake encounter in which you may either try to kill the snake (fight) or run away (flight) because of your fright or fear.

When your muscles stay contracted the blood flow to your muscles decreases. This cuts off the oxygen supply to your muscles. Without oxygen, your muscles begin to hurt. When you are under stress, the muscles around your ribcage become contracted and you don't breathe as deeply. At this time you may want to concentrate and take a deep breath to increase the oxygen into your bloodstream so that your muscles may have adequate oxygen.

You must learn to stop pain before it becomes chronic. When you begin to experience pain, there are things that you can do to decrease your muscle tension and pain. Here are some physical therapy techniques that you can do to decrease your pain: When sitting at a desk or at a computer, have a friend or relative observe your posture to make sure it is correct. Position your computer monitor at a height that is eye level so that you do not have to look down or up. If you have lower back pain, you may want to put a pillow between the chair back and your back. This will provide you some support for the curve in your lower back.

When you are driving, keep your seat back from the steering column. The length of your seat and the adjustment of your automobile seat should have enough flexibility so that your knees can be kept at a 90 degree angle to your hips. At work, use a telephone headset if you have to use a telephone frequently. If you use a regular telephone receiver, you may bend your neck to the right or left, which over time can cause you to have muscle strain and in turn cause you significant pain.

Over a long time, you can develop a chronic pain syndrome as a result of your habits. Do you slouch when you sit or stand? Prolonged slouching over several years can make some of your muscles contract while the opposite muscles can become longer. This could cause chronic muscle pain. For example, if you slouch over a computer you can put pressure on the discs in your neck and back that act as absorbers. Slouching can cause these discs to rupture.

You must attempt to balance the muscles in your body. In other words, you want equal stress on both sides of your body; this is accomplished by correct posture. This will decrease your pain associated with increases in your stress levels. When you feel pain, you must listen to your body and not ignore the pain. Attempt to do something with respect to your posture or position to decrease your pain. Your therapist will show you stretching exercises that will be safe for you to do based on your overall health. You may want to do these exercises periodically throughout the day. Do stretching exercises in the morning and before you go to bed at night. If you have an acute injury, you can use a cold pack for 10 to 12 minutes to decrease tissue swelling following the injury. You can take a package of frozen food out of your freezer and apply it over your area of pain. You should wrap the frozen food package in a towel to prevent a cold injury to your skin.

You should not use cold packs if you have chronic muscle spasm pain. The cold can decrease the blood flow to the muscle and in turn decrease oxygen, which may increase your muscle contraction and worsen your pain. For chronic muscle or joint pain, use a heat pack. Be careful not to burn your skin with a heat pack. Wrap the heat pack in a towel to prevent a heat injury to your skin. While using heat or cold packs, remember to breathe deeply. Take a deep breath in through your nose and hold it for several seconds and then blow out through your nose. Also remember to oxygenate the injured area every four or five minutes by removing the hot or cold pack. Learn to manage your pain with breathing and exercise techniques. Pregnant women have been shown to decrease their labor pain by doing certain breathing exercises.

Neck pain is a common occurrence in almost everyone. Be sure that you always use proper posture techniques. Also pay attention to your neck position when you are using a telephone. Deep breathing before and after completing your exercises is important. If you feel that your neck is stuck or "catches" in a certain position when doing exercises, that cause may be related to a joint in your neck. The bones in your neck and back stack on top of each other like Lego blocks. Sometimes these joints can get out of position, especially if you slouch over a computer all day. Your physical therapist may be able to help you with this misalignment of your neck.

Pain in your lower back is also common. The vast majority of people who go to a pain-medicine doctor have pain in their lower back. Eighty percent of people living in the United States will experience back pain in their lower back at some point in their lives. Stress in your life can be a cause of significant back pain because it tightens your back muscles.

Throughout your spine there are a large number of bones that are separated from one another by discs that work as shock absorbers. These joints throughout your back are called facet joints. Between the two bones, a small joint is formed which allows your back bones to have smooth spinal movement. This is the maneuver that enables you to bend forward, bend backward, and twist to the right and left sides. There are holes in each bone that allow the nerves in your spine to go to your arms and legs and occasionally to your internal organs. Your spine is kept in place by the muscles in your lower back, which enables you to maintain your posture as well as give you stability in your back when you move. Ligaments attach the bones in your back, neck, and mid back to each other. Your ligaments and muscles are necessary to give your back stability and to enable you to position your spine correctly.

If you slouch or have bad posture, these elements of your back can become out of alignment. Your muscles then can pull to one side and stretch on the opposite side of your back. Remember, if you slouch over a chair for a long period of time, your spine is going to adapt to these positions. Just changing your posture, therefore, will not relieve you of your pain. If you sit hunched over a desk all day, your ability to stand or sit upright will be compromised. Slouching puts more pressure and stress on the discs of your back than any other posture. When you are sitting for any length of time, you should stand for 10 minutes each hour to take the pressure off the discs in your lower back.

If you sit in an abnormal position for a long length of time over months and years, the joints in your back that fit together like Lego pieces wear away, the joints calcify, and the alignment of your spine becomes abnormal. Note your position now while you are reading this book. When sitting for any length of time, put a pillow behind your back in the lower part of your chair to relieve some of the stress on your back.

Good posture is important to help prevent back pain. You should adjust your chairs and car seat to keep your mid back in a straight position. If you sit in an improper position, such as bending over a computer, you may injure the area where your ribs attach to your breastbone. This can cause you to have an aching chest pain, which you may confuse with a heart attack. It is important that you always attempt to sit up straight.

There have not been many studies that address physical therapy and ethnicity. However, physical therapy in general does help people manage pain in most people. Community programs which utilize physical therapy students and volunteer faculty could be effective and be a solution to health care access.

References

1.   Park J, Manotas K, Hooyman N. Chronic pain management by ethnically and racially diverse older adults: pharmacological and nonpharmacological pain therapies. Pain Manag. 2013;3(6):435-454.

2.   Ingram M, Ruiz M, Mayorga MT, Rosales C. The Animadora Project: identifying factors related to the promotion of physical activity among Mexican Americans with diabetes. Am J Health Promot. 2009;23(6):396-402.

3.   Gagnon CM, Matsuura JT, Smith CC, Stanos SP. Ethnicity and interdisciplinary pain treatment. Pain Pract. 2014;14(6):532-540.

4.   Shavers VL, Bakos A, Sheppard VB. Race, ethnicity, and pain among the U.S. adult population. J Health Care Poor Underserved. 2010;21(1):177-220.

5.   Castaneda C, Layne JE, Munoz-Orians L, et al. A randomized controlled trial of resistance exercise training to improve glycemic control in older adults with type 2 diabetes. Diabetes Care. 2002;25(12):2335-2341.

6.   Manson J, Rotondi M, Jamnik V, Ardern C, Tamim H. Effect of tai chi on musculoskeletal health-related fitness and self-reported physical health changes in low income, multiple ethnicity mid to older adults. BMC Geriatr. 2013;13:114.

7.   Dutton GR, Johnson J, Whitehead D, Bodenlos JS, Brantley PJ. Barriers to physical activity among predominantly low-income African-American patients with type 2 diabetes. Diabetes Care. 2005;28(5):1209-1210.

8.   Zatzick DF, Dimsdale JE. Cultural variations in response to painful stimuli. Psychosom Med. 1990;52(5):544-557.

9.   Healey WE, Reed M, Huber G. Creating a community-physical therapy partnership to increase physical activity in urban African-American adults. Prog Community Health Partnersh. 2013;7(3):255-262.

10.   Wyatt B, Mingo CA, Waterman MB, White P, Cleveland RJ, Callahan LF. Impact of the Arthritis Foundation's Walk With Ease

Program on arthritis symptoms in African Americans. Prev Chronic Dis. 2014;11:E199.

9. Alternative Medicine

The use of alternative medicine among the public has increased rapidly over the last few decades. There has been a significant increase in professional interest in the area of alternative medicine. Some health plans have now announced their intention to incorporate payment for some alternative medicine practices into their insurance coverage. Some managed care corporations have revealed their intentions to include alternative medicine practices for payment. Some state governments are considering legislation pertaining to the practice of alternative medicine by health-care professionals. Younger, well-educated individuals with significant acculturation levels, and have stayed in the US for a relatively short period of time preferred alternative medicine.[1] Younger women are more likely to use CAM than older women.[2]

If you are going to use a natural substance or therapy, you are responsible for your own care. You must not self-diagnose. You must discuss your symptoms of pain with your physician before taking any nutritional supplement. Remember, medicine is a drug used to treat disease and is manufactured for this purpose. A supplement is not manufactured as a treatment disease. A vitamin is a supplement and is not used to treat a disease per se. The use of complementary and alternative medicine (CAM) is likely to vary among racial/ethnic groups because its use is related to cultural and health beliefs.[3] Evaluation of CAM use in ethnically diverse populations should recognize ethnic-specific modalities and variation across ethnicity. Racial and ethnic differences in CAM use in women are minimal, and approximately one third of all treatments used were rated "very effective" by users.[4]

There are risks and benefits that you should be aware of when using alternative medications and therapies to manage your pain. In addition, the alternative medications you take could react with the prescription medications your doctor has given you and cause you even more problems. If in doubt, consult the Physician's Drug Reference for herbal medicines. This will advise you about safe doses and any precautions and drug interactions that you may need to be aware of.

In 1994, Congress passed the Dietary Supplement Health and Education Act. In passing this act, Congress recognized that many individuals believed that dietary supplements offered health benefits. The bill gave dietary supplement manufacturers freedom to produce more products and to provide information about their products' health benefits. The Food and Drug Administration (FDA), on the other hand, is responsible for overseeing any claims by the dietary supplement manufacturers to the truthfulness of these claims. The Federal Trade Commission regulates the advertising of all of the dietary supplements. You should be aware that the quality control standards for natural substances are a problem within this industry. Some of the manufacturers of these products will not have the amount of substance in the natural medication as stated on the container label.

You must do your own research to determine whether the natural substance that you are taking has an accurate dosage as stated on the container label for the product. Remember the chemical can be actually less than what the label states. A good rule of thumb for you to consider is that if one product is much cheaper than an identical product, you may want to consider purchasing the more expensive product. The reason for this is that companies that follow appropriate standards usually have their own quality-control systems in effect. As a result, they will probably have a higher overhead and will have to charge more for the natural medication.

The NIH does award grants for the study of research in complementary as well as alternative medicines (CAM). Clinical trials are being done throughout the United States with respect to complementary and alternative medicines. You may want to participate in one of these trials. Trials with respect to herbal medicines are an important part of the medical research process. The results from clinical trials can define better ways to treat your painful conditions. Individuals with OA commonly use CAM. Use of these therapies varies by racial/ethnic group. Some CAMs may be effective for symptom relief, while others may interact with prescription medications, suggesting that routine queries by physicians concerning CAM use would be beneficial.[5] Some CAMs may be effective for symptom relief, while others may interact with prescription medications.

A clinical trial is a research study in which a therapy is tested on individuals to ensure that what is being tested is safe and effective. Always remember that clinical trials have risks. Before participating in a clinical trial, discuss this trial with your primary care physician. To find out about ongoing clinical trials go to www.nccam.nih.gov. You also may want to access the National Library of Medicine online (www.pubmed.com). PubMed contains a database from which you can search for "complementary medicine" to find citations to recently published scientific articles on this subject.

Men and women use conventional medicine at about the same rate. In the United States and Canada, studies have shown that women use complementary and alternative "medical care" more than men. These women generally tended to have higher incomes and were more educated than the general population. Healthcare providers must understand how African Americans decide what to believe about CAM modalities to improve their health[6] For example the prevalence of type 2 diabetes among non-Hispanic African American adults aged 20 years and older is 11.4%, compared to 8.4% non-Hispanic whites.[7] Given the high rate of diabetes in this population, it is important to determine whether African Americans use complementary and alternative medicine (CAM), and if so, what kind.

Racial/ethnic differences in self- reported health problems and herbal use as a self-care practice between white American and African-American older women, and between herbal users and nonusers.8 African-American herbal users indicated a higher number of combination products than African-American nonusers.

Homeopathic specialists prescribe dilutions of natural substances from plants, minerals, and animals. Homeopathy has been around for more than 200 years. About 500 million people around the world receive homeopathic treatment each year. The World Health Organization has recommended that homeopathy is a system of traditional medicine that should be integrated with conventional medicine, which is considered the traditional approach to medicine.

It is important to know that the U.S. Food and Drug Administration recognizes homeopathic remedies as official drugs and regulates their manufacture. This is unlike the herbs used for medicinal use. Homeopathy qualities of medicine are used frequently by conventional physicians in Europe. In Britain, homeopathy is a part of the national health system.

The basic principles of homeopathy are that a disease can be destroyed and removed by a type of medicine that is able to produce the disease in humans. In other words, a substance that in large doses would produce symptoms of a disease can be used in very minute doses to cure it. In conventional medicine, this is called the theory of antibiotics. Homeopathic practitioners adhere to the fact that the more a substance is diluted, the more potent it is. In conventional medicine, it is believed that a higher dose of the medicine will lead to a greater effect.

The purpose of diluting out substances in homeopathic medicine is to avoid side effects. Homeopathic practitioners adhere to the fact that illness is different for every person. Homeopathic treatments are unique for each patient. Homeopathic medicine emphasizes that patients are individuals and have individual signs and symptoms of an illness and should be treated only on an individual basis. The entire individual is treated, which includes the physical, psychological and spiritual portions of each person.

Naturopathic medicine treats disease by using your body's natural ability to heal itself. Naturopathic practitioners invoke healing processes by using a variety of treatment options based on your particular needs. In naturopathic medicine, disease symptoms are a sign of your body's attempt to heal itself naturally. Naturopathic medicine gets its data from Chinese, Native American, and ancient Greek cultures. Naturopaths recommend healing of the person and not the disease. Naturopathic medicinal treatments will include doses of natural substances that are much higher than those used by practitioners of homeopathic medicine

Even though your primary care physician may not "believe" in complementary and alternative medications, you should not be afraid to approach your doctor with the fact that you are taking herbal medications. This is important not only because of possible drug interactions, but because some substances such as garlic and gingko can decrease your blood's ability to form a blood clot normally. This could result in excessive bleeding.

It is extremely important if you are about to have a surgical procedure that you let your surgeon know you are taking an herb that can thin your blood. You surgery may need to be delayed until your blood's ability to form a normal clot has been restored. The use of prayer was a major factor in differences between blacks and whites in CAM use.[9] Herb use is more common among Asians than non-Hispanic Whites, particularly among the elderly.[10]

Be aware that when you are using alternative medicines that these medicines are not strictly controlled with respect to dosage and the amount of drug in a pill, capsule, or tea. All plants have different amounts of substances in them. A true dose of a medication is unknown in many instances. You should look carefully at the label before taking one of these substances and not take more than the label recommends. The overall drug interactions of herbal substances have not been established because they are not required to be strictly studied by the FDA.

To best choose a natural product to decrease your pain, you should know which chemicals in the body produce pain. With this knowledge, you can pick the analgesic best suited to relieve your pain. If you have joint pain, for instance, you will want to use an alternative medicine that has anti-inflammatory properties. If you are injured or have inflammation, your body makes a variety of chemicals that transmit pain impulses to a pain-processing center in your brain. These chemicals include the prostaglandins, cytokines, substance P, glutamic acid, and nitric oxide.

Nitric oxide is a gas that is a pain chemical transmitter in your nervous system. This should not be confused with nitrous oxide, which is used for pain control in dental procedures. A placebo-controlled study means that one group in a study receives a sugar pill while the other group receives the study drug. In theory, the group receiving the drug should get better relief than the sugar pill group.

Cannabinoids are another natural substance for the control of pain. State legislation throughout the United States will eventually make a decision on the use of cannabinoids for medical purposes. Marijuana has been used since antiquity. In 1942, marijuana was reported to be a dangerous, harmful, and addictive drug. In 1970, marijuana was classified as a highly addictive drug with no accepted medical use. However, in 1996, voters in Arizona and California passed referenda to legalize marijuana for medicinal use. The expression of the cannabinoid receptors is dependent on gender and ethnic background.[11]

There has been a recent discovery of two cannabinoid receptors, CB-1 and CB-2. Now the scientific medical community is interested in this substance. Cannabinoids are now reported to have therapeutic value as pain relievers. This means that marijuana could help you with your pain in many situations. There have not been any controlled clinical trials for the use of this drug.

Cannabinoids do exhibit some anti inflammatory properties. However, they are no more effective than the current anti-inflammatory medications available. If you suffer from pain involving your nerves, such as shingles or reflex sympathetic dystrophy, you may be able to note some pain relief with the use of marijuana.

To date the safety and efficacy of marijuana has not been found. In 1997, the American Medical Association House of Delegates recommended to allow adequately designed controlled studies of cannabinoids with respect to their effect on pain as well as other illnesses.

This recommendation was adopted by the AMA House of Delegates as a policy during the 2001 AMA Annual Meeting.

In New York, clear differences exist in the price per gram between the purchases of commercial (average 8.20 dollars/g) and designer (average 18.02 dollars/g) marijuana. [12] Designer purchases are more likely to be made by whites, downtown (Lower East Side/Union Square area), via delivery services, and in units of 10 dollar bags, 50 dollar cubes, and eighth and quarter ounces. Commercial marijuana purchases are more likely to be made by blacks, uptown (Harlem), via street dealers, and in units of 5 dollar and 20 dollar bags. Imported commercial types Arizona and Chocolate were only found uptown, while designer brand names describing actual strains like Sour Diesel and White Widow were only found downtown.

To date there have been no adequate studies demonstrating the effectiveness of complementary and alternative medicines in men and women. The only information available is the fact that women are more likely to use complementary and alternative medicine than men.

Acupuncturists practice alternative medicine methods. Acupuncture is used in traditional Chinese medicine. It involves inserting fine needles into the body at specific points that have been found to be effective in the treatment of specific health problems. The purpose of acupuncture is to balance the body's flow of energies. Acupuncture can relieve pain, and those who perform acupuncture say it is able to restore health. Sometimes acupuncturists will burn herbs around a specific acupressure point for added relief.

Chiropractic medicine has been around since 1895. It is the second largest health profession in the world and one of the fastest growing. Chiropractors are aware of the possible dangers posed by conventional medical procedures. Chiropractors have found a way to approach the healing of body ailments that one that uses the body's own healing abilities to restore health. Chiropractic medicine is a science dedicated to the treatment of diseases by the manipulation of your backbone. Chiropractic medicine is based on the theory that your pain can be traced to incorrect alignment of your bones, which can cause pressure on nerves that can cause not only nerve pain but also muscle pain.

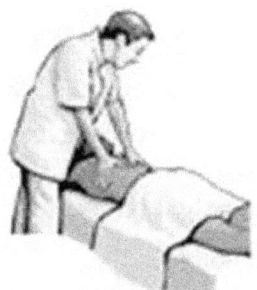

Figure 1. Chiropractic medicine.

Chiropractic medicine emphasizes individual well-being, including having a healthful diet and using natural medicines. Chiropractic therapy can be extremely effective in the management of painful conditions of the spine. Chiropractors are not allowed by law to prescribe conventional medicines, but do recommend natural substances that can promote healing of the body and prevent illnesses.

Reflexology is another method used in nonconventional medicine practice to decrease your pain. Reflexology relieves muscle stress and relaxes your muscles through the application of pressure on specific areas of your feet. Reflexology has been used for thousands of years in mideastern countries. In the early twentieth century, a doctor mapped the foot areas that related to areas of the body that affected different medical conditions. This doctor divided the body into 10 zones and he labeled parts of the foot that he believed controlled each zone. Gentle pressure on an area of the foot would generate not only pain relief but healing in general in the defined zone. These areas of pressure in your feet are called reflex points.

The philosophy of reflexology is that your body contains an energy field. When your energy field is blocked, you develop pain and/or illness. Stimulation of your foot and the nerves that end in your feet can unblock the energy flow and increase energy to various parts of your body and promote healing as well as decrease your pain. It also is believed that stimulation of your feet can release the natural painkillers in your body called endorphins. Reflexology treatment sessions can last from 30 to 60 minutes. Usually you will receive a four-week treatment program.

Reflexology can be used for the management of your back pain. Reflexologists believe that nerve endings in the feet have inner connection throughout the spinal cord and brain to reach all areas of the body. The problem with reflexology is that it has not been scientifically studied and still remains an unproven treatment regimen for the management of your pain.

A therapeutic massage can significantly help you control your pain, especially if you have muscle spasms. Massage therapy can decrease your stress as well as decrease your headaches and pain associated with whiplash injuries. Massage therapy promotes generalized body relaxation.

Massage is the application of touch to your muscles or ligaments that does not cause you to move or change position of a joint. Massage therapy can decrease your lower back pain as well as your neck pain. It also has been effective to reduce pain associated with sciatica. Massage therapy can decrease the pain associated with tension headaches.

There are different types of massage therapy. The Swedish massage is the most common form of massage therapy in the United States. Swedish massage works on the superficial layers of the skin as well as the superficial muscles of your body. Swedish massage promotes relaxation and improves circulation in your superficial muscles. Another type of massage is deep-tissue massage. This is more direct pressure on the deeper muscle layers of your body.

Deep tissue massage is highly effective for the treatment of lower back pain. Sports massage combines Swedish massage with deep-tissue massage. This type of massage therapy can decrease your pain following a vigorous athletic workout. It may not be a good idea to use therapeutic massage if you have certain forms of cancer, heart disease, or some infectious diseases.

Another method to help you control your pain is aromatherapy. Women have a better perception of smell than men. Therefore, women are more likely to use aromatherapy because they have better results from this method than men. For hundreds of years, oils extracted from plants have been used to relieve pain. During your first session with an aromatherapy specialist, the specialist will select the oil that is appropriate for relieving your pain. You may have a treatment for up to nine minutes. Aromatherapy stimulates pleasure centers in your brain from nerves in the nose that senses smell. Aromatherapy can be used to improve your quality of life and provide you with some relaxation. It has been used for pain management during childbirth. It can be used if you have arthritis, back pain, neck pain, and other chronic pain syndromes.

Aromatherapy is reportedly effective for the treatment of muscle pain as well as pain that originates from a nerve injury. You must not use any of the aromatherapy oils if you are allergic to the herbs from which the oils were derived. If you have trouble breathing, you should not use aromatherapy. Some aromatherapy can cause drowsiness.

Sage, rosemary, and juniper oils may increase uterine contractions if you are pregnant. You should not use these oils during pregnancy. Essential oils such as clove, cinnamon, and thyme can have anti-inflammatory properties and are useful in decreasing your joint pain if you have arthritis. Aromatherapy can be used in the following preparations: nose drops, air sprays, steam tents, candles, and drops in your bath.

White women with Multiple Sclerosis are more likely to use CAM. The longer that people had MS and the less satisfied they were with conventional health care the more likely they were to use CAM therapies.[13] The most common reasons for using CAMs was the desire to use holistic health care and dissatisfaction with conventional medicine. Ingested herbs were the most frequently used CAM modalities, followed by chiropractic manipulation, massage and acupuncture. Women were 25% more likely than men and whites were 30% more likely than non-whites to use CAM therapies. There was no significant relationship between the frequency of use and the reported efficacy of the CAM techniques.

With respect to age, ethnicity and gender, It has been shown that 27.7% of older adults use CAM, with the highest level of use among Asians (48.6%), followed by Hispanics (31.6%), Whites (27.7%), and Blacks (20.5%). [14] Asian elders have significantly greater odds than Whites of using any CAM, alternative medical system, biologically based therapies, and mind-body medicine and lower odds of using body-based and manipulative methods.

Hispanic elders have greater odds than Whites of using any CAM and biologically-based therapies. Black elders differ significantly from Whites only in their lesser use of body-based and manipulative methods. With respect to back pain, Hispanic ethnicity and female gender were the best predictors of CAM use.[15] Blacks were more likely than Whites to utilize CAM.

Overall, who uses CAM depends on the modality; however, education, pain severity, and pain duration are persistent correlates of CAM usage regardless of the therapy considered. Blacks used less biofeedback/relaxation and manipulation services than Whites. Aging was related to more acupuncture, but less biofeedback/relaxation use.[16]

References

1.   Kim J, Chan MM. Factors influencing preferences for alternative medicine by Korean Americans. Am J Chin Med. 2004;32(2):321-329.

2.   Adler SR. Complementary and alternative medicine use among women with breast cancer. Med Anthropol Q. 1999;13(2):214-222.

3.   Hsiao AF, Wong MD, Goldstein MS, et al. Variation in complementary and alternative medicine (CAM) use across racial/ethnic groups and the development of ethnic-specific measures of CAM use. J Altern Complement Med. 2006;12(3):281-290.

4.   Factor-Litvak P, Cushman LF, Kronenberg F, Wade C, Kalmuss D. Use of complementary and alternative medicine among women in New York City: a pilot study. J Altern Complement Med. 2001;7(6):659-666.

5.   Katz P, Lee F. Racial/ethnic differences in the use of complementary and alternative medicine in patients with arthritis. J Clin Rheumatol. 2007;13(1):3-11.

6.   Jones RA, Taylor AG, Bourguignon C, et al. Complementary and alternative medicine modality use and beliefs among African American prostate cancer survivors. Oncol Nurs Forum. 2007;34(2):359-364.

7.   Jones RA, Utz S, Wenzel J, et al. Use of complementary and alternative therapies by rural African Americans with type 2 diabetes. Altern Ther Health Med. 2006;12(5):34-38.

8.   Yoon SL. Racial/Ethnic differences in self-reported health problems and herbal use among older women. Journal of the National Medical Association. 2006;98(6):918-925.

9.   Woodward AT, Bullard KM, Taylor RJ, et al. Complementary and alternative medicine for mental disorders among African Americans, black Caribbeans, and whites. Psychiatr Serv. 2009;60(10):1342-1349.

10.   Tanaka MJ, Gryzlak BM, Zimmerman MB, Nisly NL, Wallace RB. Patterns of natural herb use by Asian and Pacific Islanders. Ethn Health. 2008;13(2):93-108.

11.   Ottani A, Giuliani D. Hu 210: a potent tool for investigations of the cannabinoid system. CNS Drug Rev. 2001;7(2):131-145.

12.   Sifaneck SJ, Ream GL, Johnson BD, Dunlap E. Retail marijuana purchases in designer and commercial markets in New York City: sales units, weights, and prices per gram. Drug Alcohol Depend. 2007;90 Suppl 1:S40-51.

13.   Nayak S, Matheis RJ, Schoenberger NE, Shiflett SC. Use of unconventional therapies by individuals with multiple sclerosis. Clin Rehabil. 2003;17(2):181-191.

14.   Arcury TA, Suerken CK, Grzywacz JG, Bell RA, Lang W, Quandt SA. Complementary and alternative medicine use among older adults: ethnic variation. Ethn Dis. 2006;16(3):723-731.

15.   Cherniack EP, Ceron-Fuentes J, Florez H, Sandals L, Rodriguez O, Palacios JC. Influence of race and ethnicity on alternative medicine as a self-treatment preference for common medical conditions in a population of multi-ethnic urban elderly. Complement Ther Clin Pract. 2008;14(2):116-123.

16.   Ndao-Brumblay SK, Green CR. Predictors of complementary and alternative medicine use in chronic pain patients. Pain Med. 2010;11(1):16-24.

10. Adjuvant Medications

Adjuvant drugs are medications used to facilitate the effects of other pain medications such as opioids and nonsteroidal anti-inflammatory drugs. Antidepressant medications and anticonvulsant medications may be used as adjuncts to opioid pain medications such as morphine, Oxycontin etc. and nonsteroidal anti-inflammatory drugs (or NSAIDs) such as Motrin and Naprosyn for the control of pain. Anticonvulsant medications not only treat mood disorders but also many pain symptoms. A combination of these drugs is also useful for the management of pain associated with nerve hyperirritability. There have not been many ethnic-gender age studies on the medications. As a result, currently available evidence on this issue is sparse.

The earliest antidepressant that was studied and was used for pain management was amitriptyline. This medication is called a tricyclic antidepressant because of its chemical structure. Amitriptyline and other antidepressant drugs generally increase the neurotransmitter chemicals norepinepherine and serotonin in the central nervous system. By increasing these chemicals, pain can be significantly decreased. Antidepressant drugs can decrease pain intensity from unbearable to more bearable, although they will not completely resolve pain. Side effects such as dizziness and sedation caused by higher doses of tricyclic antidepressants cause doctors to increase doses of antidepressants only very gradually over several weeks. Initially only low doses of antidepressants such as a tricyclic are needed. However, the dose needed to control pain will usually need to increase over time.

A tricyclic antidepressant used commonly for pain is amitriptyline (Elavil). This agent can cause constipation and dry mouth, and some patients complain of dizziness when they stand quickly.

Sedation and tremors may also be seen, and weight gain and sexual dysfunction have been reported. Some people even complain of a craving chocolate. An overdose of tricyclic antidepressants or related drugs may cause a dangerous and even fatal abnormality of heart rhythm. Tricyclic antidepressants in combination with opioids can cause more constipation than either of the drugs used alone. No antidepressant should be stopped without the advice of a doctor. When stopped suddenly, anxiety, vivid dreams, nausea, vomiting, and dizziness may result.

Because of the frequent side effects associated with tricyclic antidepressants, a newer class of antidepressant drugs called selective serotonin reuptake inhibitors (SSRIs) with fewer side effects are starting to take their place. Some of the tricyclic antidepressant drugs may have an effect on acid production in the stomach. Some of these drugs can actually decrease acid production and be of some benefit in patients who suffer from ulcers, reflux, or gastritis.

Another class of antidepressants is monoamine oxidase inhibitors (MAOIs). This class is used for significant depression and is not usually used for pain management. These drugs have a high incidence of side effects; overdoses can be lethal. These drugs increase the appetite of some patients. This class of drug increases the concentration of epinephrine, norepinephrine, and dopamine in the central nervous system, and when combined with foods such as cheese and wine high in tyramine may cause severe hypertension. For this reason, MAOIs should not be used by people with preexisting hypertension.

Side effects of MAOIs include constipation, nausea, vomiting, dry mouth, drowsiness, and dizziness. Sexual dysfunction may occur. If an MAOI is taken with meperidine (Demerol), a significant and potentially lethal elevation in body temperature can occur. MAOIs can also be associated with liver damage. Blood tests of liver function, therefore, should be monitored for anyone taking this medication. Examples of MAOIs include Marplan and Parnate. The only time that a pain-management doctor sees a patient taking these drugs is when a patient is referred by another doctor who was treating the patient for severe depression.

A more recently developed class of antidepressant drugs is the selective serotonin reuptake inhibitors (SSRIs). The first of this class was fluoxetine (Prozac), introduced in 1987. Overall, this class of drugs causes fewer side effects than the tricyclic antidepressants or the MAOIs. The SSRIs exert their pain modulating and antidepressant effect by increasing serotonin levels in the central nervous system. This neurochemical is extremely valuable in reducing pain. Other SSRIs include paroxetine (Paxil) and sertraline (Zoloft).

Another antidepressant drug is venlafaxine (Effexor), which has been studied for its pain-modulating effects in chronic pain. This particular selective serotonin reuptake inhibitor has been shown to be effective in the control of pain in many painful disorders. The selective serotonin reuptake inhibitor class of drugs can cause nausea and diarrhea. Jitteriness and lack of sleep have also been reported as side effects in a small number of patients. Other individuals complain of sedation. If sedation is a problem, the medication should be taken only in the evening. The drug can be used as a nonaddicting sleep aid. A decreased libido is occasionally associated with this class of drugs. Be aware that SSRIs can decrease the efficacy of the opioid analgesics hydrocodone or oxycodone if taken in combinations with these agents.

Lexapro does not interfere with the transformation of oxycodone and hydrocodone to morphine. Consequently, its use with these drugs will not decrease the efficacy of the opioid prescribed. Patients must be told that the selective serotonin reuptake inhibitors can cause generalized muscle pain in a small number of patients. Muscle pain is not associated with tricyclic antidepressant use.

Trazodone (Desyrel) is essentially in its own antidepressant class and is known as an atypical antidepressant. Like other classes of antidepressants, this drug exerts its effect by increasing serotonin in the brain and spinal cord. It is not as potent as the tricyclic antidepressants but it does cause drowsiness and may be used to enhance sleep. Side effects include dizziness and dry mouth. Priapism, a painful, persistent erection, is one of the most serious side effects and may precipitate a visit to an emergency room for treatment. The incidence of priapism in males is 1 in 10,000. The drug should be stopped immediately if there is any change in erectile function.

Studies have demonstrated that antidepressants can lessen the pain of the following syndromes in many patients: phantom pain, acute herpes zoster, post-herpetic neuralgia, cancer pain, cluster headaches, migraine headaches, reflex sympathetic dystrophy, and tension-type headaches. Is one class of antidepressant more effective than another? The drug of choice depends on the incidence of side effects.

Anticonvulsant medications, which are used to treat seizures, may also be effective in the management of pain. They are most effective in treating pain related to direct injury of either a peripheral nerve or the brain and spinal cord. Anticonvulsant medications may also be useful for the treatment of some types of cancer pain, headaches, reflex sympathetic dystrophy, phantom pain, post-herpetic neuralgia, and trigeminal neuralgia. Common anticonvulsant drugs used for the treatment of pain include gabapentin (Neurontin), carbamazepine (Tegretol), valproic acid (Depakote), clonazepam (Klonopin), phenytoin (Dilantin), and lamotrigine (Lamictal).

Neurontin is the most frequently prescribed anticonvulsant medication because it has the least side effects. It is also the most studied anticonvulsant for the management of pain. Neurontin and other anticonvulsants relieve severe, lancinating pain.

All anticonvulsant medications can cause lethargy and drowsiness, but gabapentin has the lowest incidence of these side effects. Anticonvulsant medications exert their effects on the chemicals that transmit impulses in the central and peripheral nervous systems. By increasing "neurotransmitting" chemicals, such as GABA, pain impulses are less readily transmitted from the peripheral nerves to the brain. As a result, less pain is experienced. Several anticonvulsant drugs affect the movement of sodium into and out of the nerve cell. By inhibiting sodium from going into the neuron, a hyper excited nerve can be made less irritable, decreasing the transmission of pain impulses down the nerve.

All the anticonvulsant medications can have side effects such as lethargy, fatigue, confusion, or sedation, and may have interactions with other medications. For this reason, when someone has been prescribed an anticonvulsant, he or she must tell his or her pain-medicine doctor. The potential for drug interactions is important with any drug. Tegretol (carbamazipine) can cause anemia as well as decrease platelets in a patient's bloodstream. For this reason, any patient taking Tegretol should have periodic laboratory tests done.

Topamax (topiramate) is an anticonvulsant medication that has found recent use for weight loss. Some doctors also prescribe this medication for the management of pain associated with reflex sympathetic dystrophy. Patients may experience trouble with concentration or memory with this agent, a side effect that occurs equally in men and women.

With respect to ethnicity, diet-drug pharmacokinetic interactions may occur during co-exposure to gabapentin and mushroom constituents. The pharmacokinetics of gabapentin in Chinese subjects who received a diet rich in shiitake mushrooms can be affected by these mushrooms. There were no significant pharmacologic consequences between the mushroom and drug however.[1]

With respect to gender specificity, there appears to be no significant gender differences when men and women take gabapentin. In many instances, a patient's ability to excrete drugs is decreased due to a patient's age. Gabapentin dosage should be decreased for elderly patients (both men and women) because of their decreased ability to excrete the drug in the urine. Male sex may be possible risk factors for the development of addictive behaviors related to pregabilin (Lyrica).[2] No clinically important differences in the pharmacokinetics of pregabalin due to race or gender have been observed. The pharmaceutical effects of pregablin were shown to be independent of gender, race, age, female hormonal status, daily dose, and dosing regimen.3

Gender and race differences in antidepressant treatments, including responses and side effects, have been studied. Because of the breakdown in the liver and the absorption of the drugs from the gastrointestinal tract into the blood, women have higher blood concentrations of tricyclic antidepressants such as amitriptyline than men. As a result, gender-specific recommendations for the prescribing of tricyclic antidepressants should be considered. Men are more responsive to selective serotonin reuptake inhibitors. Men have lower blood levels than women, but a greater affect is noted in men than in women.

Some studies note that women may better respond to selective serotonin reuptake inhibitors than tricyclic antidepressants. In another, men responded more to a tricyclic than to a selective serotonin reuptake inhibitor. Women taking selective serotonin reuptake inhibitors are more likely to report side effects of nausea and dizziness, whereas men reported increased urinary frequency and sexual dysfunction.

Differential effects of chlorpromazine (thorazine), imipramine hydrochloride (Tofranil), and a placebo were examined in black and white depressed patients.[4] The major study findings were the differential effects of the active drugs for Black men and women. Chlorpromazine was the most efficacious treatment for Black women, whereas imipramine was most efficacious for black men. Black patients also evidenced a higher improvement rate at one week, than did the white patients.

Evidence has further been published which depicts that black patients need lower doses of tricyclic antidepressants than White patients to attain a similar response in the treatment of major depression.[5] Black patients might need lower doses of selective serotonin re-uptake inhibitor antidepressants than white patients to attain a similar response in the treatment of major depression.

With respect to tricyclic antidepressants, women complain more of nausea, whereas men report increased urinary frequency and sexual dysfunction. Men appear to respond quicker to a tricyclic antidepressant than women. The exact mechanism responsible for differences in males and females is unknown. One hypothesis suggests selective serotonin reuptake inhibitors are important for female biophysiology but are not as important for males.

Preliminary studies report that estrogen, a female hormone, enhances serotonin activity. This has led to the finding that hormone replacement therapy in postmenopausal women enhances selective serotonin reuptake inhibitor efficacy. The consensus among doctors knowledgeable in gender-specific medicine is that the gender and menopausal status of women should be taken into consideration when prescribing antidepressant medications.

Sex hormones such as estrogen, progesterone, testosterone, and dehydroepiandrosterone (DHE, a male hormone) have a significant effect on brain functioning through interactions with neurochemical transmitters. Alteration of these hormones will interfere with mood, behavior, and pain responses in the brain. A current study is looking at the possible antidepressant effects of hormones. The effects of hormone therapy on pain perception will also be studied. With respect to antidepressants there is a growing body of evidence6that patients from minority groups have outcomes that are similar to those of Caucasians.[6] With respect to nortriptyline-treated patients black patients had significantly higher (50%) nortriptyline plasma levels than did white patients, which may explain the more rapid response to tricyclic treatment demonstrated in Blacks. Decreased rates of nortriptyline metabolism in blacks can result in increased side effects and treatment failure if the therapeutic plasma range is exceeded.[7]

Muscle relaxants are used to treat increased contraction of muscles. When a muscle is contracted, blood flow and oxygen delivery are decreased. Reduced oxygen causes a buildup of lactic acid with sustained contraction, which can lead to burning pain. All of these events collectively result in muscle pain. Two classes of muscle relaxant medications can be taken to relieve muscle pain. One, an antispasmodic drug, is used to treat severe chronic muscle spasms; the other, a "centrally acting" muscle relaxant, works at the level of the brain and spinal cord and is useful in treating more mild muscle contractions. People with cerebral palsy, who suffer from sustained painful muscle contractions, require an antispasmodic muscle relaxant. People with episodic muscle pain are best treated with centrally acting muscle relaxants.

A muscle "spasm" is an increase in muscle tone not under the control of the affected individual that increases during movement of the muscle. It is mostly seen with stretching of the muscle. Muscle spasms result from decreased transmission of nerve impulses to the muscle. People with spinal cord injuries can have muscle spasms even though the nerves to the muscles are damaged. Antispasmodic drugs can act within the central nervous system, especially the spinal cord, to decrease muscle contractivity and even exert a depressant effect on the muscle itself.

Examples of centrally acting antispasmodics include benzodiazopines (for instance, Valium), baclofen (Lioresal), and tizanidine (Zanaflex).

Because of the potential side effects associated with muscle relaxants in general, people suffering from pain generally attempt other modalities first. These modalities should include stretching exercises, range of motion exercises, and heat/cold packs. Water aerobics may help reduce the pain associated with muscle spasms. The heat of the water can be soothing and can directly relax tense muscles. Only when these modalities have failed should one consider the use of muscle relaxant drugs.

Valium, a benzodiazepine, exerts it effect on the central nervous system by decreasing the excitability of nerves going to the muscle. Valium is an especially effective drug for people with spinal cord injuries and resulting muscle spasms. It is also used for people with spasms from cerebral palsy and those that follow a stroke. Valium can also be used for muscle pain following an injury. Unfortunately, Valium and other benzodiazepines can cause drowsiness, dizziness, decreased muscle strength, and can be addictive.

Valium is also used for the treatment of anxiety, although anxiety and depression can also be side effects of the drug. If Valium is stopped immediately, seizures may occur. Because Valium is highly addictive, it is rarely used by pain-medicine specialists. The presence of a single-nucleotide polymorphism (G681A) of the CYP2C19 gene segregates with the impaired metabolism of diazepam and desmethyldiazepam among Chinese subjects in a gene-dosage effect manner.[8] Body fat and stature may account for inter-ethnic differences in the apparent volume of distribution of diazepam being higher in Caucasian patients compared to Chinese subjects as Valium is a highly lipid-soluble drug.[9]

Baclofen (Lioresal) is another antispasmodic drug. Like Valium, Baclofen decreases conduction in the nerves that go to muscles and is used in the treatment of painful muscle spasms associated with spinal cord injuries and other conditions. Baclofen causes less sedation than Valium; however, sedation can occur if the dose is too high. With smaller doses, side effects are few to none; the dose can then be slowly increased to allow the body to adjust to its effects. Addiction potential with baclofen is much less than with Valium. Baclofen's effects are not as long lasting as Valium's; more frequent dosing may be necessary.

Dantrolene (Dantrium) is another antispasmodic drug. Unlike the antispasmodics so far discussed, Dantrolene exerts its effects on muscle tissue, directly reducing muscle tone. Dantrolene can cause dizziness and confusion. Dantrolene is also used to decrease spasms associated with spinal cord injury and stroke. Because it results in significant muscle weakness, it is not used in patients who have to walk, including most people being treated for pain, and is mostly used in those who are bedridden. Dantrolene can cause liver injury. For this reason, patients must have periodic blood tests to measure liver function.

Tizanidine (Zanaflex) is a drug frequently prescribed by pain-management doctors. This medication works at the spinal cord level and lasts about four hours, reducing muscle spasms and also decreasing sharp and burning pain. It can boost the effects of opioid drugs. Like most muscle relaxants, Zanaflex has side effects, including dry mouth, fatigue, and occasionally dizziness. It can also decrease blood pressure. If the medication is abruptly stopped, an elevation in blood pressure may occur, which can be pronounced in people who already have high blood pressure. Unlike Valium and baclofen, Zanaflex can decrease muscle spasms without causing muscle weakness.

Zanaflex decreases transmission of impulses in the nerve fibers that transmit pain from the arms and legs to the spinal cord and ultimately the brain, making it effective not only by decreasing muscle spasm but also by inhibiting firing of the nerves that transmit pain impulses. The drug does not interfere with day-to-day life because it causes little sedation and dizziness. The absence of muscle weakness makes it safe to use in people who need to get about for work and so on. This medication may cause headaches, dry mouth, and, rarely, hallucinations. Patients may want to suck on ice cubes or chew sugarless chewing gum to counter the drying effects. Because this medication can decrease blood pressure, people taking it should have their blood pressure carefully monitored, especially if they are taking antihypertensive drugs.

As previously stated, the centrally acting muscle relaxants are used for more mild muscle pain or spasms. These agents include carisoprodol (Soma), chlorzoxazone (Paraflex), cyclobenzaprine (Flexeril), methocarbamol (Robaxin), and metaxalone (Skelaxin). All drugs decrease pain by decreasing muscle spasms. Use of these drugs should include physical therapy for individuals with acute muscle injuries if the pain persists for more than two weeks. Heat and cold packs should also be used in combination with these medications. These centrally acting muscle relaxant drugs are useful in situations where there has been a muscle strain in addition to pain and swelling in the muscle tissues.

All of the mild muscle relaxants are effective, but Flexeril is most effective for chronic use. Soma may cause sedation. It has abuse potential and has a street value among substance abusers. A reduction in dose or dosing frequency should be considered when prescribing these drugs in the elderly and in patients with liver disease.[10] Cyclobenzaprine can cause cyclobenzaprine-induced delirium in elderly patients.[11]

Flexeril, which is chemically related to the tricyclic antidepressants, has antidepressant activities in addition to its effects on decreasing muscle spasms, and is an excellent medication to induce sleep. It does not decrease muscle strength and is not effective for spasticity associated with strokes or spinal cord injuries. Flexeril reduces the number of pain impulses that reach the pain center in the brain. Flexeril is recommended for short-term use. Long-term use studies remain to be completed. Side effects include drowsiness and dry mouth. Flexeril and other muscle relaxants should not be used with alcohol. Alcohol should not be consumed when any medication is used.

Soma will relax muscles somewhat through its effects on the central nervous system, causing sedation, which relaxes muscles. It is not useful for treating spasms associated with spinal cord injury or strokes. This drug can cause mental irritability and difficulties with sleep (despite causing drowsiness and dizziness). People should not drive or operate machinery when taking any muscle relaxant medications because it can decrease their overall response time.

Skelaxin is a muscle relaxant that is prescribed by many pain-medicine doctors. It has the fewest side effects of all the mild centrally acting muscle relaxing medications. It can be used safely in geriatric patients (because these patients can become easily sedated). This drug causes minimal sedation or dizziness. Dizziness is to be avoided, especially in elderly patients because a fall can cause a hip fracture or other bone fracture because their bones are brittle. In some patients, it may cause gastrointestinal upset, including nausea and vomiting.

Muscle relaxants can be beneficial in muscle-overuse injuries. Another study has demonstrated the beneficial effects of a muscle relaxant on overuse injuries especially in females. An overuse injury is a result of chronic overuse rather than from a single traumatic event. With overuse, there is an accumulation of muscle damage that is a result of insufficient recovery time from minor muscle injury.

Chronic muscle use can result in microscopic injury to the muscle tissue. The repair of the muscle tissue or ligament tissue may be incomplete before further use occurs. The effect of increased mechanical stimulation can stimulate pain receptors in muscle tissue. Females suffer more frequent ligament injuries or muscle injuries than males, especially during certain times of the menstrual cycle. It is known that ligaments in pregnant patients are lax during pregnancy.

Female hormone levels contribute to the laxity of the ligaments. An increase in hormones during pregnancy has been shown to decrease the pain associated with rheumatoid arthritis. Women may be more prone to overuse injuries because of the differences between males and females with respect to hormonal factors and connective tissue stress tolerances. Flexeril appears to be the muscle relaxant that is most studied for the treatment of these injuries.

With respect to gender specificity, studies have demonstrated that women may have a more profound response to benzodiazapines than males. Valium can enhance the chemicals in the brain and spinal cord that can inhibit pain impulses. Valium in high enough doses may also suppress seizures. With respect to the control of seizures, there are no gender differences between males and females. On the other hand, it is the effects on pain that are more pronounced in the female patients. The exact cause is not known but may be hormonal related. Gender has no effects on the breakdown of Zanaflex in the liver, the effects of the drug on receptors or on the excretion of the drug by the kidneys.

While no differences in the pharmacokinetics of dosage requirements of antipsychotic drugs have been demonstrated among black, Hispanic, and white persons, Asians seem to have a lower threshold for both the therapeutic and adverse effects of antipsychotic drugs than do Caucasians. Use of lower than usual initial dosages of antipsychotic drugs in Asian patients appears to be prudent.

Higher plasma benzodiazepine concentrations and lower drug clearance observed in Asians compared with Caucasians are consistent with clinical observations of lower dosage requirements for Asian patients; smaller than usual dosages of these agents are recommended for Asian patients. Interracial pharmacokinetic and pharmacodynamic differences for psychotropic drugs can affect clinical outcomes.[12]

References

1.   Toh DS, Limenta LM, Yee JY, et al. Effect of mushroom diet on pharmacokinetics of gabapentin in healthy Chinese subjects. Br J Clin Pharmacol. 2014;78(1):129-134.

2.   Gahr M, Freudenmann RW, Hiemke C, Kolle MA, Schonfeldt-Lecuona C. Pregabalin abuse and dependence in Germany: results from a database query. Eur J Clin Pharmacol. 2013;69(6):1335-1342.

3.   Bockbrader HN, Burger P, Knapp L, Corrigan BW. Population pharmacokinetics of pregabalin in healthy subjects and patients with chronic pain or partial seizures. Epilepsia. 2011;52(2):248-257.

4.   Raskin A, Crook TH. Antidepressants in black and white inpatients. Differential response to a controlled trial of chlorpromazine and imipramine. Arch Gen Psychiatry. 1975;32(5):643-649.

5.   Varner RV, Ruiz P, Small DR. Black and white patients response to antidepressant treatment for major depression. Psychiatr Q. 1998;69(2):117-125.

6.   Lesser IM, Myers HF, Lin KM, et al. Ethnic differences in antidepressant response: a prospective multi-site clinical trial. Depress Anxiety. 2010;27(1):56-62.

7.   Ziegler VE, Biggs JT. Tricyclic plasma levels. Effect of age, race, sex, and smoking. JAMA. 1977;238(20):2167-2169.

8.   Qin XP, Xie HG, Wang W, et al. Effect of the gene dosage of CgammaP2C19 on diazepam metabolism in Chinese subjects. Clin Pharmacol Ther. 1999;66(6):642-646.

9.   Kumana CR, Lauder IJ, Chan M, Ko W, Lin HJ. Differences in diazepam pharmacokinetics in Chinese and white Caucasians--relation to body lipid stores. Eur J Clin Pharmacol. 1987;32(2):211-215.

10.   Winchell GA, King JD, Chavez-Eng CM, Constanzer ML, Korn SH. Cyclobenzaprine pharmacokinetics, including the effects of age, gender, and hepatic insufficiency. J Clin Pharmacol. 2002;42(1):61-69.

11.   Engel PA, Chapron D. Cyclobenzaprine-induced delirium in two octogenarians. J Clin Psychiatry. 1993;54(1):39.

12.   Bond WS. Ethnicity and psychotropic drugs. Clin Pharm. 1991;10(6):467-470.

11. Non-steroidal Anti Inflammatory Drugs

Like opioids, Nonsteroidal Anti-Inflammatory Drugs (NSAIDs) are a class of drugs that have similar chemical structures and properties and are effective for many forms of pain. Unlike opioids, NSAIDs do not cause addiction. NSAIDs can have serious side effects, including bleeding from the stomach and intestines, and are responsible for as many as 10,000 deaths per year when used in prescribed doses. Nonsteroidal anti-inflammatory drugs (NSAIDs) can decrease your pain if you suffer from the following: rheumatoid or osteoarthritis, headaches, menstrual pain, or generalized acute and chronic pain.

Aspirin is the prototype NSAID. Approximately 2,400 years ago, Hippocrates prescribed bark from a white willow tree to his patients for various painful ailments. NSAIDs have progressed since the time of Hippocrates' work. Aspirin was the first NSAID. The active ingredient of willow bark is salicin. This is a bitter-tasting chemical. Chemists took salicin and converted it to salicylic acid in the nineteenth century. It was noted then that salicylic acid could decrease fever. In the late 1880s, a 29-year-old man named Felix Hoffmann changed the chemical structure of salicylic acid. His research resulted in what is now aspirin. It is now known that aspirin has a beneficial effect on the heart and that it can prevent heart attacks. It is now one of the first drugs of choice following a myocardial infarction.

The problem with aspirin is that it irritates the gastrointestinal tract. Over time, ibuprofen was developed. Products such as Advil and Motrin contain ibuprofen. Aspirin sales decreased in the 1970s when medical studies implicated children's aspirin as a cause of Reye's Syndrome. This disease is a complication of a flu illness and with the use of aspirin could be fatal to a child.

You should realize that NSAIDs can have side effects. The problems associated with long-term aspirin use include bleeding ulcers, gastritis, bleeding into the brain causing a stroke, and asthmatic reactions. Original aspirin studies were done on men. Current research is now being done directed toward the risk of heart attack versus stroke in men versus women. The incidence of heart attacks in men is greater than in women. In 1982, a British pharmacologist, Sir John Vane, discovered that aspirin blocked the formation of chemical substances called prostaglandins. It was noted that the prostaglandins cause pain and can be involved in fevers. Aspirin was noted to stop the enzyme that is involved in the production of prostaglandins. Further studies have recently shown that aspirin can decrease dementia associated with Alzheimer's disease.

The NSAIDs are widely used worldwide. They may be the most widely used drug in the United States. These drugs are used not only for menstrual cramps but also for arthritis, headaches, and minor muscle strains and ligament and tendon sprains. The newer NSAIDs are used for postsurgical pain and are noted to be effective for the control of pain in general. NSAIDs were not traditionally given for postoperative pain because NSAIDs can inhibit clotting mechanisms and cause you to bleed from your surgical incision. The newer NSAIDs (Celebrex and Mobic) can be given to you after surgery for pain control and you should not have any bleeding problems associated with one of these drugs.

The NSAIDs in general are classified as weak acids. This means that they are absorbed from your stomach or small intestine at different rates into your bloodstream at a rate that is dependent on the pH of your stomach or small intestine. That is why aspirin is buffered to increase its pH. You may have strained your back before. A NSAID is an excellent medication for pain control following a back sprain. Acetaminophen (Tylenol) does have some weak anti-inflammatory properties. Acetaminophen is a nonacid drug. Acetaminophen exerts it effects in the brain and spinal cord as well as in your arms and legs.

The nonsteroidal anti-inflammatory medications are usually combined with other analgesics to decrease the overall experience of your pain and suffering. These drugs are used to decrease the overall pain experience without resorting to the need for the increased use of morphine like medications. Opioid drugs act primarily in your brain and spinal cord. The nonsteroidal anti-inflammatory drugs exert their pain-relieving effects in your peripheral nervous system as well as in your brain and spinal cord. By combining these two different mechanisms, your physician can have better control of your pain that originates from the peripheral nervous system.

NSAIDs directly impact prostaglandin pathways and have been proposed as potential risk factors for spontaneous abortions.[1] Race analyses showed protection from spontaneous abortions among African Americans but no effect in Caucasians.[2] Celecoxib was as effective as naproxen in relieving OA pain in African Americans and was well tolerated. Research has shown important racial differences in pain thresholds and perceptions, but little is known about racial variations in responses to pain medications.[3]

As stated previously, prostaglandins desensitize nerves that propagate painful stimuli. When you injure your finger hammering a nail, prostaglandins are formed at the area of the tissue injury. Prostaglandins are important in many normal physiological states as well as pathological states. Prostaglandins are ultimately synthesized as a result of trauma or normal secretion from the outer aspects of various cells. The outer cover of your cells in your body is called the cell membrane. Within this cell membrane are fatty substances that contain arachidonic acid. Arachidonic acid is present in all of your cell membranes.

In response to a cell stimulus such as a hit on your finger with a hammer, the arachidonic acid in your cell membrane is released and is quickly converted to different types of prostaglandins. A chemical in your body called cyclooxygenase (COX) ultimately converts the arachidonic acid to the various prostaglandins. Your arachidonic acid formation from your cell membranes can be broken down in your body and mixed with other chemicals to form leukotrienes.

These leukotrienes are formed and released from the white blood cells. These chemicals are important in the formation of inflammation (redness, swelling, warmth) in areas of your body as well as allergic reactions. Histamine production in your body released from your body's Mast cells is also involved in allergic reactions.

There are two types of cyclooxygenase chemicals in your body called cyclooxygenase I (COX I) and cyclooxygenase II (COX II). Prostaglandins causing pain can be formed in your body as a result of tissue trauma and COX 2 activity, but your body needs "good prostaglandin" to maintain normal physiologic functions. When prostaglandins are formed, they sensitize the peripheral nerve endings to other pain-causing substances in your body, which causes enhanced pain. The prostaglandins do not cause pain themselves but make the nerve endings more sensitive to other pain-producing chemicals such as bradykinins in your body. Occasionally the pain can become more pronounced than one would expect with a normal painful stimulus such as the hammer hitting your finger. The prostaglandin can make your skin much more sensitive than the pain usually associated with a hammer blow.

Prostaglandin inhibition in the brain and spinal cord produces pain relief. In the past decade, the two structures of cyclooxygenase were discovered. The two cyclooxygenase chemicals are called COX-1 and COX-2 enzymes. Enzymes in your body speed up biological reactions. COX-1 is present in most tissues under normal conditions. COX-2 is formed following tissue trauma. The older NSAIDs decrease the effects of both COX-1 and COX-2 activity. Side effects exhibited by NSAIDs are the result of inhibition of the COX-1 chemicals. Recently, NSAIDs have been developed that are specific for the COX-2 chemicals. These new drugs do not inhibit the COX-1 chemicals. This is significant because you need a normal level of COX-1 enzymes in your body.

Prostaglandins in females can be associated with primary dysmenorrhea. There are two types of prostaglandins can that can cause strong contractions of the muscle of the uterus. Prostaglandins can furthermore decrease the calibers of arterial blood vessels in tissue, which causes a decreased blood flow as well as decreased oxygen to tissue. A decrease in oxygen to tissue will result in pain. Dysmenorrhea seen in female patients is a result of increased pain in the pain-containing nerves in the uterus as well as increased muscle contractions and decreased blood flow to the tissue.

NSAIDs are divided into different classes of NSAID, depending on the drug's chemical structure. There are three classes of NSAIDs. The first are the carboxylic acid and enolic acid groups. This general class includes ibuprofen, naproxen, indomethacin, and ketorolac. The second are the benzene sulfonic acid derivatives such as Celebrex. The third group is the thenol group, which includes acetaminophen. In spite of having different chemical structures, all these medicines do provide anti-inflammatory effects. You should be aware that acetaminophen has only mild anti-inflammatory properties.

The advent of cyclooxygenase-2 inhibitors is important because NSAIDs are the most commonly used analgesics worldwide. Prostaglandins can be formed within minutes following tissue injury. The problem with the COX-2 enzyme inhibitors is that some moderate pain requires inhibition of both COX-1 and COX-2 enzymes. Recent studies report that the COX-2 enzyme may be involved in some forms of cancer. COX-1 and COX-2 may also be involved in the formation of atherosclerotic plaque. COX inhibition may provide you with relief or even prevention of plaques and cancer. COX-2 inhibitors have been approved by the FDA for the treatment of individuals with osteoarthritis as well as rheumatoid arthritis. Celebrex has been approved by the FDA for the treatment of patients suffering from acute muscle and bone pain.

COX-2 inhibitors are useful in the treatment of dysmenorrhea, which can be disabling in female patients. The NSAIDs are extremely useful for the management of your joint pain. Arthritic entities that can be successfully treated include osteoarthritis as well as rheumatoid arthritis and ankylosing spondylitis.

Other uses for NSAIDs that you might find useful include the treatment of migraine headaches as well as tension headaches. NSAIDs can be used for pain management in cancer patients who have mild to moderate pain. If the pain progresses, opioid medications can be added. NSAIDs are especially useful in bone pain. Some tumors can invade your bone. This pain can be agonizing. In addition to the treatment of arthritic conditions such as osteoarthritis and rheumatoid arthritis, it is possible that the COX-2 inhibitors may provide protection against some forms of cancer as well as Alzheimer's disease.

Women can experience painful menstrual periods. The pain can be sharp, intermittent, or dull and aching. The pain is usually in the pelvic area or lower abdomen. Painful menstruation affects about 40 percent of menstruating women. Ten percent of these women are incapacitated for one to three days. Painful menstruation is the leading cause of lost time from school and work among women of childbearing age. Pain associated with menstruation may precede the actual menstruation by several days. The pain usually subsides as the menstruation subsides.

Mild pain during menstruation is normal, but excessive pain is not. Severe menstrual pain that disrupts normal activities is called dysmenorrhea. There are two types of dysmenorrhea. Primary dysmenorrhea is menstrual pain that occurs in normal healthy women. Secondary dysmenorrhea is menstrual pain that is associated with an underlying disease such as endometriosis, fibroids, and so forth.

Prostaglandins are causative chemicals associated with primary dysmenorrhea. Prostaglandin levels are much higher in women with severe menstrual pain than women who have only mild pain. Use of nonsteroidal anti-inflammatory drugs has a success rate of 80 percent. NSAIDs have been shown to be useful in the management of the pain associated with dysmenorrhea. Because the NSAIDs are used only for a short period of time, an older NSAID or a newer COX-2 inhibitor can be used for this painful condition.

Female hormones are believed to be responsible for the increased production of prostaglandins in women who suffer from dysmenorrhea. Patients with dysmenorrhea sometimes require opioids, however, the initial analgesic chosen should be a NSAID. Oral contraceptives also are sometimes indicated for the management of the severe pain.

You should not use NSAIDs if you have of any of the following: A history of a gastrointestinal bleed, A history of a peptic ulcer or gastrointestinal intolerance to these medications, A bleeding history or a history of bruising easily, If you are taking blood thinners, A history of kidney disease or If you are a geriatric patients.

Prostaglandins can cause a decrease in the blood flow to your kidneys and disrupt renal function. In kidney failure, sodium and water retention occur, causing you to appear swollen. Potassium can be elevated in your bloodstream as well. If your potassium becomes too high, your heart rhythm can be adversely affected. Overall hypertension may occur, which can cause you to have severe headaches. Ultimately, chronic use of nonsteroidal anti-inflammatory drugs can cause significant damage to your kidneys.

You should ensure that your physician assesses kidney function every six months. The development of more recent NSAIDs does not spare the effects of NSAIDs on your kidney function. The effect of NSAIDs on your kidneys can occur within a few days from the time that you begin to take the drug. Again, have your kidney functions tested periodically.

Liver damage can occur following chronic nonsteroidal anti-inflammatory use, and you must be aware of this side effect. Liver damage occurs in approximately 3 percent of patients receiving NSAIDs. Therefore, liver function tests must be performed periodically if you are taking NSAIDs long term. If the whites of your eyes become yellow, notify your physician immediately. Nonsteroidal anti-inflammatory drugs increase the activity of your "bad" prostaglandin.

This particular prostaglandin sensitizes your tissues to the pain effects of other chemicals from the nerve endings. Nonsteroidal anti-inflammatory drugs have "ceiling effects." Ceiling effect means that if your pain is decreased with a certain dose of NSAID, for example, any higher dose will not give you greater pain relief. If you have severe pain, your doctor can increase the dose until you experience pain relief.

Even though nonsteroidal anti-inflammatory drugs are used for inflammatory pain such as arthritis, the Food and Drug Administration (FDA) has approved some of the NSAIDs for mild to moderate pain. Ketarolac can be used in the recovery room after surgery and can be administered in your muscle or in your vein. There also is an oral form of the drug that can be used by you for pain management. You should not use this medication for more than three to five days because of the possible serious side effects to your liver.

Motrin, Advil, and Nuprin are trade names for ibuprofen. These drugs are approved for the use in pain management. Nalfon can also be used strictly for pain management in situations where noninflammatory pain is present. If you suffer from fibromyalgia, for example, which is not an inflammatory disease, some of the NSAIDs are approved for pain control.

If you do not want a narcotic like drug, one of the NSAIDs can be used. Dolobid and Naproxen are two brand name drugs that you can use for pain control. Diflunisal (Dolobid) has a longer duration of action than aspirin and longer than many of the other NSAIDs. It is effective for pain management and has a longer duration of action than the ibuprofen drugs or the fenoprofen drugs. Naproxen has also been successfully used for generalized pain.

Prostaglandins can cause you to have a fever. NSAIDs can be effective in decreasing your fever. NSAIDs do affect the smooth muscle of the uterus as well. Prostaglandins can also relax the muscle in the lungs. Some prostaglandins inhibit gastric acid secretion in the stomach and make mucus secretion, which is another protective mechanism for the stomach. Other prostaglandins can increase gastrointestinal motility.

The "good" prostaglandins can regulate the blood flow to the kidneys as well as sodium/potassium exchange. If the sodium/potassium exchange is compromised, you may retain sodium as well as fluid, which can increase your blood pressure. The "bad" prostaglandins can sensitize nerve endings to pain. As you can see, the many types of prostaglandins have many different functions. This is why you and your physician need to select the right drug for your pain.

These drugs can also cause effects such as peptic ulcer disease as well as gastritis and belching. NSAIDs can also cause you to experience diarrhea. Rarely have NSAIDs been implicated in kidney failure. NSAIDs decrease your blood's ability to form a blood clot. However, this may not be an entirely adverse event, because the use of an NSAID could protect your heart from a heart attack. NSAIDs have been reported to adversely affect the liver. You could develop jaundice from chronic use of NSAIDs.

NSAIDs should not be used if you have a fractured bone. The use of NSAIDs may delay healing of your fracture. NSAIDs may affect cartilage repair in your joints if you suffer from osteoarthritis. If you have pain associated with osteoarthritis, it is recommended that the newer COX-2 enzyme inhibitors be prescribed.

With respect to gender specificity, previous studies directed at the more traditional NSAIDs reveal that male patients respond better to the effects of the traditional NSAIDs than females. The problem with earlier studies is that most of the original studies were done on male patients. In female patients, production of estrogen, the female hormone, may increase the number of prostaglandins present at any one time. This increase in any number of prostaglandins may attenuate the efficacy of NSAIDs.

There is evidence that disparities in the treatment of pain occur because of differences in race. In a previous study done in 2005, racial differences in opioid use for chronic nonmalignant pain were noted while there were no differences by race in the use of other treatment modalities such as physical therapy and nonsteroidal anti-inflammatories or in the use of specialty referral. Equal treatment by race occurs in nonopioid-related therapies, but white patients are more likely than black patients to be treated with opioids.[4]

Minorities with osteoarthritis were prescribed NSAIDs with less COX-2 selectivity and lower days' supply than whites. Further research should address underlying reasons and whether these differences impact outcomes such as pain control, side effects and cost-effectiveness of care.[5] The American Heart Association recommended aspirin for the primary prevention of coronary heart disease.[6] Regular aspirin use in adults at increased and high risk for coronary heart disease remains suboptimal in different races. Important racial/ethnic disparities exist for unclear reasons.[7]

Due to their risk profile NSAIDs are less appropriate due to high incidence rates and drug-related risk patterns in elderly patients.[8] Acetaminophen, metamizol and flupirtin may be recommended instead. Avoiding NSAIDs whenever possible, substituting less toxic COX-2 inhibitors, monitoring risk, and providing co therapy with proton pump inhibitors, or misoprostol may decrease NSAIDs associated morbidity and mortality in the patient population.[9]

Aging is accompanied by changes in physiology, resulting in altered pharmacokinetics and pharmacodynamics.[10]   Decreased drug clearance may be related to decreases in hepatic mass, enzymatic activity, blood flow, renal plasma flow, glomerular filtration rate, and tubular function associated with aging. Older people are more likely to experience adverse gastrointestinal and renal effects related to NSAIDs. The use of aspirin for prevention of cardiovascular disease increases the toxicity of NSAIDs.

Older people have more illnesses than younger patients and therefore take more medications, increasing the possibility of drug-drug interactions with NSAIDs. Adverse drug reactions related to multiple medication interactions are common causes of hospital admissions and may have important consequences.[11] Older patients statistically take more medications than younger patients. The most important determinant for adverse drug reaction related hospital admissions is the number of drugs taken.1[2] Adverse drug reactions may therefore be expected in older individuals. Topical diclofenac sodium 1% gel is a treatment is generally well tolerated for arthritic joints because uptake is less than oral medications.[13] A careful management of therapeutics regimens by means of educational campaigns for patients and guidelines for doctors finalized to avoid excessive drug prescription.

References

1.   Essex MN, O'Connell M, Bhadra Brown P. Response to nonsteroidal anti-inflammatory drugs in African Americans with osteoarthritis of the knee. J Int Med Res. 2012;40(6):2251-2266.

2.   Velez Edwards DR, Hartmann KE. Racial differences in risk of spontaneous abortions associated with periconceptional over-the-counter nonsteroidal anti-inflammatory drug exposure. Ann Epidemiol. 2014;24(2):111-115 e111.

3.   Gagnon CM, Matsuura JT, Smith CC, Stanos SP. Ethnicity and interdisciplinary pain treatment. Pain Pract. 2014;14(6):532-540.

4.   Chen I, Kurz J, Pasanen M, et al. Racial differences in opioid use for chronic nonmalignant pain. J Gen Intern Med. 2005;20(7):593-598.

5.   Dominick KL, Baker TA. Racial and ethnic differences in osteoarthritis: prevalence, outcomes, and medical care. Ethn Dis. 2004;14(4):558-566.

6.   Sanchez DR, Diez Roux AV, Michos ED, et al. Comparison of the racial/ethnic prevalence of regular aspirin use for the primary prevention of coronary heart disease from the multi-ethnic study of atherosclerosis. Am J Cardiol. 2011;107(1):41-46.

7.   Brown DW, Shepard D, Giles WH, Greenlund KJ, Croft JB. Racial differences in the use of aspirin: an important tool for preventing heart disease and stroke. Ethn Dis. 2005;15(4):620-626.

8.   Burkhardt H, Wehling M. [Non-opioid pain medication in the elderly]. Schmerz. 2015;29(4):371-379.

9.   Akhtar AJ, Shaheen M. Upper gastrointestinal toxicity of nonsteroidal anti-inflammatory drugs in African-American and Hispanic elderly patients. Ethn Dis. 2003;13(4):528-533.

10.   Barkin RL, Beckerman M, Blum SL, Clark FM, Koh EK, Wu DS. Should nonsteroidal anti-inflammatory drugs (NSAIDs) be prescribed to the older adult? Drugs Aging. 2010;27(10):775-789.

11.   Ventura MT, Laddaga R, Cavallera P, et al. Adverse drug reactions as the cause of emergency department admission: focus on the elderly. Immunopharmacol Immunotoxicol. 2010;32(3):426-429.

12.   Vandraas KF, Spigset O, Mahic M, Slordal L. Non-steroidal anti-inflammatory drugs: use and co-treatment with potentially interacting medications in the elderly. Eur J Clin Pharmacol. 2010;66(8):823-829.

13.   Baraf HS, Gold MS, Petruschke RA, Wieman MS. Tolerability of topical diclofenac sodium 1% gel for osteoarthritis in seniors and patients with comorbidities. Am J Geriatr Pharmacother. 2012;10(1):47-60.

12. Opioids

Pain is often poorly managed, highlighting the need to better understand and treat patients' pain. Research suggests that pain is assessed and treated differently depending on patient sex, race, and/or age.[1] Opioids are a class of drugs which depress the central nervous system to relieve pain. An opioid is a drug that acts similarly to morphine. Some opioids are found naturally in the environment, whereas others are made in a lab. A narcotic is a similar type of medication. However, it applies to drugs similar to morphine as well as to any type of substance that could cause you to become dependent on it. Attention been focused on the importance of interethnic differences as determinants of individual variability in drug responses.[2] Ethnicity for example has been shown to be an important determinant of the disposition and effects of morphine.

Opioids bind themselves to receptors on nerves in your body that are located in your central nervous system and in the peripheral nerves in your arms and legs. When an opioid attaches to one of your receptors like the mu receptor, it turns it on. When the receptor is turned on the number of pain sensations that reach your brain are lessened. This receptor blocks painful impulses. An opioid is a chemical that binds to opioid receptors, which are widely distributed in the central and peripheral nervous system and gastrointestinal tract. The different effects elicited by activation of these receptors are due to their specific neuronal and extra neuronal distribution.

The painkiller effect of opioids is induced by the synergy of the two events, namely reduction of pain threshold and emotional detachment from pain. Three major types of opioid receptor, m, d and k (mu, delta and kappa), were defined pharmacologically several years ago. All 3 receptors produce analgesia when an opioid binds to them. However, activation of k receptors does not produce as much physical dependence as activation of m receptors. Morphine and most other pain medications bind to the mu receptor.

Burorphanol (Stadol) binds to the kappa receptors. Naloxone and Naltrexone antognize the mu receptors. Dynorphin occupys the receptors. Opioids inhibit pain neurotransmitter chemical release, and this is considered to be their major effect in the nervous system. Genetic, environmental, and demographic factors work together to control adverse and reinforcing opioid responses, but contribute differently to specific responses.[3] For example, meperidine produces fewer side effects than morphine during short-term use. The risk of respiratory depression increases substantially after 60 years of age. Women have nausea and vomiting more often than men.[4] The effect of race deserves further investigation.

Opioid drugs can either be classified as weak or strong, depending on how they interact with the opioid receptors in your body. Codeine and propoxyphene (Darvon) are considered weak opioids. All others are considered strong opioids. All opioid drugs provide pain relief by decreasing the amount of chemicals in your body that attach to pain receptors that transmit pain. With this decrease your overall pain impulses are dampened or may not even reach your brain at all. Pain management is an important part of prehospital care, yet few studies have addressed the effects of age, sex, race, or pain severity on prehospital pain management. A previous study suggests that Caucasians are more likely than African-Americans or Hispanics to receive prehospital analgesia for blunt trauma injuries.[5]

Some opioid medications can alter your mood or occasionally cause you to experience euphoria or excitement. Changes in the chemicals that exist in your brain cause these types of mood changes. When you take opioids over a large time span of weeks or months, you can build up a tolerance to the effect of the opioids. When you become tolerant to the opioid, its ability to provide pain relief is decreased. Tolerance and dependence are induced by chronic exposure to morphine and other opioids more than any other group of drugs. Tolerance means that higher doses of opioids are required to produce an effect. When the degree of tolerance is very marked, the maximum response attainable with the opioid is also reduced. Tolerance is mainly due to receptor desensitization.

Although dependence usually accompanies tolerance, they are distinct phenomena. Dependence is masked until the opioid drug is removed from its receptors, either by stopping the drug or by giving an opioid receptor antagonist such as naloxone. A withdrawal or abstinence response then occurs. The withdrawal response is very complex and involves many brain regions. Dependence occurs much more rapidly in the body. Tolerance and dependence are induced by chronic exposure to morphine and other opioids more than any other group of drugs.

Tolerance means that higher doses of opioids are required to produce an effect. When the degree of tolerance is very marked, the maximum response attainable with the opioid is also reduced. Tolerance is mainly due to receptor desensitization induced by functional uncoupling of opioid receptors from G-proteins, thus uncoupling the receptors from their effector systems. However, the mechanism of this desensitization is still not fully understood.

Although dependence usually accompanies tolerance, they are distinct phenomena. Dependence is masked until the opioid drug is removed from its receptors, either by stopping the drug or by giving an opioid receptor antagonist such as naloxone. A withdrawal or abstinence response then occurs. The withdrawal response is very complex and involves many brain regions. Dependence occurs much more rapidly than tolerance

Opioid drugs can be further classified into three categories: agonist, antagonist, and mixed agonist/antagonist. Agonist drugs such as morphine attach to two of the three opioid receptors in your brain and spinal cord to provide pain relief by switching the receptors on. Antagonist drugs bind to all three types of receptors throughout your body. When they bind to the receptor, they do not switch the receptor on. The mixed agonist/antagonist drugs stimulate activities at the opioid receptors, but do not allow them to be switched on.

Morphine is classified as a naturally occurring agonist drug. It has been made into a slow-release formula. The slow-release morphine (MS Contin) needs to be taken only every 12 hours. It allows a gradual release of morphine as the pill passes through your stomach and intestine. Other drugs like Oxycontin and Nucynta ER are made into slow release forms. Ethnicity influences the response to morphine. Native Indians for example, are more susceptible to morphine depression of the respiratory drive than Caucasians.[6] Morphine may be administered after surgery by patients for pain control. One study identified no statistically significant difference in either opioid prescribing or self-administration between Hispanic and White post-operative patients.

Codeine is considered a weak agonist drug and is not commonly used for severe pain management. It is often used for mild pain, whereas morphine is used for more severe types of pain. Codeine also is less likely to cause addiction than other opioids. When codeine enters your body, it is converted into morphine, which produces its pain-relieving effects.

An example of a synthetic opioid is methadone. Methadone lasts a long time in the body. This drug offers an advantage to patients because less-frequent dosing is required. Methadone is an excellent medication for use in patients who have some component of their pain that is related to nerve inflammation such as shingles or reflex sympathetic dystrophy. Meperidine (Demerol) can cause seizures if it is administered for a long time in patients. The medication fentanyl was originally used for anesthesia during surgery. However, fentanyl can now be administered by a patch or by a lozenge. It also is available in a sucker form for administration. Fentanyl is one of the most powerful drugs that have been mentioned.

Tramadol (Ultram) is a synthetic chemical similar to codeine. It also increases serotonin and norepinephrine in your brain and spinal cord. These are two chemicals within the central nervous system that decrease feelings of depression. Serotonin and norepinepherine also decrease the number of pain impulses that ultimately reach your brain. Tramadol also can be combined with acetaminophen (Ultracet) to provide mild pain-relieving effects.

Butorphanol (Stadol nasal spray) and nalbuphine (Nubain) are agonist/antagonist drugs. Butorphanol is available as a nasal spray and is now in a generic form. Nalbuphine is another agonist/antagonist drug that is available only intravenously.

Side effects of opioids can include drowsiness, alteration in mood, and mental clouding. If the dosage is too high, your ability to concentrate can be affected. Opioid drugs can decrease your breathing rate. Opioids can cause constipation. They cause constipation by decreasing the ability of the stomach and bowel to push food through to the rectum. Some of the agonist drugs also can cause hives. Animal studies have demonstrated the differences between males and females with respect to responses to opioids. Male rats have demonstrated greater pain relief with morphine than female rats following painful stimuli.

In another laboratory study, there were no sex differences reported with fentanyl and buphrenorphine. The same types of effects have been found in people. Gender-specific issues exist with respect to opioids. Men respond better to some opioids than women. For example, women have more side effects than men do while taking Oxycontin. It is interesting to note that when a placebo (sugar pill) is given to men and women in clinical drug studies, their response to the placebo is equal.

The difference between the effects of opioids on men and women may be related to the different sex hormones that are located on your receptors. Receptors on cells differ between men and women. One study has shown that when the female hormone estrogen is given to males and the male hormone androgen is given to women, the effects are different from when female hormones are given to women and male hormones are given to men. This observation implies that your receptors are affected by your sex hormones.

The amount of drug and the frequency of dosing also should differ between men and women. Examinations of pharmacological textbooks as well as the Physician's Desk Reference do not specify gender differences in the dosing and frequency of dosing. These factors need to be addressed with future studies. More women are addicted to cocaine than men. The reason for this observation may be due to the effects of female hormones on the addictive pathway in the female central nervous system.

It is concluded that sex hormones influence the effects of many drugs. The menstrual cycle, pregnancy, and menopause can each affect how a particular drug reacts in a female body. Female patients must tell their pain-medicine doctor that they are taking hormone replacement. This is imperative because hormone replacement therapy can alter drug interactions in women. Pain medications such as hydrocodone contain acetaminophen. Acetaminophen in addition to hydrocodone is an analgesic. Acetaminophen is inactivated 50 percent more in women who are taking an oral contraceptive. Analgesic effect of an opioid containing acetaminophen may, therefore, be decreased.

Most pain-medicine doctors require that a patient sign a contract when the patient is admitted into the doctor's practice. The contract states that the patient will obtain pain-relieving medications from only one doctor and will use only one pharmacy. These contracts are usually mandated by state medical boards.

Natural and semisynthetic opioid analgesics, such as hydrocodone, morphine, and oxycodone, were involved in multiple drug-poisoning deaths.[8] During the past decade, adults aged 55-64 and non-Hispanic white persons experienced the greatest increase in the rates of opioid-analgesic poisoning deaths. Ethnicity influences the response to morphine. Native Indians are more susceptible to morphine depression of the ventilatory response than Caucasians.

Narcotic analgesic doses in one hospital for an entire postoperative period revealed that male patients received significantly larger initial doses than female patients.[9] There was no gender difference in the total dose received postoperatively. White patients received significantly more total postoperative narcotic analgesics than ethnic minority patients. Results from another study generally indicated that for pressure and ischemic pain, African American subjects showed greater analgesic responses to both medications compared with non-Hispanic whites.[10]

African American children 11experienced significantly more postoperative pain than Caucasian children in one hospital as measured by postoperative opioid requirements.[11] Although Caucasian children received relatively less opioids perioperatively, they had significantly higher opioid related adverse effects. African American children with obstructive sleep apnea were more likely to have prolonged post anesthesia recovery unit stay due to inadequate pain control. Caucasians are more likely than African-Americans or Hispanics to receive prehospital analgesia for blunt trauma injuries. In addition, patients with whom paramedics spend more time and for whom a pain score is recorded are more likely to receive analgesia. The CYP2D6 enzymes that metabolize some pain medications has metabolic activity that ranges considerably within a population and includes ultra-rapid metabolizers , extensive metabolizers, intermediate metabolizers and poor metabolizers. There is a considerable variability in the CYP2D6 allele distribution among different ethnic groups, resulting in variable percentages of PMs, IMs, EMs and UMs in a given population. This implies that better pain assessments need to be used to adequately treat patients of different ethnic groups and that the appropriate doses of medications be prescribed to patients suffering from severe pain.

Women and men respond differently to pharmaceuticals as well as alcohol. The number of adverse effects related to pain management with opioids is more serious in women than men. The differences are related to the way in which drugs are taken up from your stomach and your small intestine into your bloodstream, the effect of the breakdown of the liver, and the elimination of the drugs through the kidneys. With these facts in mind, you would expect that the amount of drug and the frequency of dosing should differ between men and women.

With respect to illicit drugs, the electric activities within a man's brain when measured by the electroencephalogram (EEG) are changed by cocaine abuse while there are no changes when a woman abuses cocaine. Women are less likely than men to experience symptoms of paranoia when smoking cocaine as compared to men. Women who take amphetamines perceive the effects of the drug differently than men.

To address drug addiction, the "exposure" theory of addiction was postulated in the 1970s. The conclusions of the study resulted from animal studies. Animals were placed in isolated cages and allowed access to addictive drugs. The animals were taught in the laboratory to be able to self-administer intravenous opioids.

The investigators of the study concluded that exposing an animal to an opioid for a long period of time would definitely cause addiction. After the 1970s, the exposure theory was challenged. Investigators demonstrated that rats placed in a nonisolated setting did not develop an addictive behavior. The animals were offered a choice between a morphine solution and water. These investigators reported that it takes more than exposure to an addictive opioid to cause addiction.

Methadone pharmacology can be affected by genetics. Treatment of opiate use disorders with methadone is complicated by wide interindividual variability in pharmacokinetics. Population pharmacokinetics is a valuable method for identifying the influences on methadone pharmacokinetic variability.[12]

Gender may affect side effects of narcotic prescriptions in emergency rooms. Narcotic analgesia is commonly given in emergency departments. Narcotic-induced nausea and vomiting is thought to be a common occurrence. The nausea and vomiting was associated with female sex and the intensity of the pain with a higher pain intensity causing more pain.[13] A comparative study of other pain medications versus narcotics for incidence of induced nausea and emesis would be useful.

Basic laboratory researchers in the field of addiction medicine have discovered an addictive pathway in an animal brain. This pathway can be turned on by chemicals associated with addiction. Some individuals who may be a result of genetics may have a greater or lesser sensitivity to the affects of substances on this addictive pathway. This is the reason why a small percentage of individuals are at an increased risk for developing an addictive behavioral pattern.

It can be difficult for a doctor to evaluate whether your pain is real. Most pain doctors think that it is most ethical to err on the side of pain relief and to prescribe opioid medications in a controlled environment rather than withhold pain-relieving drugs from an individual who is suffering. Patient should be evaluated on a case-by-case basis. The American Society of Addiction Medicine, the American Pain Society, the American Academy of Pain Medicine, and the United States Federation of State Medical Boards have declared that the use of opioids for the treatment of noncancerous pain is appropriate in individuals who are properly evaluated.

These organizations also have declared that a patient history of previous substance abuse is not a contraindication for the prescribing of opioid drugs. These organizations have furthermore outlined the responsibilities of doctors for prescribing opioid medications.   A multicenter study to better understand emergency department (ED) pain management practices was done and examined the influence of patient and provider gender on analgesic administration. Female physicians were more likely to administer analgesics than male physicians. Provider gender as opposed to patient gender appears to influence pain management decisions in the ED.[14]

Studies have found that living in a rural community in the US is associated with health care disparities. Rural residents have higher odds of having n opioid prescription than similar non-rural adults.[15] The overall consequences of increased opioid prescribing on rural communities.

Home remedy use is an often overlooked component of health self-management, with a rich tradition, particularly among African Americans and others who have experienced limited access to medical care or discrimination by the health care system. This fact needs to be taken into consideration if a patient seeks medical attention in an emergency room. African American elders reported greater use than white elders; women reported more use for a greater number of symptoms than men. The home remedy use has the potential to interfere with medical management of pain in some instances.

Race, sex, and poverty are associated with the use of diagnostic cardiac catheterization and coronary revascularization during treatment of acute myocardial infarction (AMI).[16] Medical therapies including opioids (morphine) are currently underused in the treatment of black, female, and poor patients with AMI.[17]

The demand for an increased use of opioids exists. However, this demand comes at a time when the United States is confronted with widespread drug abuse and drug trafficking. An examination of the history of opioid use over the centuries demonstrated that there have been periods of liberal opioid use for the treatment of pain that were followed by periods that prohibited the prescribing of opioids. It is felt that this is a result of the adverse consequences associated with opioids. In today's medical environment, doctors must use opioids for their pain relieving qualities but at the same time minimize adverse effects of the drugs that may result from their chronic use.

Public, patient, and self-education is the key to eliminating fears associated with opioid addiction. As long as you do not have a substance-abuse disorder, the likelihood that you will become addicted to opioids is extremely rare. The American Pain Society is requesting that legislatures avoid making policies that establish barriers to keep opioid drugs from the people who need them.

The fact that some people abuse opioids should not be a barrier to keeping opioids from people who actually need them. Everyone needs to be educated about the important role of opioid drugs in pain management and ethnic; gender and age considerations must be .taken into consideration when a physician prescribes a medication.

References

1. Wandner LD, Torres CA, Bartley EJ, George SZ, Robinson ME. Effect of a perspective-taking intervention on the consideration of pain assessment and treatment decisions. J Pain Res. 2015;8:809-818.

2. Zhou HH, Sheller JR, Nu H, Wood M, Wood AJ. Ethnic differences in response to morphine. Clin Pharmacol Ther. 1993;54(5):507-513.

3. Angst MS, Lazzeroni LC, Phillips NG, et al. Aversive and reinforcing opioid effects: a pharmacogenomic twin study. Anesthesiology. 2012;117(1):22-37.

4. Cepeda MS, Farrar JT, Baumgarten M, Boston R, Carr DB, Strom BL. Side effects of opioids during short-term administration: effect of age, gender, and race. Clin Pharmacol Ther. 2003;74(2):102-112.

5. Young MF, Hern HG, Alter HJ, Barger J, Vahidnia F. Racial differences in receiving morphine among prehospital patients with blunt trauma. J Emerg Med. 2013;45(1):46-52.

6. Cepeda MS, Farrar JT, Roa JH, et al. Ethnicity influences morphine pharmacokinetics and pharmacodynamics. Clin Pharmacol Ther. 2001;70(4):351-361.

7. Adams RJ, Armstrong EP, Erstad BL. Prescribing and self-administration of morphine in Hispanic and non Hispanic Caucasian patients treated with patient-controlled analgesia. J Pain Palliat Care Pharmacother. 2004;18(2):29-38.

8. Ruhm CJ. Drug poisoning deaths in the United States, 1999-2012: a statistical adjustment analysis. Popul Health Metr. 2016;14:2.

9. McDonald DD. Gender and ethnic stereotyping and narcotic analgesic administration. Res Nurs Health. 1994;17(1):45-49.

10. Sibille KT, Kindler LL, Glover TL, et al. Individual differences in morphine and butorphanol analgesia: a laboratory pain study. Pain Med. 2011;12(7):1076-1085.

11.   Sadhasivam S, Chidambaran V, Ngamprasertwong P, et al. Race and unequal burden of perioperative pain and opioid related adverse effects in children. Pediatrics. 2012;129(5):832-838.

12.   Bart G, Lenz S, Straka RJ, Brundage RC. Ethnic and genetic factors in methadone pharmacokinetics: a population pharmacokinetic study. Drug Alcohol Depend. 2014;145:185-193.

13.   Zun LS, Downey LV, Gossman W, Rosenbaumdagger J, Sussman G. Gender differences in narcotic-induced emesis in the ED. Am J Emerg Med. 2002;20(3):151-154.

14.   Safdar B, Heins A, Homel P, et al. Impact of physician and patient gender on pain management in the emergency department--a multicenter study. Pain Med. 2009;10(2):364-372.

15.   Prunuske JP, St Hill CA, Hager KD, et al. Opioid prescribing patterns for non-malignant chronic pain for rural versus non-rural US adults: a population-based study using 2010 NAMCS data. BMC Health Serv Res. 2014;14:563.

16.   Rathore SS, Berger AK, Weinfurt KP, et al. Race, sex, poverty, and the medical treatment of acute myocardial infarction in the elderly. Circulation. 2000;102(6):642-648.

17.   Xu C, Zhang Y, Zheng H, Loh HH, Law PY. Morphine modulates mouse hippocampal progenitor cell lineages by upregulating miR-181a level. Stem Cells. 2014;32(11):2961-2972.

13. Topical Medications

Another way of delivering medication is through a patch, cream, spray etc. placed on your skin over the site of your pain. Because analgesic patches have fewer side effects and fewer drug interactions than some oral medications, you may find that a patch will work better for you. The problem with any topical analgesic however, is that it is hard to control and regulate the dose of medication that you receive.

Pain relievers that can be applied directly to your skin are available for the control of a variety of your pain syndromes. These topical pain relievers are a noninvasive and convenient method for delivering pain-relieving medication to you. This is especially important and beneficial if you are not able to take medications by mouth. Topical pain relievers include complementary and alternative medications as well as conventional medications. Topical analgesics can be used to relieve minor pain from muscle soreness to major pain from cancer. The stronger versions of topical analgesics are prescription-only.

Topical forms of analgesics, or pain relievers, have been used throughout human history. The use of ointments for medicinal purposes is mentioned in the Bible on many occasions. The purpose of a topical analgesic is to transmit a medication through your skin for the effect of pain relief. The amount of drug that actually gets through your skin is determined by the amount of pressure applied as you rub it over your skin, the area of your skin covered by the drug, the way in which the drug is dissolved, and the use of dressings over your skin.

Analgesics are available in ointments, creams, and gels. They also may be placed in patches that may be applied to your skin. The advantage of topical analgesics is that they can be placed on the skin over the site of your pain. When compared to oral medications, you will have a lower blood level of the drug and will have fewer side effects and fewer drug interactions. People who are allergic to the adhesives on patches, for example, should avoid them. Anyone who is sensitive to the active ingredient in an oral pain reliever should not try it in topical form either.

Ointments are semisolid preparations that melt at body temperature and spread easily. Ointments are not routinely used in the practice of pain medicine unless the ointment is specially compounded by a pharmacy. Ointments are defined in three categories based on your skin penetration. One type of ointment does not penetrate beyond the external layer of your skin called the epidermis. Ointments of this class can be used for the treatment of sunburn. A second type of ointment penetrates to the internal layer of your skin called the dermis. The third type of ointment actually goes through your skin to the nerves and ligaments and in some instances into your bloodstream.

Substances applied on your skin can evaporate. You do not want your analgesic drug evaporating from your skin. Your pharmacist will add substances such as glycerin to the ointment to keep this evaporation from happening. Ointments can be prepared by your pharmacist or purchased over the counter or by prescription; ointments should be packaged in tubes. Some ointment preparations will contain absorption enhancers. Absorption enhancers make it easier for the drug to be absorbed through your skin. Azone and DMSO can both enhance the absorption of ointments through your skin.

Creams are opaque, thick, liquid substances that consist of medications dissolved in a cream base that usually vanishes through the skin. They are less of a liquid consistency than ointments. The term cream is used to describe a soft type of preparation that is less affected by your body temperature than ointments. The therapeutic difference between creams and ointments is that creams penetrate deeper than ointments. The pharmacological effect of lidocaine topical cream is superior a comparison with a placebo.[1]

Gels are a drug-delivery system that usually contain penetration enhancers and are usually used for administering anti-inflammatory medications. The anti-inflammatory medication must be absorbed through your skin to provide you with pain relief. Gels are useful treatment methods if you have arthritic and/or muscle pain. Gels usually are thicker than creams or ointments and are usually clear, unlike creams and ointments. The concentration of medication in gels is usually no greater than 2 percent.

For example, lidocaine, which is a numbing medicine for the control of pain, is dispensed as a 2 percent gel. However, the cream is available in a 5 percent concentration. This is because medications are usually absorbed through the skin better if used in gel form. Gels usually have clarity and sparkle. They maintain their thickness even with an elevated body temperature. Some gels have been developed to be given nasally. Some drugs are absorbed better through the nose than through the skin. Gels are usually dispensed in tubes or squeeze bottles.

Another delivery system for analgesics is a transdermal patch, which contains medication that is transmitted directly through your skin.

A patch containing a medication is placed on your skin and remains there for a specified time so that the drug within the patch can be delivered through your skin to your bloodstream. Local anesthetics such as lidocaine, capsaicin cream, and fentanyl, a potent opioid medication, are some of the medicines that can be delivered through your skin using a transdermal drug delivery system. These patches should be applied only to areas on your skin that have no blisters or open areas such as a cut. The patches are made of adhesive materials. You should not use the patch if you are allergic to some adhesives. With respect to the patches, the amount of drug that is absorbed from the patch is directly related to the length of the application of the patch, as well as the area of your skin to which it is applied.

The advantage of the patch is that it gives you a continuous flow of analgesic medications. When you take a pill, after it leaves your stomach or intestine and enters into your bloodstream, you receive a high concentration of the drug initially. As the drug is distributed to other tissues in your body, your blood level concentration of the drug will decrease. Once your body breaks down the drug, you will no longer have an analgesic effect of that particular drug. However, when using a patch, you will have a continuous release of the drug from the patch into your bloodstream. You will have constant pain relief without the peaks and valleys of the drug concentration in your bloodstream associated with oral medications.

Women use these medications more than men. However, there have been no good studies comparing the effects of topical analgesics on men as compared to women or on older or ethnic group individuals. As new topical analgesics are being developed, it is anticipated that a gender analysis will be a part of the topical analgesic drug study.

Natural compounds such as herbs or leaves and roots also can be used to treat your pain topically. Aloe Vera can be used to decrease your pain if you have sunburn. Use of this natural topical product for the treatment of various medical conditions was discovered in 1935. This drug is effective for the treatment of skin inflammation as well as minor burns. There are no side effects nor are there are any known drug interactions.

Capsaicin is a drug that has been extensively studied in both the clinical and laboratory settings. Capsaicin is the active component of chili or red peppers. Capsaicin can be put on your skin over your joints if you have joint pain. The capsaicin first stimulates the small pain-transmitting fibers by depleting them of the neurotransmitter substance P.

After the substance P has been depleted, you will have a block of the pain fibers that cause burning pain sensations. Observations in Hispanic individuals demonstrated that they did not have mouth or stomach pain after ingesting red peppers. The reason is the depletion of the substance P in the nerve endings in these areas following continual exposure to red peppers.

A study was performed in African Americans, East Asians, Hispanics and Caucasians.[2] Warmth sensation and heat pain detection thresholds, as well as pain intensity, were measured before and after application of capsaicin or placebo on forearms along with skin blood flow and the extent of the flare reaction. In African Americans the heat pain detection threshold, pain intensity and skin blood flow did not change significantly after capsaicin application, while in the other three ethnic groups a significant change occurred characterized by hyperalgesia and vasodilatation.

The number of fentanyl-related deaths has increased over the past 20 years, corresponding to both statewide increases in the medical use of fentanyl and the abuse of prescription opioids. The demographics of these fentanyl-related overdoses showed that subjects were more likely to be female, white non-Hispanic, and older than those in previously described overdose deaths.[3]

Substance P also is present in your joints throughout your body. For this reason, capsaicin can be an effective pain reliever for the treatment of pain associated with osteoarthritis and rheumatoid arthritis. It may take a week for you to feel the pain-relieving effects of capsaicin. As substance P is being depleted from your nerve endings, you nerve endings still manufacture substance P. As a result, it will take several days to deplete enough of the substance P to provide you with pain relief. Once you discontinue use of this cream, your nerves will replenish substance P and your pain may return.

You may have a brief burning sensation following the use of capsaicin. You should be warned to avoid contact with your eyes and genital areas. It is recommended that you use rubber gloves when applying the capsaicin cream. You should use the capsaicin cream no more than three times a day. Various concentrations of capsaicin exist. Begin with a small concentration that contains 0.025 percent capsaicin. You may eventually increase your capsaicin dose to 0.075 percent capsaicin.

Menthol is oil that is one component of peppermint oil. This oil in a cream base can significantly decrease your pain. When you place a menthol preparation on your skin, the menthol will feel cold to your nerve endings. While you feel the cold, your pain-stimulating nerves will be depressed. Following the initial cool sensation, you will feel a period of warmth. Menthol products can be used for the treatment of pain associated with arthritis, muscle pain, and tendonitis. Application of a menthol-containing cream may be of benefit to you if you suffer from tension headaches. It can be rubbed around the neck muscles just below the skull. It can be an extremely effective method for the treatment of your headaches.

Another topical medication used to prevent pain is EMLA cream. It is used as a numbing agent more than it is used for reducing pain. This is a cream consisting of lidocaine and prilocaine, which are both numbing agents. This local anesthetic combination is packaged in tubes. There also is an EMLA cellulose disc that can be applied over your painful area.

The purpose of this medication is to provide pain relief over the area of the skin. It is used in children to reduce the pain of starting intravenous lines. Some pain-management doctors advocate its use to decrease the pain associated with reflex sympathetic dystrophy or the pain associated with shingles. This cream should be placed on an intact skin area. The EMLA should be applied under a bandage for at least 60 minutes to provide relief over the painful area of your skin. This cream is not recommended if you have an allergy to lidocaine or prilocaine. If you have the blood disorder methemoglobinemia you should not use this cream. It is recommended that you not use this medication if you are taking heart medication. The local anesthetics in this cream can interact with some heart medicines.

Many individuals with osteoarthritis also have other chronic, comorbid conditions, such as obesity, hypertension and diabetes, which can compound the risk for developing cardiovascular adverse events that have been associated with specific analgesics. [4] Pharmacotherapy may be complicated by genetic factors that may influence drug metabolism in certain individuals. These risks may vary according to race and ethnicity.

Black and Hispanic populations are known to have a higher prevalence of cardiovascular risk factors and disease, and a substantial proportion of black and Hispanic individuals possess genotypes of the cytochrome P450 2C9 enzyme involved in the metabolism of many NSAIDs and the CYP2D6 enzyme involved in metabolism of the dual opioid agonist/norepinephrine-serotonin reuptake inhibitor tramadol. As a result, the efficacy and safety of available analgesics may vary between patients in different racial and ethnic groups. Particular emphasis is given to the place of topical NSAIDs and capsaicin in the management of OA patients for whom systemic exposure to available pharmacotherapy poses particular risk.

Another analgesic cream that is available is a combination of methyl salicylate and menthol. This is a cream that is effective for the temporary relief of arthritis and pain in your muscles. You should not use this medicine if your skin is sensitive to the oil of wintergreen. You should apply this cream around the sore areas on your body. You should not apply this cream more than three times a day. Do not place this cream over areas of the skin that are broken because it will cause extreme discomfort to that area.

Steroid creams are sometimes used for the treatment of joint pain. Topical steroids are anti-inflammatory agents. Pramoxine hydrochloride is a topical anesthetic agent that sometimes is combined with steroids to attempt to manage pain. This cream provides a temporary relief from pain. You should not use this cream if you are allergic to any of the substances in the cream such as the steroid or the pramoxine. If you develop a rash or blistering, you must stop using the cream. You should not use this cream more than three times a day.

Nonsteroidal anti-inflammatory agents (NSAIDS) that are commonly taken by mouth for the treatment of bone, joint, and muscle pain may be placed into a cream by your pharmacist. For these drugs to give you pain relief, they must penetrate your skin and enter your bloodstream. These creams should not be used more than three times a day. Side effects with the nonsteroidal anti-inflammatory creams are the same as with the NSAIDs taken by mouth. However, the side effects of the topical NSAIDS are less than the oral NSAIDS.

The side effects of any NSAID can include stomach upset and allergic reactions. If the dose is high enough, it could affect your liver and kidneys. The ketoprofen gel and the diclofenac gel can relieve some joint pain. Aspirin creams also may provide you with some pain relief when applied over your painful joints or muscles.

Flector Patches contain diclofenac, a nonsteroidal anti-inflammatory drug (NSAID). Diclofenac works by reducing substances in the body that cause pain and inflammation. The Flector patch is used to treat pain caused by minor sprains, strains, or bruising. The diclofenac in Flector patches can increase your risk of fatal heart attack or stroke, especially if you use it long term or take high doses.

Starting at 30 weeks gestation, Flector Patch and other NSAIDs should be avoided by pregnant women as premature closure of the ductus arteriosus in the fetus may occur. The diclofenac sodium patch provides clinically relevant pain relief in patients with acute traumatic injuries.5 The diclofenac sodium patch provides clinically relevant pain relief in patients with acute traumatic injuries. Maximum effects versus placebo are detected at 2 - 3 days post-injury.[5]

A study confirmed the beneficial pain intensity reducing efficacy of Ketospray 10% associated with good local tolerability of 7 days treatment course.6 A new topical diclofenac sodium solution (Pennsaid) containing the absorption enhancer dimethyl sulfoxide-was evaluated for the relief of the symptoms of primary OA of the knee.[7] Topical diclofenac is effective in the treatment of the symptoms of primary OA of the knee.

Amitriptyline, which is an antidepressant, has pain-relieving properties when applied topically. Amitriptyline cream may be advantageous if you do not want to take amitriptyline pills by mouth. The amitriptyline cream will not help you if you are suffering from significant depression, but can be helpful in decreasing your pain. Some people complain of being tired while taking amitriptyline. However, amitriptyline cream can contribute to pain relief in fibromyalgia and the topical application may be a way of avoiding significant side effects that can be associated with oral use.

The transdermal Fentanyl patch system has become popular since it was introduced in the 1980s. This strong opioid medication was used initially for cancer pain management and then for noncancerous, chronic pain management. The fentanyl is able penetrate your skin easily. Fentanyl is 70 times more potent than morphine. It produces less histamine release from cells in your bloodstream and causes less itching than morphine. The fentanyl patch is primarily used for chronic or cancer-related pain. A fentanyl patch can be used for most moderate to severe pain syndromes.

The number of fentanyl-related deaths has increased over the past 20 years, corresponding to both statewide increases in the medical use of fentanyl and the abuse of prescription opioids. The demographics of these fentanyl-related overdoses showed that subjects were more likely to be female, white non-Hispanic, and older than those in previously described overdose deaths.[3]

In the fentanyl patch, the medication exists as a gel in a drug reservoir. Between this reservoir and your skin is a release membrane that has various-size holes that regulate the amount of fentanyl that is delivered to your skin. The larger the size of the holes in the patch causes more fentanyl to be distributed through your skin. The adhesiveness around the patch keeps it in place. When the fentanyl patch is placed on your skin, the drug diffuses through the holes in the release membrane to the surface of your skin. It then goes to the outer layer of your skin and is deposited in a storage area.

From the storage area, it is gradually absorbed into your bloodstream. This is the reason that it takes at least an hour before the fentanyl has begun to enter your bloodstream. You will probably not notice any pain-relieving effects from this drug delivery system for about six hours. The patch is usually removed every three days. After the patch is removed, you will still have some drug that remains in the storage area under your skin. If you remove the patch and do not replace it, you will still receive Fentanyl for hours after the patch has been removed.

Fentanyl patches come in different concentrations. The concentrations correlate with the area of the skin to which they are applied. The effectiveness of the patch is not affected by placing it on your chest, your back, or your upper arm. An increase in temperature will cause the medication to be rapidly delivered from the patch to your bloodstream. Your skin's thickness also can affect the amount of fentanyl that is absorbed through your skin. The thicker your skin, the slower the rate of delivery of the fentanyl will be. The patch should not be applied over broken skin because the blood level of fentanyl can be significantly raised. The patch can cause a decrease in breathing and even death if you receive a significantly high dose of the fentanyl.

If you have significant vomiting associated with your severe pain, you cannot keep oral medications in your stomach. Therefore, they are not absorbed into your bloodstream and you receive no pain relief from the medicine. If this is the case, consult with your doctor about possibly using the fentanyl patch for pain control. There is no upper limit as to the number of fentanyl patches that can be worn at one time. Some cancer patients require more than one patch at a time.

Side effects of the patches containing fentanyl include nausea, constipation, and sleepiness. Be aware that the patch can cause reactions to your skin related to the adhesive used in the patch. If you notice an irritation on your skin related to the patch, stop using the patch. If you have difficulty with the patch sticking to your skin, you can secure the edges of the patch with adhesive tape. You should not use the fentanyl patch if you are allergic to adhesives.

Occasionally, you may need medication for breakthrough pain, an episode of temporary pain, if you do something to aggravate your chronic pain syndrome. For example, if you are using the patch for chronic pain and you go into your garden and do lifting, pushing, or digging, you may cause the onset of temporary pain on top of your chronic pain. At that time, an oral medication can be taken for treatment of your breakthrough pain.

With respect to gender specificity, the fentanyl patch appears to work just as well in men as it does in women. The fentanyl patch has been successful for the management of cancer-related pain and chronic pain syndromes and has paved the way for further research into the utilization of other opioid drugs for the management of chronic pain.

Another popular patch that is readily available by prescription from your pain-management doctor is the lidocaine-containing patch. The lidocaine transdermal drug-delivery system exerts a significant amount of its pain-relieving effects by releasing a small amount of lidocaine into your bloodstream. There also is an effect on the nerves under your skin that are transmitting pain. This patch is used for the treatment of post-herpetic neuralgia, a long-lasting pain that is a result of shingles. Approximately 1 million people develop shingles every year. Twenty percent of these individuals will develop post-herpetic neuralgia, which is an extremely painful syndrome.

The U.S. Food and Drug Administration has approved the use of the lidocaine patch for the treatment of the severe pain following the onset of shingles. Shingles is an infection caused by the chicken pox virus. You may have had chicken pox as a child. However, the virus remains inactive in your nervous system for many years. At some time in your life, this virus can become reactivated and travel via nerves to certain areas of your skin, causing you to have severe pain.

When the virus reaches your skin, you may develop blisters that can be severely painful as well. After the blisters have disappeared, you may have persistent pain. This pain is call post-herpetic neuralgia. You may feel as if your body is on fire in the areas affected by the post-herpetic neuralgia. Your skin may become extremely sensitive to touch. In many instances there is no cure for this pain. Often your doctor will try to treat the symptoms of your pain to provide you relief. The lidocaine patch has been demonstrated in clinical studies to significantly decrease pain following the outbreak of shingles.

The lidocaine patch contains 5 percent lidocaine. The lidocaine essentially does not reach your bloodstream like fentanyl does in the fentanyl patch delivery system. The lidocaine penetrates your skin just enough to reach the nerve endings that are transmitting your pain. As a result, there are minimal side effects from the use of this patch other than from the adhesive layer of the patch. The amount of the lidocaine that is absorbed from the Lidoderm is related to the length of application over your skin.

The patch should be used for 12 hours over your painful area and then removed for 12 hours. If an irritation or a burning sensation occurs around the adhesive aspect of the patch, you should discontinue use of the patch. None of the patches mentioned in this chapter should ever be reused.

The lidocaine patch has a polyester felt backing covered with a polyethylene film release liner. Prior to applying the patch on your skin, the release liner must be removed. Be aware that the patch does contain methylparaben, which is found in many suntan lotions. Do not use the Lidoderm patch if you have allergies to any suntan lotions that contain this chemical.

There does not appear to be any gender specificity related to the lidocaine in the patch. However, the incidence of shingles is higher in women than it is in men. You should not use the Lidoderm patch if you are using a heart drug to control your heartbeat. Even though the amount of lidocaine that you can absorb is small, it can interfere with some heart medicines. If you are using heart medications, discuss any potential drug interactions with you doctor. If you become lightheaded following application of the patch, you must stop using the patch immediately.

Clonidine is another transdermal medication. This patch is applied weekly to an area of your skin. The clonidine patch inhibits the release of norepinephrine, which is a pain transmitter. The clonidine patch also is used for the treatment of hypertension. If you have neuropathic pain (pain from a nerve that is diseased) or reflex sympathetic dystrophy, the clonidine patch may provide you with significant pain relief. It also can be successfully used if you have pain following shingles. The application of the clonidine patch can be most useful for pain associated with a nerve injury or inflammation of a nerve. The patch comes in different doses. The usual dose is the 0.1 milligram patch that is administered weekly.[8] Patients who described their pain as sharp and shooting may have a greater likelihood of responding to clonidine.[9]

EMLA cream is a topical emulsion composed of prilocaine and lidocaine, and produces complete anesthesia of intact skin following application.[10] For the optimum effect, EMLA cream must be applied and covered with an occlusive dressing for 60 minutes. Many individuals with osteoarthritis also have other chronic, comorbid conditions, such as obesity, hypertension and diabetes, which can compound the risk for developing cardiovascular adverse events that have been associated with specific analgesics, most notably nonselective nonsteroidal anti-inflammatory drugs. Pharmacotherapy may be further complicated by genetic factors that may influence drug metabolism in certain individuals. These risks may vary according to race and ethnicity.

Black and Hispanic populations are known to have a higher prevalence of cardiovascular risk factors and disease, and a substantial proportion of Black and Hispanic individuals possess genotypes of the cytochrome P450 (CYP) 2C9 enzyme involved in the metabolism of many NSAIDs and the CYP2D6 enzyme involved in metabolism of the dual opioid agonist/norepinephrine-serotonin reuptake inhibitor tramadol. As a result, the efficacy and safety of available analgesics may vary between patients in different racial and ethnic groups. This review article focuses on racial and ethnic differences in cardiovascular risk and genetic factors altering drug efficacy and safety and evaluates the pharmacologic options that can be used for the management of OA in these populations. Particular emphasis is given to the place of topical NSAIDs and capsaicin in the management of osteoarthritis patients for whom systemic exposure to available pharmacotherapy poses a particular risk.[4]

References

1. Yaacob HB, Noor GM, Malek SN. The pharmacological effect of xylocaine topical anaesthetic--a comparison with a placebo. Singapore Dent J. 1981;6(2):55-57.

2. Wang H, Papoiu AD, Coghill RC, Patel T, Wang N, Yosipovitch G. Ethnic differences in pain, itch and thermal detection in response to topical capsaicin: African Americans display a notably limited hyperalgesia and neurogenic inflammation. Br J Dermatol. 2010;162(5):1023-1029.

3. Krinsky CS, Lathrop SL, Crossey M, Baker G, Zumwalt R. A toxicology-based review of fentanyl-related deaths in New Mexico (1986-2007). Am J Forensic Med Pathol. 2011;32(4):347-351.

4. Balmaceda CM. The impact of ethnicity and cardiovascular risk on the pharmacologic management of osteoarthritis: a US perspective. Postgrad Med. 2015;127(1):51-56.

5. Mueller EA, Kirch W, Reiter S. Extent and time course of pain intensity upon treatment with a topical diclofenac sodium patch versus placebo in acute traumatic injury based on a validated end point: post hoc analysis of a randomized placebo-controlled trial. Expert Opin Pharmacother. 2010;11(4):493-498.

6.   Fulga I, Lupescu O, Spircu T. Local tolerability and effectiveness of Ketospray(R) 10% cutaneous spray solution. Panminerva Med. 2012;54(1 Suppl 4):23-33.

7.   Roth SH, Shainhouse JZ. Efficacy and safety of a topical diclofenac solution (pennsaid) in the treatment of primary osteoarthritis of the knee: a randomized, double-blind, vehicle-controlled clinical trial. Arch Intern Med. 2004;164(18):2017-2023.

8.   Motsch J, Kamler M. [Alpha 2-adrenergic agonists. Use in chronic pain--a meta-analysis]. Schmerz. 1997;11(5):339-344.

9.   Byas-Smith MG, Max MB, Muir J, Kingman A. Transdermal clonidine compared to placebo in painful diabetic neuropathy using a two-stage 'enriched enrollment' design. Pain. 1995;60(3):267-274.

10.   Farrington E. Lidocaine 2.5%/prilocaine 2.5% EMLA cream. Pediatr Nurs. 1993;19(5):484-486, 488.

14. Invasive Treatments

There is currently insuffient evidence to comment on diversity in injection therapies. The spinal epidural injection procedures using steroids mixed either with local anesthetics or normal saline have an effect in reducing pain and improving functional activities in some patients.[1] Epidural steroid injections (ESI) can be helpful for hastening recovery from radiculopathy following disc herniation and can provide temporary relief for patients with chronic radicular pain. There is little evidence that they are of benefit for patients with back pain or neural claudication associated with spinal stenosis. There is little evidence that they reduce the need for spine surgery or that they improve long-term outcomes.

In April 2014, the Food and Drug Administration (FDA) issued a Drug Safety Communication requesting that corticosteroid labeling include warnings that injection of corticosteroids into the epidural space of the spine may result in rare but serious adverse events, including loss of vision, stroke, paralysis, and death. [2] Neurological and other complications of epidural steroid injections have been widely discussed in recent years. Consequently, the US FDA issued a warning about serious neurological events, some resulting in death, and consequently is requiring steroid label changes.[3] Furthermore, multiple disasters have been described in recent years with transforaminal (placing the needle where the nerve exits the spinal canal) epidural injections.[4] They are utilized extensively even though their effectiveness has been debated.

Recent studies document a 629% increase in Medicare expenditures for epidural steroid injections; a 423% increase in expenditures for opioids for back pain; a 307% increase in the number of lumbar magnetic resonance images among Medicare beneficiaries; and a 220% increase in spinal fusion surgery rates.[5] It is important that patients understand the risks and benefits of these procedures and that we do everything possible to prevent rare but catastrophic neurological complications. Epidural steroid injections have a moderate short-term effect in the management of low-back pain with radiculopathy. Severe neurological complications can however occur.[6]

The Dr. Oz Show on May 6, 2013 commented on the potential danger of ESI therapy .Epidural steroid injections have become the most common procedure doctors do for low back pain – done nearly 9 million times a year, according to an analysis of Medicare records. ESIs are not

FDA approved. The steroids used in epidural steroid injections are FDA-approved for your muscles and joints, but the FDA has never approved the injections for spinal use.

Epidural steroid injections are promoted as a less invasive alternative to back surgery, but there are potential problems when doctors work so close to your spinal cord, even if they're using needles instead of knives. It's impossible to get a grip on the number of injuries and deaths due to ESIs because doctors are not required to report them. A relatively high rate of inadvertent intradiscal injections occurs in the performance of the retrodiscal approach for transforimanil epidural epidural injections.[7]

In addition to arachnoiditis, other serious epidural steroid injection complications include meningitis, paralysis and death. In 2012, more than 700 people contracted meningitis or other infections and 50 later died after doctors performed epidural steroid injections using steroids tainted with fungus. There is anecdotal evidence that multiple intrathecal steroid injections may be associated with neurological dysfunction as well.[8]

If a doctor accidentally places the steroid solution into a patient's artery, that can create a blockage, cause a stroke, and cause death. The risk rises when ESIs are performed by poorly trained doctors. The number of epidural steroid injections performed has surged, rising 271% from 1994 to 2001 according to an analysis of Medicare claims. In fact, today, general practitioners, physician assistants, dentists and chiropractors have started offering ESIs.

Some doctors spend just one weekend learning the delicate procedure at training centers that teach cosmetic injections like Botox and fillers, but also teach doctors how to poke around people's spines. One weekend training center advertises epidural steroid injections as "lucrative specialty options" that "create dramatic earnings for your practice."

Several studies over the decades have concluded that injecting steroids epidurally works no better than injecting saline, a placebo. Other studies have shown that receiving epidural steroid injections does not help a patient avoid back surgery and may even increase surgery rates. ESIs are best suited for a diagnosis of radiculopathy, a pinched or inflamed nerve root with pain radiating down your leg. This diagnosis only fits a small minority of patients.

Most insurance companies also take this approach, paying for epidural steroid injections only for patients who have "radiating pain" or "radiculopathy." When performed by experienced interventionalists, major complications are probably rare and it could take years for a significant complication to occur.9 ESI can give a transient benefit in pain relief, compared with placebo at up to 3 weeks following the procedure.[10]

If you are considering an ESI: Confirm your diagnosis. Make sure that you have the one diagnosis that may respond to ESIs: a pinched or inflamed nerve with radiating pain. This is sometimes called a "herniated" or "bulging" disc with "radiculopathy" or "sciatica." Only get an injection if you are seeing zero progress after this conservative wait-and-see period. Look for an experienced doctor. If you are going to try an epidural steroid injection, choose a doctor who is board certified in a relevant specialty and had extensive ESI training, rather than a weekend course. It is imperative that any provider who performs ESIs know the risks, benefits, complications, and contraindications for this procedure.[11]

Avoid doctors who automatically recommend an entire course of steroid shots rather than trying just one to see if it will help you.. Most ESIs today are performed under "fluoroscopic guidance," kind of like a live X-ray, so that the doctor can position the needle correctly in the epidural space before releasing the medication. Insist on this as part of your treatment. Use of radiographic guidance with adherence to specific recommended practices when performing epidural corticosteroid injections should lead to a reduction in the incidence of neurologic injuries.[12]

The Food and Drug Administration has just issued a Medwatch Alert warning that Epidural steroid injections or "ESIs" for back and neck pain can be extremely dangerous. However, it is believed that epidural steroid injections are safe and effective when administered by a Fellowship trained, Board Certified Interventional Pain Management doctor.

One of the major concerns in the medical field at the moment is some doctors not having enough training when it comes to various pain management techniques. Quite a few doctors are learning how to give these shots through weekend courses. Board Certified Pain Management Doctors on the other hand, go through years of training to master these procedures. It is important for patients to choose the most qualified and experienced doctor when considering treatment.

Limited research suggests that repeat injections may improve outcomes, but the evidence is insufficient to make any conclusions. There does not appear to be any evidence to support the current common practice of a series of three injections.[13] If you're suffering from back pain that hasn't improved from conservative methods, take a judicious approach when considering epidural steroid injections and understand that their benefits may be limited .

The ASA Committee on Pain Medicine, in their 2010 Statement on Anesthetic Care during Interventional Pain Procedures for Adults, wrote: "It is the opinion of the Committee that the majority of minor pain procedures, under most routine circumstances, do not require anesthesia care other than local anesthesia." The use of sedation and anesthesia must be balanced with the potential risk of harm from doing pain procedures in a sedated patient, especially those undergoing cervical spine procedures.[14] Despite these policy statements, an increasing number of patients receive sedation for interventional pain procedures. [15] In the treatment of lumbar spinal stenosis, epidural injection of glucocorticoids plus lidocaine offered minimal or no short-term benefit as compared with epidural injection of lidocaine alone.[16]

There is a limited body of evidence to support the use of epidural injections in spinal stenosis in elderly patients.[17] However, epidural steroid injections have been reported to provide limited improvement in short-term and long-term benefits in lumbar spine patients.[18]

Your spine has joints on each side called facet joints. These joints can cause back pain. Therapeutic lumbar facet joint interventions are implemented to provide long-term pain relief after the facet joint has been identified as the basis for low back pain. The therapeutic lumbar facet joint interventions generally used for the treatment of low back pain of facet joint origin are intraarticular facet joint injections, lumbar facet joint nerve blocks, and radiofrequency neurotomy.

The injection of local anesthetic and/or steroids into the facet joint is being practiced widely worldwide as a means of treating patients in whom it is believed the facet joint is the cause of the symptoms of their back pain. There is good evidence for the use of conventional radiofrequency neurotomy, and fair to good evidence for lumbar facet joint nerve blocks for the treatment of chronic lumbar facet joint pain resulting in short-term and long-term pain relief and functional improvement. [19] Bone scanning with SPECT imaging can help identify patients with low back pain who would benefit from facet joint injections.[20]

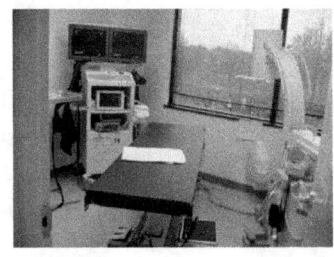

Figure 1. Injections should be done with X ray guidance.

The efficacy of injection therapy in general is however controversial.[21] Facet joint, epidural injections and trigger point injections have not clearly been shown to be effective and can consequently not be recommended.[22] There is no scientific evidence on the effectiveness of spinal stenosis surgery as well. Surgical discectomy may be considered for selected patients with sciatica due to lumbar disc prolapses that fail to resolve with the conservative management.

Facet joint injections may be done with the local anesthetic and steroid placed within the joint (intraarticular facet joint injections) or at the nerve where it enters the facet joint (medial branch blocks). With intraarticular facet joint injections, the evidence for short- and long-term pain relief is limited for cervical pain and moderate for lumbar pain.[23] For medial branch blocks, the evidence is moderate for short- and long-term pain relief. For medial branch neurotomy, the evidence is moderate for short- and long-term pain relief.

Myofascial pain syndrome is a common nonarticular local musculoskeletal pain syndrome caused by myofascial trigger points located at muscle, fascia, or tendinous insertions, affecting up to 95% of people with chronic pain disorders.24 Injections into muscles are called trigger points. Fixed-location treatment with Botulism toxin of patients with upper back myofascial pain syndrome did not lead to a significant improvement in one study. Trigger point injections can be beneficial in both the acute and the persistent phases.in whiplash injuries. However, there is insufficient evidence to support or refute the use of trigger point injections for chronic lower back pain without radiculopathy.[25]

There is insufficient evidence to support the use of injection therapy in subacute and chronic low-back pain.[21] However, it cannot be ruled out that specific subgroups of patients may respond to a specific type of injection therapy.

References

1.   Song SH, Ryu GH, Park JW, et al. The Effect and Safety of Steroid Injection in Lumbar Spinal Stenosis: With or Without Local Anesthetics. Ann Rehabil Med. 2016;40(1):14-20.

2.   Kennedy DJ, Levin J, Rosenquist R, et al. Epidural Steroid Injections are Safe and Effective: Multisociety Letter in Support of the Safety and Effectiveness of Epidural Steroid Injections. Pain Med. 2015;16(5):833-838.

3.   Manchikanti L, Benyamin RM. Key safety considerations when administering epidural steroid injections. Pain Manag. 2015;5(4):261-272.

4.   Zhu J, Falco FJ, Formoso F, Onyewu O, Irwin FL. Alternative approach for lumbar transforaminal epidural steroid injections. Pain Physician. 2011;14(4):331-341.

5.   Deyo RA, Mirza SK, Turner JA, Martin BI. Overtreating chronic back pain: time to back off? J Am Board Fam Med. 2009;22(1):62-68.

6.   Benoist M, Boulu P, Hayem G. Epidural steroid injections in the management of low-back pain with radiculopathy: an update of their efficacy and safety. Eur Spine J. 2012;21(2):204-213.

7.   Levi D, Horn S, Corcoran S. The Incidence of Intradiscal, Intrathecal, and Intravascular Flow During the Performance of Retrodiscal (Infraneural) Approach for Lumbar Transforaminal Epidural Steroid Injections. Pain Med. 2015.

8.   Abram SE. Epidural steroid injections for the treatment of lumbosacral radiculopathy. J Back Musculoskelet Rehabil. 1997;8(2):135-149.

9.   Derby R, Lee SH, Kim BJ, Chen Y, Seo KS. Complications following cervical epidural steroid injections by expert interventionalists in 2003. Pain Physician. 2004;7(4):445-449.

10.   Price C, Arden N, Coglan L, Rogers P. Cost-effectiveness and safety of epidural steroids in the management of sciatica. Health Technol Assess. 2005;9(33):1-58, iii.

11.   Snarr J. Risk, benefits and complications of epidural steroid injections: a case report. AANA J. 2007;75(3):183-188.

12.   Rathmell JP, Benzon HT, Dreyfuss P, et al. Safeguards to prevent neurologic complications after epidural steroid injections: consensus opinions from a multidisciplinary working group and national organizations. Anesthesiology. 2015;122(5):974-984.

13. Novak S, Nemeth WC. The basis for recommending repeating epidural steroid injections for radicular low back pain: a literature review. Arch Phys Med Rehabil. 2008;89(3):543-552.

14. Hodges SD, Castleberg RL, Miller T, Ward R, Thornburg C. Cervical epidural steroid injection with intrinsic spinal cord damage. Two case reports. Spine (Phila Pa 1976). 1998;23(19):2137-2142; discussion 2141-2132.

15. Schaufele MK, Marin DR, Tate JL, Simmons AC. Adverse events of conscious sedation in ambulatory spine procedures. Spine J. 2011;11(12):1093-1100.

16. Friedly JL, Comstock BA, Turner JA, et al. A randomized trial of epidural glucocorticoid injections for spinal stenosis. N Engl J Med. 2014;371(1):11-21.

17. Abdulla A, Adams N, Bone M, et al. Guidance on the management of pain in older people. Age Ageing. 2013;42 Suppl 1:i1-57.

18. Liu K, Liu P, Liu R, Wu X, Cai M. Steroid for epidural injection in spinal stenosis: a systematic review and meta-analysis. Drug Des Devel Ther. 2015;9:707-716.

19. Falco FJ, Manchikanti L, Datta S, et al. An update of the effectiveness of therapeutic lumbar facet joint interventions. Pain Physician. 2012;15(6):E909-953.

20. Pneumaticos SG, Chatziioannou SN, Hipp JA, Moore WH, Esses SI. Low back pain: prediction of short-term outcome of facet joint injection with bone scintigraphy. Radiology. 2006;238(2):693-698.

21. Staal JB, de Bie RA, de Vet HC, Hildebrandt J, Nelemans P. Injection therapy for subacute and chronic low back pain: an updated Cochrane review. Spine (Phila Pa 1976). 2009;34(1):49-59.

22. van Tulder MW, Koes B, Seitsalo S, Malmivaara A. Outcome of invasive treatment modalities on back pain and sciatica: an evidence-based review. Eur Spine J. 2006;15 Suppl 1:S82-92.

23. Boswell MV, Colson JD, Sehgal N, Dunbar EE, Epter R. A systematic review of therapeutic facet joint interventions in chronic spinal pain. Pain Physician. 2007;10(1):229-253.

24. Malanga GA, Cruz Colon EJ. Myofascial low back pain: a review. Phys Med Rehabil Clin N Am. 2010;21(4):711-724.

25. Watters WC, 3rd, Resnick DK, Eck JC, et al. Guideline update for the performance of fusion procedures for degenerative disease of the lumbar spine. Part 13: injection therapies, low-back pain, and lumbar fusion. J Neurosurg Spine. 2014;21(1):79-90.

15. Neck Pain

At any given time, neck pain affects 10 percent of the general population in the United States. Neck pain is a frequent reason why patients seek medical attention. A reported survey of 10,000 adults in the United States discovered that 34 percent of responding individuals experienced neck pain during the previous year of the survey. Chronic neck pain was reported in 17 percent of women and 10 percent of men in a similar study. Another study evaluated 8,000 adults, and chronic neck pain was identified in 13.5 percent of female respondents as compared to 9.5 percent of males.

Most of your neck pain is self-limited and does not usually require seeing a doctor for the management of your pain. However, if you have serious cervical spine problems such as that seen rheumatoid arthritis, notify your doctor if you have the sudden onset of significant neck pain that does not go away within two or three days. Neck pain is caused by conditions that compress nerves or irritate the outer part of discs that are cushions between the bones in your neck. Ligaments in the front and in the back of your bones in your neck can cause pain because they have many pain fibers within these ligaments. These ligaments are called the anterior and posterior longitudinal ligaments.

Where the bones of your neck stack on top of each other like Lego blocks, they form a joint called a facet joint. The outer capsule of this joint has a rich supply of pain fibers. The outer capsule holds the top and bottom of the facet joint together not unlike a clamshell. If this capsule is pulled or stretched by an injury, the parts of the joint loosen making the joint unstable. This instability can cause spine pain. If your neck becomes misaligned, you can also develop significant neck pain. Over time, the bones and joints in your neck can wear out as well. This is called degenerative disc or joint disease or in medical terms is called osteoarthritis. The disc between your bones can rupture. Your facet joints in your neck can deteriorate and be a cause of your chronic neck pain. Your neck muscles can become tense and cause you neck pain.

There are seven separate bone segments in your neck. These bones are held together by ligaments and stack on top of each other and form joints with the analogy of joints formed by Lego blocks. The lining of these joints can wear out. These joints contain a lubricating fluid that helps you turn and move your neck up and down. These joints in your neck not only limit your neck motion but also allow your neck to move in many planes. Try and put your ear on your shoulder. You facet joints limit your movement so your neck will not bend too far. The muscles and ligaments in your neck can have many pain nerve endings. These nerves transmit pain impulses following trauma or if you slouch and have poor neck posture. Irritation or injury to muscles or ligaments in your neck as well as the discs and joints in your neck can cause you to have neck pain.

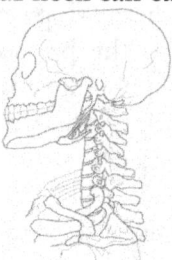

Figure 1. The neck protects the spinal cord from injury.

The bones in your neck protect your spinal cord and the nerves that come off of your spinal cord. The nerves that come off of your spinal cord pass through holes in the bones in your neck. If these nerves are compressed by narrowing of the hole where the nerve exits from the bone in your neck, it can cause you to have significant pain. If the nerve is compromised by bones in your neck, you can have weakness as well as pain in your arms.

You should see that there are many causes of neck pain because there are many structures in your neck and each of these structures has pain fibers and one or all of them can cause you to have neck pain. Neck pain can come not only from the degeneration of discs in your neck or the degenerating facet joints in your neck, but also can arise from infections or tumors of structures in your neck.

Neck pain in general does not occur as often as lower back pain. Therefore, the overall cost of neck pain to society is much less than that of lower back pain. There are fewer work days lost and less medications prescribed in patients with neck pain as opposed to lower back pain. Your head weighs between 10 and 12 pounds. The bones in your neck are relatively small in comparison to your head. Your neck muscles are necessary to hold your head in a proper position. Your neck muscles must be strong to hold your head up. Try holding a bowling ball vertically for as long as you can. You will notice that your arm muscles get tired easily.

The same analogy is true with respect to your neck muscles tiring from holding your neck up.

If you experience stress in your neck, it can cause you to have not only neck pain but also the headaches. Headaches may begin in your neck and go to the top of your head. At times if your neck is tense you can have difficulty turning it. If you are beginning to experience neck pain, evaluate your posture both sitting and standing in the mirror. Poor posture can lead to muscle spasms as well as dislocation and misalignment of your facet joints. If you have the onset of numbness of your arms, notify your doctor immediately. You also must be aware that nerves in your neck that come off of your spinal cord also can cause pain elsewhere in your body. The pain that is perceived elsewhere that comes from your nerves in your neck is called referred pain. For example, pain in your shoulder may be referred from nerves in your neck.

The bones in your neck that are called vertebral bodies contain many pain fibers. Each bone is wrapped by a tissue called a periosteum. If you fracture one of the bones in your neck, you can have severe pain. The tissue wrapper around your neck bones can be injured. The fracture of a bone in your neck can cause abnormal stress to the ligaments, muscles, and joints around the fracture as well as injury to your periosteum. Osteoporosis, which is a weakening of your bones with a loss of your bone density, can cause small, tiny fractures in the bones of your neck and in turn can be a cause of your pain. Osteoporosis can be a source of severe neck pain.

Discs are cushions between the bones in your neck. These discs act as shock absorbers in between your bones. The cushions are important because without them your neck bones would stack on top of each other. Remember the periosteum and the pain fibers contained in the periosteum? Without these cushions you would have terrible pain.

In the very center of your disc in your neck is a thick fluid like substance called a nucleus pulposus. This fluid ball is surrounded by an outer tough fiber called an annulus. Annulus is Latin for "outer ring." A fluid nucleus acts as a ball bearing when you bend your head forward and backward or from side to side. It also is a ball bearing when you rotate your neck. The annulus around your disc acts as a ligament that prevents your neck from having excessive motion. Otherwise your bones would sit on a fluid-filled ball. You can imagine that your neck would not be very stable. Excessive motion in your head and neck would make you function as a Slinky toy. Your annulus at its outer layer has many pain fibers.

To find out if your pain is coming from the disc in your neck, a doctor can place a needle in your disc. After the needle has been properly placed, fluid can be injected into your disc. If the injected fluid into your disc reproduces your neck pain, this is a good indication that your disc in your neck is the cause of your pain syndrome. If your pain is from your disc you will need physical therapy to strengthen the neck muscles which hold your discs in place.

Neck pain makes up a significant portion of the complaints confronting your doctor as well as your physical therapist and your pain doctor. If you have a job that requires you to repetitively look at the ceiling, which happens if you are a painter, your job may be a source of your neck pain. Magnetic resonance imaging (MRI) and computerized tomography scanning (CT) can help your doctor identify any bone or disc abnormalities that may be a source of your neck pain. Be aware, however, that an abnormal imaging study does not necessarily mean that you will have neck pain. It is possible that you can have a ruptured disc in your neck and you may not experience any neck pain.

There is a normal C-shaped curve in your neck. Your neck bones form a C curve with the C part of the curve located in the middle of your neck. The C curve is called a lordosis. The curve is sharper at the lower level of your neck. The curve in your neck determines your posture. If you have a neck injury, the muscles in your neck may pull your neck in a straight line and the curve is obliterated. If you have an x-ray following an injury, your doctor will note that your neck is straight as opposed to being curved. Your neck supports your head. Your brain controls most of your total body functions. If your neck becomes lopsided, you can compress a nerve that goes to one of your organs and could affect the function of one of your organs. For example, a spinal cord injury could affect your diaphragm and make it difficult for you to take a breath. Your head always needs to be supported in the proper position to allow you to have normal motion.

The discs in your neck have a normal blood supply when you are a toddler until you become a teenager. These discs are nurtured with oxygen and sugar in your bloodstream until your blood supply shuts off, which occurs when you reach adolescence. Your blood vessels essentially become obliterated at this time. By your 30s, the discs in your neck have no blood flow. Therefore, the nutrition to your discs must come from the ends of the bones in your neck. The bones in your neck are like sponges soaked with your blood. Pressure gradients will provide your discs with nutrition. Your disc essentially acts like a sponge and takes the blood that it needs from the bones in your neck.

When your disc eventually begins to lose fluid, it will deteriorate. The very center of your disc, called the nucleus pulposus, is 80 percent water. Substances in this liquid environment can attract fluid into your discs to keep your discs well hydrated. Eventually this hydration will dry up. As you get older, the ends of your neck bones calcify. When this happens, less blood flow is available for your discs as the blood cannot get out of your vertebrae to hydrate your disc. Your disc will essentially dry out. Your disc becomes wafer thin and does not provide you with a nice cushion. As a result, you will begin to experience some degree of neck pain. One way to slow it down is to exercise, stop smoking, and watch your posture.

The outer ring of your disc, called the annulus, will contain the nucleus pulposus within its structure. Think of this anatomy as a jelly doughnut. The jelly in the doughnut is held in place by the outer doughnut ring. Be aware that a basic law of physics states that the nucleus pulposus, which is a liquid, cannot be compressed. Therefore, any pressure applied to your disc at any point can cause the nucleus pulposus to spread outward and even rupture through the outer annular ring. As an example, you can compress a foam pillow to make the pillow smaller during compression. But, compressing a liquid will not decrease its size (volume). Your disc jelly will not become smaller in its dimensions under pressure. Consequently when this liquid mass is attempted to be compressed, it will push through the outer ring of your disc.

When this happens, you suffer what is called a disc herniation or rupture. The nucleus pulposus material contains acids. When this disc material does come out of the annulus, the surrounding tissues can be become swollen and red from the acidic liquid. This is the reason that your doctor may do a cervical epidural steroid injection on you. The purpose of this method is to decrease the swelling of your tissue and nerves caused by the acidic nucleus pulposus contents. The acid will make your nerves extra sensitive to irritability, which will cause you to experience pain.

In front of the bones in your neck is a ligament that runs vertically. In the back of the bones in your neck is another ligament that also runs vertically. These ligaments are called longitudinal ligaments. These ligaments run all the way from the base of your skull to your lower back and contain many pain fibers. The ligament in the back of your bones limits your ability to bend your head forward. If you bend too far, the ligament transmits pain signals to your brain telling you to stop this movement. The front ligament and the joints in your neck keep you from bending your neck backward too far. Sometimes your neck can be bent backward following a whiplash injury and can cause you significant pain.

To better understand the concept of a whiplash injury, consider that your head is like a bowling ball attached to a flexible whip called your neck. At the time of an accident your bowling ball flies away from the traumatic event but fortunately or unfortunately it is still connected to your neck. This connection causes your neck and head to snap like a whip which can cause an injury not only to your neck but also to your brain.

Not only does your neck go forward and backward, it also rotates to the right and the left. You also can place your ear toward your shoulder, which is called lateral flexion of your neck. When you have neck pain, inform your health-care giver as to what movement or movements cause you to have neck pain. Remember to keep a pain diary. When you bend your head forward, your discs can be compressed. This also occurs when your neck goes backward. However, forward movement of your neck can cause your discs to rupture. This is sometimes caused in motor vehicle accidents if your vehicle strikes an object from the front. This can cause your neck to bend forward, which in turn can compress the nucleus pulposus in your disc and can cause a disc herniation.

If you run your fingers along the center of the back of your neck, you will feel bony objects. If you look at someone from behind, you will notice an area that sticks out from their neck in the center. These bony prominences are called spinous processes. The one that sticks out the most is the bony prominence of the seventh cervical vertebra. In between these spinous processes are ligaments that hold the spinous processes together from top to bottom. These ligaments keep your head from going too far forward. An injury can disrupt or tear these ligaments, which can cause you to have pain. Always remember that pain can be a warning to you and can be a protective mechanism for you telling you to decrease your movement. The joints in your neck that are called facet joints will keep your neck from going backward too far.

Your spinal cord and the nerves that come capsule that encloses your facet joint contain many pain fibers. Excessive strain of this capsule will cause you to experience pain. The pain tells you not to move your neck anymore because of the chance that you could cause a worse injury if you continue to move your neck. Your muscles off of your spinal cord can be sources of neck pain.

When you bend your head forward or bend your head backward, your spinal cord will move up and down a short distance because it is somewhat elastic. This means that the nerves that go through the holes in your neck bones also move along with spinal cord movements. If the holes in your neck bones decrease in diameter as is seen in arthritis, movement of these nerves across a small hole can cause irritation in your nerves and make them swell and become extra sensitive to irritability. You can then experience pain in your arms.

Occasionally, if you have arthritis, the small bony growth that forms anywhere around the holes in the bones of your neck can irritate or compress one of your nerves. This bone growth is called an osteophyte. Osteophytes themselves are not painful. However, when they brush over your nerves or ligaments, they can cause you to have neck pain. Osteophytes, if they occur, are usually pointed. If one of your nerves brushes up against one of these osteophytes, or if the osteophytes compress your nerves, you may experience mild to moderate pain.

Steroid injections in and around your nerves can decrease the swelling of the nerve and decrease your pain. Sometimes your doctor may give you oral steroids. The problem with oral steroids is that they can cause you to have a significant weight gain. The injection places a tiny amount of steroids at the area of your pain. Oral steroids have to go to your stomach and pass out of your gastrointestinal system to reach your bloodstream. The total amount of the steroid that will reach your swollen nerves will vary. This is why pain medicine doctors advocate the use of special needles to place steroids at the level of your nerve swelling. The amount of drug placed at your nerve is more reliable than that given by mouth.

The muscles of your neck can be a source of your pain. The neck muscles are probably the most common cause of your neck pain. There are two groups of muscles in your neck. There is a group that bends your head forward, and there is a group of muscles that extends your head backward. Most of the muscles in your neck are located toward the back of your neck. These are the muscles that bend your head backward. If you have poor posture, the muscles in the back of your neck can become longer or can become shorter. When this happens, the short muscles in your neck lose blood flow, causing you to have pain.

If you are at work and have poor posture, persistent compression of your neck muscles can cause pain. The muscles in the front of your spinal cord bend your head forward. The muscles under the base of your skull and above your mid-back pull your head backward. A strain of any of these muscles can also cause you to experience neck pain. If you slouch over a computer or workbench, you may compress your neck muscles and shorten them. Your neck will eventually conform to this posture. This is the reason why you have to have good posture. The muscles in your neck need to be strong to protect the nerves coming off your spinal cord from injury from excessive head movement, which happens in a whiplash injury. Major muscles that pull your neck backward are located just under the base of your skull, and another group is located right above your lungs. The muscles that pull your neck forward are located in the front and middle of your neck.

The muscles in the base of your skull can compress a nerve that comes off of your spinal cord and travels to the top of your head. This is called the occipital nerve. If this nerve is compressed by a tight muscle, you can develop a headache called an occipital headache. If you put some heat over the muscle that is compressing this nerve, it can relax the muscle and relieve your headache.

Your posture can be influenced by work demands. If you have to paint overhead daily, you may develop weakness in the discs in your neck that could eventually rupture. Be aware of what tissues cause you to have neck pain. Your cervical disc is a common cause of neck pain. The anterior longitudinal ligament in front of the bones in your neck contains many pain fibers. The posterior longitudinal ligament also has pain fibers. The nerve roots coming off of your spinal cord that run through the holes in your neck bones also can be a source of your neck pain.

Coverings of the facet joints in your neck called facet joint capsules can be a source of your pain as well. Because there are so many structures that can cause pain in your neck, your health-care provider will try to isolate the tissue or tissues that contribute to your pain syndrome. This is not a precise science and x-rays, CT scans, and MRIs may need to be performed by your doctor following your history and physical examination. Sometimes laboratory tests taken from your blood are needed to rule out rheumatoid arthritis, which can cause significant neck pain.

Electromyography and/or nerve conduction tests consist of needles placed in the muscles and nerves of your upper arms and legs. The electromyography study can enable your doctor to determine if you have compression of one of the nerves that goes from your spinal cord to your fingers. Another way of diagnosing your pain is for your doctor to inject a numbing medicine in each of your tissues to see if your pain can be decreased. This series of injections can help to diagnose the cause of your pain.

When you become older than 35 years of age, you may develop degenerative disc disease in your neck. Degeneration of your neck is called spondylosis. Degenerative disc disease of the cervical spine causes more neck pain and upper-extremity nerve pain than does a disc herniation. Men have a higher incidence of cervical spondylosis than women. In one study, the evidence of spondylosis was noted to be 60 percent in women but 80 percent in men. These findings were before the age of 49 years. However, at age 70 or greater there was a 95 percent incidence of degenerative disc disease in men and women. With degenerative disc disease, your disc becomes narrow. Think of a normal disc as a jelly donut; a degenerated disc is more like a thin communion wafer.

Diagnosis of spondylosis is made by x-ray but also can be seen on an MRI. Degeneration of your disc can cause calcification of the ends of your neck bones. As stated previously, there is decreased blood flow to your discs following puberty. Your discs normally obtain blood from the spongy vertebral bodies. However, if the end plates are calcified, your discs cannot receive hydration and nutrition. As a result, your discs essentially dry out, also called dessication.

If you do develop degenerative disc disease of your neck, which most of us do when we are over age 50, you can have decreased range of motion about your neck. The decreased range of motion around your neck is an early indication that you are developing degeneration of the discs and joints in your neck. You will have trouble turning your head and attempting to look behind you. Looking up or down also can be difficult as well as painful. Attention to your neck posture and doing daily range-of-motion exercises for your neck can reduce the progression of degenerative disc disease involving your neck. For example, move your neck up and down, put your ears on your shoulders, and turn your head to the right and left as far as you can.

If you have a severe state of contractions of a muscle in your neck, you may have severe pain. This prolonged contraction of a neck muscle is called torticollis. This usually occurs on one side of your neck. Your head is usually twisted to one side with your chin pointing to the opposite side. Torticollis usually results from disease or an injury to your brain or spinal cord. Injuries to the muscles of your neck can also be a cause of torticollis as well. Sometimes an injection of botulism toxin into your muscles can provide temporary relief.

Women have more neck pain than men. The incidence of neck pain increases with age. Whiplash injuries can cause neck pain as well and are more common in women than in men. Furthermore, repetitive activities in a workplace setting can be a source of neck pain. Unfortunately, you can have neck pain for a long time. It is not self-limiting as some other types of pain syndromes are. Neck pain is a symptom of problem processes going on in your neck.

Women are more prone to neck pain because they have smaller necks and it makes them vulnerable to the onset of pain. Remember that the neck must hold a 10- to 12-pound head. A smaller neck receives more stress from the head than a larger neck. It also has been hypothesized that men are more stoic than women and do not report their neck pain as often as women. Because of their smaller necks, women are more prone to suffer severe whiplash injuries than men. Not only do men have larger necks than women, but the overall body mass of the neck is more than a woman's.

Be aware that women can suffer neck injuries in beauty parlors and hair salons.[1] When you bend your head backward into a sink to have your hair washed, the angle of the compression of the neck sometimes causes a disc in your neck to rupture. Some people also pass out when their head is bent backward because of compression of arteries that go to the brain that are present in the back of the neck.

The slender column of your neck is the most vulnerable part of your spine. Your mid back and lower back are protected by more tissue mass. You must keep your muscles strong. Your physical therapist or chiropractor can give you sets of exercises to safely do to strengthen your neck muscles. To prevent neck pain, you must move your neck. Your facet joints are designed to provide your head and neck with movement. The joints get nutrition through movement. If you have experienced neck pain before, complete range of motion exercises with your neck. For example, move your head up and down followed by attempting to place your ears on your shoulders. These maneuvers will provide increased blood flow to your facet joints.

Remember that sitting in a position over a desk or work table for a long time can cause you to have pain. Not moving your head and neck can cause your pain. When you do not move your neck, the lubricant in your facet joint can dry out. When this occurs you will have difficulty moving your neck. When you are working at a computer, remember to keep your eyes looking straight ahead. This will keep your neck in proper alignment. When you are sleeping, you must not place your head on a big, fluffy pillow. This could cause your neck to become misaligned. There are pillows available that are made specifically for neck comfort. You may be interested in purchasing one of these pillows.

If you are riding in a vehicle, you should raise your head rest to the position that meets the back curve of your skull to help prevent whiplash. If you have an onset of pain, you may want to take a long hot shower, letting the shower water bathe your neck. This method may provide you with pain relief if your pain is not from a recent injury. If have had a recent injury, you should apply ice packs on your neck pain. You should wrap ice or a package of frozen vegetables in a towel. Press the cold substance to the painful area on your neck for about 10 minutes. You should not let the cold packs numb your neck.

You also should remember that strenuous working postures can cause you to have significant neck pain. For example, if you paint frequently overhead, make sure that you take a break every hour or two and do range-of-motion exercises for your neck. You must remember that high levels of psychological stress in your workplace also can contribute to your neck pain. If you are in a stressful situation at work, talk to your supervisor to see if there is something that can be done to lessen your stress level.

Treatment of neck pain for men and women will be determined on an individual basis by your doctor or therapist. Be sure that you follow the doctor's or therapist's instructions carefully so that you do not injure yourself further. If your pain does not get better during your treatment, be sure to discuss this with your doctor or therapist so that he or she can perform further examinations and discuss other treatment options with you. The hyperextended neck position during hair shampoo treatment in a beauty parlor may be a risk factor for cerebellum vascular insufficiency. 2 Public education should lead to avoidance of this position during hair shampoo treatment at hair dressing salons.

With respect to ethnicity and neck pain, a study published in 2010 reported that care seeking was similar among races (83% white, 85% black, 72% Latino).[3] Uses of opioids were also similar between races, at 49% for whites, 52% for blacks, and trended lower at 35% for Latinos. There were few racial/ethnic differences in care seeking, treatment use, and use of narcotics for the treatment of chronic back and neck pain.

The issue of racial and ethnic disparities in neck and back pain prevalence and care reveal that few disparities were found recently. Care quality issues may affect all ethnic groups similarly. Previous findings of disparities in chronic-pain management may be decreasing. Severe headache or migraine is often associated with other common pains, seldom existing alone. It is common to have headaches with neck pain. Severe headache or migraine is often associated with other common pains, seldom existing alone. Two or more comorbid pains are common, similarly affecting gender and racial/ethnic groups.[3] race itself does not appear to be a causative factor. Cervical arthrosis is a common condition. Cervical arthrosis is independent of race and sex.[4]

Epidural injections have been used since 1901 in managing low back pain and sciatica. Spinal pain, disability, health, and economic impact continue to increase, despite numerous modalities of interventions available in managing chronic spinal pain. Studies show the efficacy of epidural injections in managing a multitude of chronic spinal conditions.[5]

The procedure is a safe and an effective treatment for patients with cervical pain syndromes. The success rates show that a large percentage of the patients may obtain relief from radicular symptoms and avoid surgery for the follow-up period which is up to 12 months.[6] Translaminar cervical epidural injections are relatively safe procedures. These injections place the steroid in the hole in the bone of your spine where the nerve emerges.[7] Although repeat injections may be necessary in some patients, excellent short-term clinical results can be achieved.

Cervical facet joint (the joints where your neck bones stack on top of each other) injections are effective and well tolerated for the treatment of cervicogenic headache and neck pain. The procedures provided significant and prolonged pain relief in the majority of patients treated.[8] Ultrasound-guided trigger point injections may help confirm proper needle placement within the cervicothoracic musculature.[9] The use of ultrasound-guided trigger point injections in the cervicothoracic musculature may also reduce the potential for a pneumothorax by an improperly placed injection. Lower cervical intramuscular anesthetic injection may be an effective treatment for head or face pain as well.[10]

New, population-based data on the issue of racial and ethnic disparities in neck pain prevalence and care. Reveal that few disparities were found and that care quality issues may affect all ethnic groups similarly. Previous findings of disparities in chronic-pain management may furthermore be decreasing.[3]

Your pain doctor might inject corticosteroid medications near the nerve roots, into the small facet joints in the bones of the cervical spine or into the muscles in your neck to help decrease your pain. Numbing medications, such as lidocaine, also can be injected to relieve your neck pain. Rarely is surgery needed for neck pain. If conservative care is not effective, surgery might be an option for relieving nerve root or spinal cord compression.

References

1.   Zangbar B, Pandit V, Rhee P, Haider AA, Khalil M, Joseph B. Beauty parlor stroke syndrome: a rare entity in a trauma patient. Am Surg. 2015;81(3):E120-122.

2.   Endo K, Ichimaru K, Shimura H, Imakiire A. Cervical vertigo after hair shampoo treatment at a hairdressing salon: a case report. Spine (Phila Pa 1976). 2000;25(5):632-634.

3.   Carey TS, Freburger JK, Holmes GM, et al. Race, care seeking, and utilization for chronic back and neck pain: population perspectives. J Pain. 2010;11(4):343-350.

4.   Master DL, Eubanks JD, Ahn NU. Prevalence of concurrent lumbar and cervical arthrosis: an anatomic study of cadaveric specimens. Spine (Phila Pa 1976). 2009;34(8):E272-275.

5.   Kaye AD, Manchikanti L, Abdi S, et al. Efficacy of Epidural Injections in Managing Chronic Spinal Pain: A Best Evidence Synthesis. Pain Physician. 2015;18(6):E939-E1004.

6.   Beyaz SG, Eman A. Fluoroscopy guided cervical interlaminar steroid injections in patients with cervical pain syndromes: a retrospective study. J Back Musculoskelet Rehabil. 2013;26(1):85-91.

7.   Strub WM, Brown TA, Ying J, Hoffmann M, Ernst RJ, Bulas RV. Translaminar cervical epidural steroid injection: short-term results and factors influencing outcome. J Vasc Interv Radiol. 2007;18(9):1151-1155.

8.   Zhou L, Hud-Shakoor Z, Hennessey C, Ashkenazi A. Upper cervical facet joint and spinal rami blocks for the treatment of cervicogenic headache. Headache. 2010;50(4):657-663.

9.   Botwin KP, Sharma K, Saliba R, Patel BC. Ultrasound-guided trigger point injections in the cervicothoracic musculature: a new and unreported technique. Pain Physician. 2008;11(6):885-889.

10.   Mellick GA, Mellick LB. Regional head and face pain relief following lower cervical intramuscular anesthetic injection. Headache. 2003;43(10):1109-1111.

16. Back Pain

Back pain has many causes. You could be experiencing pain in your back as a result of injury, stress, poor posture, or even aging. Many people experience back pain, and there are treatment methods available that could help ease that pain. It is important to note that the onset or worsening of back pain can be prevented by utilizing proper posture techniques and performing stretching exercises. The majority of patients seen in most pain clinics have complaints of pain in their lower back. Do you know why lower back pain is so common?

Our backs are made up of a large number of bones called vertebrae that are separated from one another by discs. These discs act as shock absorbers. Between each bone in our spine, the bones stack on top of each other like Lego blocks and form joints called facet joints. The purpose of the bones in your spine is to protect your spinal cord from injury. There are foramina, which are holes in each vertebra. The nerves off of your spinal cord go through these holes and go to your arms, legs, and organs within your body.

Your spine is kept in place by muscles in your back that maintain your posture. Your muscles also make your back stable during movement. You have many muscles in your back. Any one of these muscles can cause you to have lower back pain. In addition to muscles, you have ligaments that attach each bone in your spine to both the one above and the one below. Ligaments also are necessary to give your back stability. Your ligaments contain pain fibers and can be a source of your back pain.

Most of your lower back pain and any associated disability associated with your lower back is usually mechanical in nature. This means that there is usually an abnormal alignment of your bones and/or joints that can cause you to have significant lower back pain. You have five bones in your lower back that are called lumbar vertebrae. Your spine functions to support you when you are standing, walking, bending, pushing, and pulling. Your back must perform repetitive tasks on a daily basis without failure.

Most of your everyday back pains are not serious. Your back pain is most probably related to a muscle strain or a ligament sprain from doing an activity that you are not used to doing. You should never ignore your back pain. You should be concerned if your back pain goes into your legs. If your back pain is associated with weakness of your legs or numbness or difficulty walking, you need to see a doctor. If you have damage to your spinal cord, you may become paralyzed. If this happens, you may lose all control of your bowel and bladder. If you lose control of your bowel and/or bladder you need to immediately see your doctor.

Back pain is the most expensive and common industrial- or work-related injury. Back pain is the most common cause of disability for workers younger than age 45. In 90 percent of working people, back pain limits working activity for usually less than 30 days. Five percent of people who have back pain have weakness, loss of sensation, or loss of reflexes in a leg. Two percent of people with back pain may end up needing surgery. Back pain is the most common cause of activity limitation in the working population between ages 18 to 55 in the United States. Back pain is responsible for 15 percent of work absenteeism in developed countries. Approximately 5 percent of the work force is disabled by back pain yearly. Attempts to prevent back pain have not been proven to be effective.

The rate of surgery for back pain in the United States is greater than in most other countries. The reason for this finding is probably due to the large number of surgeons in the United States when compared to other countries. Following the onset of back pain, there can be a recurrence of lower back pain in a person within 1 year and a 75 percent recurrence in a person's lifetime. Sixty-five percent of patients usually recover from an episode of back pain within six weeks. At 12 weeks, 85 percent of those with back pain are essentially pain free.

If you have pain for more than 12 weeks, it is unlikely that you will receive significant relief of your back pain. If you have been off of work for more than 26 weeks, you will probably not be able to return back to work. Studies have shown that if you have been off of work for 104 or more weeks, you will not return back to work. If you receive compensation from a workmen's compensation insurance carrier or compensation following a motor vehicle accident, your chances of returning to work are significantly decreased.

Lower back pain is the cause for approximately 20 percent of all industrial injuries. Back pain amounts to 50 percent of the cost of all work-related injuries. Only 10 percent of the injuries account for 80 percent of the total cost due to disability. If you are over 50 years of age, you can expect to have problems with your back and also have limitations in your activity due to back pain.

Back pain from heavy physical work is common by age 50. Even people who have not done heavy physical work can begin experiencing increased back pain by age 50. You should realize that it will be difficult to decrease your back pain if you have become inactive. For this reason, you should do aerobic exercise to prevent back pain. You also can use exercise to treat back pain. The muscles in your back must be strong in order to support your back. This is the reason that you must do regular exercise activity.

Your lower back is made up of five bones called lumbar vertebrae. The lower part of your back below these bones is called the sacrum. It is made up of five fused bones. Your pelvis anchors here. Your tailbone is called a coccyx. If you sit in a chair correctly or in the seat of your car correctly, you are keeping all of these bones properly aligned. Each bone then bears the full weight of the bone above it. It is reported that proper alignment of your back can help build bone mass. This is important if anyone in your family has a history of osteoporosis.

Cushions that are called discs are located between the bones in your back. These discs are prone to injury as well as to wear and tear. As you grow older, your discs lose their elastic properties and they become thinner and can become wafer thin. As the discs in your back decrease in height, your overall height decreases. If you are over 40, you may have noticed that you are beginning to decrease with respect to your height.

As your discs begin to shrink, pressure from the bones above and below can cause your discs to press outward. This is called a disc bulge. Sometimes a disc bulge can press on one of your nerves. A disc bulge is not a disc rupture. However, a disc bulge can press on one of your nerves coming off of your spinal cord and can cause you significant pain. If your pain persists and you develop numbness, you may ultimately have to have surgery to remove a portion of this bulge off of your nerve.

In the very center of your disc is a thick liquid. Liquids cannot be compressed. If you bend a certain way or attempt to lift a heavy object in an awkward position, the fluid inside of your disc can burst through the outer ring of your disc. This is called a disc herniation or ruptures and can cause you significant pain. The liquid material that bursts outside of your disc is highly acidic. This acid content can cause your nerves, your ligaments and your muscles to become swollen and inflamed and you can develop severe pain.

Discography is a way of diagnosing whether or not that you have disc-related pain. An MRI and CT scan can show a disc herniation. However, these imaging studies cannot define pain. A discogram is an injection of material into your disc. The pressure in your disc is then measured. You should have a relatively high pressure when material is injected into the center of your disc. If your disc leaks, the leakage of the acidic nucleus pulposus can cause you to have pain. When your nucleus pulposus leaks out of your disc it hardens just like glue out of its tube.

Sciatica is a pain that is felt in your back and the outer side of your thigh, leg, and foot. It is usually caused by degeneration of one of the discs between your back bones. When the disc protrudes laterally off to the side, it can compress the nerves in your lower back. Usually the last two or three nerves are compressed on the side of your pain Furthermore, it can be brought on if you are performing an awkward lifting position or if you are doing a twisting movement such as raking the leaves.

People who have sciatica usually have stiff backs and have pain when they attempt any movement. You may have numbness in your leg as well as weakness associated with your sciatica. Bed rest for 24 hours may decrease your pain. If you have significant weakness and pain, nonsteroidal anti-inflammatory medication can help. If this medication does not provide you with relief, your pain-medicine doctor may want to inject the sciatic nerve with some numbing medicine and a steroid. If you still have pain after conservative treatments have been done, a surgeon may need to do a surgical procedure to get either a muscle or disc off of your nerve to relieve your pain.

Where your backbone and pelvis meet, they form a joint called the sacroiliac joint. Your sacroiliac joint can be a source of your back pain. This joint has a thick capsule that has strong ligaments both in the front and the back of your joint. Other ligaments also help to form and support this joint. The joint is C shaped.

As you become older, the cartilage that attaches to your pelvic bone degenerates faster than the cartilage in your sacrum. As a result this joint can become unstable. It can be a cause of your pain as well. Related to hormone changes that occur during pregnancy, the ligaments becomes loose. This is the reason that many pregnant women experience pain in their sacroiliac joint that can last after the birth of their baby until the ligament becomes stronger.

Sometimes the pain from your sacroiliac joint can cause pain to go down your leg. You may notice pain in your back when you roll over in bed or when you get out of a car. Furthermore, you can have pain when you go up or down steps. If the muscle over your sacroiliac joint is tender, it can cause you to have pain. The diagnosis of this problem can be done by examination. A bone scan is helpful in diagnosing sacroiliac arthritis.

During this procedure, a very small dose of a radioactive dye is injected into your veins. After the radioactive dye has had time to go to your joints, pictures are taken with a camera of your sacroiliac joint. If you have arthritis, there will be darkened areas in your joints that will show up on the scan. Usually plain x-rays are not sufficient to diagnose problems with your sacroiliac joint.

The treatment of this problem consists of physical therapy. A type of Velcro belt called an SI belt can be used to hold your joint in place. If you have no relief from these methods, your pain-medicine doctor can inject a steroid and local anesthetic into your joint under x-ray needle guidance. These methods should rid you of your pain. If your pain does persist, destruction of the nerves that goes to your joint can be done with heat. This is called a rhizotomy.

Occasionally, a surgeon may have to stabilize your joint surgically. Nonsteroidal anti-inflammatory medications also can be very helpful for the management of pain in your sacroiliac joint. Because the pain involves a joint, muscle relaxants may not be of any benefit. If you have a disc herniation, the disc herniation can be diagnosed by a CT scan or an MRI. In some instances, you may need to seek chiropractic therapy to realign your back. If the bones in your back are properly aligned, your nerves should be able to transmit normal impulses to your muscles to allow your muscles to function in an optimal fashion. If there is some entrapment of your nerves, or pressure on your nerves by adjacent body structures, your nervous system cannot function properly.

If you are overweight and don't exercise and don't use proper posture, your back muscles and discs will become progressively weaker. You will then be prone to a disc rupture. The weakness in your discs does not just happen overnight. This weakness progresses over time due to the lack of activity as well as other factors. This is the reason why you need to maintain a healthful lifestyle that includes exercise. Preventative pain medicine is just as important as the treatment of pain problems.

Changes in the architecture of your discs and joints due to wear and tear are called osteoarthritis. This is the most common form of arthritis and it affects approximately 21 million Americans. Arthritis can cause the diameter of your spinal column to decrease. Your spinal column is hollow in the center. Your spinal cord runs vertical within the hole in the spinal column.

If you begin to experience osteoarthritis, the hole in the vertebral body in which the spinal cord is placed can narrow and can eventually put pressure on your spinal cord, which can cause you to have significant pain. The holes in the bones in your spine allow your nerves from your spinal cord to go to your arms, legs, and organs. These nerves can cause pain in your extremities or organs. However, these nerves also can control muscle movement in your arms and legs. With osteoarthritis, the holes in which your nerves emerge from the spinal cord can decrease their diameter. When this happens, one or more of your nerves can be compressed, which can cause you pain, numbness, and weakness.

After the age of 30, your bones gradually lose calcium. The loss of calcium can decrease your bone mass, especially in your vertebral bodies. This is called osteoporosis. Osteoporosis is seen more commonly in women than men. In females, the loss of the female hormone called estrogen, which occurs at menopause, will accelerate this bone loss. The loss of calcium in bone mass in your vertebral bodies can collapse them and cause a fracture of your vertebrae. These fractures are called compression fractures. The height of your vertebral bone decreases. Osteoporosis can be very painful. Some doctors are now putting a hardening substance into the bones of the back if patients have osteoporosis and have compression fractures. This technique is referred to as vertebroplasty.

In addition to degenerative changes in the back and joints as being common causes of back pain, the most common cause of back pain is muscle tension in the lower back. Approximately 80 percent of people living in the United States will experience one incident of an aching back at some time in their lives. Be aware that stress plays a major role in the origin of your lower back pain. If you are frightened or nervous, your muscles become tense.

If you play tennis or golf, the muscles on one side of your back can become short while those on the other side become long. Tennis and golf rotate your spine in one direction in a repetitive fashion. If you sleep on one side most of the time, the muscles on that side of your spine shorten while the muscles on the other side of your spine lengthen. The muscles that are lengthened can become weak while the ones that are shortened can become tight.

Have you ever slipped on the ice and landed on your buttocks? If this has happened to you, the muscle in your lower buttocks called the piriformis muscle can spasm or can even shorten, which compresses your sciatic nerve. Injection of a local anesthetic into the muscle can relieve your pain. If your pain returns, botulism toxin (Botox), which can relax your muscle for up to three months, may be effective when followed by stretching exercises by your physical therapist.

Only rarely does a surgeon have to operate on your piriformis muscle if you have persistent sciatic pain. Sometimes chiropractic therapy can offer you a conservative alternative for the treatment of your sciatica.

Your chiropractor can treat you with methods such as heat and electrical current to decrease your need to take a pain pill.

Misalignment of your back due to poor posture or other mechanical strains such as slouching in a chair can cause you to have back pain. If you sit over a computer desk with your back rounded, your muscles are going to adapt to that position. Often the muscle fiber length will change to conform to your improper position. When this happens, your spine is going to adapt to these positions as well.

You must remember that hunching over a desk or slouching in a chair can press some muscles and elongate other muscles. Also, tendons, joints, and ligaments that support your back are affected. Some of the ligaments are stretched while some are compressed. When you slouch or when you sit rounded over, you can compress some of the facet joints while opening other facet joints.

Your lower back has a natural C curve at the lower end of your back. This normal curve is called a lordodic curve. Chronic slouching can straighten this normal C curve in your back. This misalignment will affect your discs, muscles, ligaments, and joints. Look at your posture in your mirror. If your posture is abnormal, you must correct it.

If you cannot do it yourself, you may want to visit a chiropractor or physical therapist to help you with this problem. The lower discs in your lumbar spine essentially do not have a blood supply from arteries to your disc after age 12. The blood supply of your discs must come from the ends of your vertebral bones. Most of the oxygen and sugar that goes to your discs comes from the ends of your vertebral bodies. Your discs need these nutrients.

The facet joints in your spine work to stabilize your spine. As your joints deteriorate, you will lose motion as your age increases. For some reason, the development of loss of lower back range of motion is slower in women than in men.

Spondylolisthesis can be another cause of your back pain. This occurs when one of your bones slips upon the one below it. This is usually hereditary in origin. However, when one bone slips over the other, it can cause pain in your facet joints and sometimes it can compress the nerves coming off of your spinal cord going to your legs. Usually surgery is not needed for this slippage. Your pain can be controlled with NSAIDs. Occasionally a steroid injection into your epidural space or a steroid into your facet joint can help to control your pain. Sometimes chiropractic therapy can help you in the management of your pain with this syndrome.

With respect to gender specificity, sacroiliac joint pain, which can cause significant pain in your back, is common in women during pregnancy and is a result of increased hormones secreted by a woman's body during pregnancy.1 We also have stated that with aging, women experience less pain initially than men. Osteoporosis, however, is more prevalent in women and can be a significant cause of chronic back pain. Compression of the bones in the lower back can cause fractures and is more common in postmenopausal women because their hormones have significantly declined after menopause.

Frequent upper body bending is associated with low back pain (LBP). The complex flexion movement, combining lumbar and pelvic motion, is known as "lumbopelvic rhythm". A previous study demonstrated the adverse effects of increasing age and female gender on lordosis, sacrum orientation and lumbopelvic rhythm.[2] Not only does gender affect the incidence of back pain, but age in gender also can affect the incidence of back pain.

For example, it was published in 1988 that back pain prevalence was higher among women than men at younger ages, but around age 45 the rate for back pain among men exceeded that of women. When people reach 65 years of age or over, the incidence of back pain was similar for both men and women. It is interesting to note that there is a decrease in the prevalence of back pain in women between the ages of 70 to 79.

Low back pain (LBP) is prevalent in dental hygienists.[3] Combined spine rotation and flexion, and tonic activity of the extensor musculature may be related to LBP in dental hygienists. You should now be aware that it is normal for you to have back pain as you age. You must try and minimize your pain. You should do range-of-motion exercises, take vitamins regularly, and if you smoke, you must stop.

In certain parts of the world back pain is considered a normal part of life. It is, therefore, less debilitating. In Japan, for example, few individuals complain of back pain when compared to the United States. As a result, disability related to back pain is less. The aging of the world population is a phenomenon that is growing progressively. Specific knowledge of osteoarticular disorders in the elderly in black Africa seems limited. Non-traumatic osteoarticular diseases in elderly black Africans are dominated by degenerative diseases of spine.[4]

Back rehabilitation now involves increasing activity and strengthening the muscles in your back. Following an injury, you may rest for one to two days. However, after this time you need to get active and begin doing range of motion about your back. If you injure your knee, your doctor will begin knee-strengthening exercises. Therefore, the same applies to your back. If you injure your back, the muscles that hold your back in position need to be strengthened. Inactivity weakens these muscles. Lower education levels, smoking, obesity, and inactivity contribute to the prevalence of back pain in the United States.

Treatments for your lower back pain can include physical therapy and chiropractic therapy. As mentioned previously, nonsteroidal anti-inflammatory drugs can decrease the swelling in your tissues as well as in your nerves to decrease your pain. Muscle relaxants on rare occasions can be of benefit to decrease your pain.

However, if your pain is related to muscle tension, heat and range-of-motion exercises can be extremely beneficial. If you are under stress at work or at home, attempt to alleviate your stressful situations. Remember that chiropractic therapy also can be an alternative method to significantly decrease your lower back pain.

If all conservative methods fail to provide you with pain relief, injections of numbing medicines and steroids can be performed in your muscles, your epidural space, around your nerves going to your spinal cord, and even in your facet joints. If you have compression of your nerves, surgery can provide you with benefit.

However, epidural steroids for lumbosacral radicular pain treatment is reported to be no better than an oral gabapentinin a German study.[5] Epidural injections are performed to manage lumbar central spinal stenosis pain utilizing caudal (medicine placed through the tail bone) , interlaminar (between the discs), and transforaminal (into the hole where the nerve exits the spine), approaches.

Significant improvement in patients suffering with chronic lumbar spinal stenosis with caudal and interlaminar epidural approaches with local anesthetic only, or with steroids with the interlaminar approach providing significantly better results.[6] Other investigators have shown the efficacy of epidural injections in managing a multitude of chronic spinal conditions as well.[7]

It is important for the pain management that a higher average skin to lumbar epidural space distance is noted in African Americans compared with Caucasians, Hispanics, Asians, and Indian/Pakistani/Bangladeshi/Sri Lankans.[8] It is important therefore for the doctor to choose the proper length needle when doing the steroid injection.

Active muscular trigger points which consist of injecting a painful muscle with a steroid and a numbing medication can help relieve back pain in patients presenting with radiating leg pain. Trigger point injection therapy in patients suffering from chronic lumbosacral radiculopathy can significantly improve their recovery.[9] A back brace can sometimes be used to decrease your pain. However, the problem with the back brace is that you lose range of motion about your spine. You should know that range of motion about your facet joints helps get nutrients to the joints. It is important to have nutrients in your joints to help form a lubricant within the joint that allows the joint to move freely. Furthermore, if you use a brace long term can decrease the strength in your muscles that holds your back in a vertical position.

In a study done in 1996, low back pain symptoms were reported less commonly in individuals older than age 60 years and in nonwhites compared with whites.[10] Thirty-nine percent of those with back pain sought medical care; 24% sought care initially from an allopathic physician, 13% from a chiropractor, and 2% from other providers. More prolonged pain, more severe pain, and sciatica were associated with care-seeking. Gender, income, age, rural residence, and health insurance status did not correlate with the decision to seek medical care. Younger age, male gender, and nonjob-related pain did correlate with the decision to seek care from a chiropractor. Older white men have a higher prevalence of spinal vertebral body fractures than older black men.[11]

When arthritis strikes on our facet joints it produces pain. The pain intensifies when you bend, flex, or extend your back. Lumbar arthrosis targets your lower back. The back pain intensifies by movements like arching and extending. This type is caused by disc generation and spinal stenosis. Concurrent lumbar and cervical arthrosis is a common condition. Lumbar arthrosis and advancing age are associated with cervical arthrosis independent of race and sex.[12] Lumbar arthrosis precedes cervical arthrosis in older patients.

Among veterans under age 65 reporting moderate to high levels of chronic noncancerous pain, blacks were less likely to be prescribed opioids than whites.[13] These facts underscore the challenges of eliminating racial differences in pain treatment. Previous research suggests female and black patients receive less optimal treatment for their chronic pain compared with male and white patients. Provider-related factors are hypothesized to contribute to unequal treatment, but these factors have not been examined extensively. This mixed methods investigation examined the influence of patients' demographic characteristics on providers' treatment decisions and providers' awareness of these influences on their treatment decisions.[14]

Vertebroplasty and kyphoplasty are frequently utilized in the treatment of symptomatic vertebral body fractures. While prior studies have demonstrated disparities in the treatment of back pain and care for osteoporotic patients, disparities in spine augmentation have not been investigated. Racial and health insurance status differences exist in the use of spine augmentation for the treatment of osteoporotic vertebral fractures in the United States. Among patients with spine augmentation, 75% received kyphoplasty and 25% received vertebroplasty.[15]

Care for low back pain is complex. Blacks receive less intense diagnostic and treatment approaches from MDs, although the severity of their impairment is at least as great.[16] After controlling for healthcare site, lower education, female sex, African-American race, and older age were associated with worse physical disability and all of these factors except age were associated with worse reports of low pain.[17]

With respect to work injuries and low back pain in a Workers' Compensation setting, Whites were 40% more likely than African Americans to receive a herniated disc diagnosis. Of claimants with the latter diagnosis, whites were 110% more likely than African Americans to undergo surgery. [18] Race differences in diagnosis and surgery may help to explain why African Americans, relative to whites, receive lower workers' compensation medical expenditures, disability ratings, and settlement awards.

The Missouri Division of Workers' Compensation provided information on medical and temporary disability expenditures, claim duration, final disability ratings, and settlement awards.[19] Differences remained for both injury and African Americans and lower socioeconomic status workers after controlling for injury, and for African Americans after controlling for both injury and socioeconomic status. Because Workers' Compensation mandates equal access to treatment and disability reimbursement for all injured workers, the differences observed in this study may reflect sociocultural biases in disability management among healthcare providers.

References

1.   Dawson PU, Rose RE, Wade NA. Fluoroscopy-guided Sacroiliac Joint Steroid Injection for Low Back Pain in a Patient with Osteogenesis Imperfecta. West Indian Med J. 2015;64(4).

2.   Pries E, Dreischarf M, Bashkuev M, Putzier M, Schmidt H. The effects of age and gender on the lumbopelvic rhythm in the sagittal plane in 309 subjects. J Biomech. 2015;48(12):3080-3087.

3.   Howarth SJ, Grondin DE, La Delfa NJ, Cox J, Potvin JR. Working position influences the biomechanical demands on the lower back during dental hygiene. Ergonomics. 2015:1-11.

4.   Diomande M, Eti E, Ouali B, et al. Profile of non-traumatic osteoarticular diseases in elderly black africans: about 157 cases seen in abidjan. Tunis Med. 2015;93(5):312-315.

5.   Steurer J. [Epidural steroids for lumbosacral radicular pain treatment is no better than an oral gabapentin]. Praxis (Bern 1994). 2015;104(17):926-927.

6.   Manchikanti L, Falco FJ, Pampati V, Hirsch JA. Lumbar interlaminar epidural injections are superior to caudal epidural injections in managing lumbar central spinal stenosis. Pain Physician. 2014;17(6):E691-702.

7.   Kaye AD, Manchikanti L, Abdi S, et al. Efficacy of Epidural Injections in Managing Chronic Spinal Pain: A Best Evidence Synthesis. Pain Physician. 2015;18(6):E939-E1004.

8.   D'Alonzo RC, White WD, Schultz JR, Jaklitsch PM, Habib AS. Ethnicity and the distance to the epidural space in parturients. Reg Anesth Pain Med. 2008;33(1):24-29.

9.   Saeidian SR, Pipelzadeh MR, Rasras S, Zeinali M. Effect of trigger point injection on lumbosacral radiculopathy source. Anesth Pain Med. 2014;4(4):e15500.

10.   Carey TS, Evans AT, Hadler NM, et al. Acute severe low back pain. A population-based study of prevalence and care-seeking. Spine (Phila Pa 1976). 1996;21(3):339-344.

11.   Tracy JK, Meyer WA, Grigoryan M, et al. Racial differences in the prevalence of vertebral fractures in older men: the Baltimore Men's Osteoporosis Study. Osteoporos Int. 2006;17(1):99-104.

12.   Master DL, Eubanks JD, Ahn NU. Prevalence of concurrent lumbar and cervical arthrosis: an anatomic study of cadaveric specimens. Spine (Phila Pa 1976). 2009;34(8):E272-275.

13.   Burgess DJ, Nelson DB, Gravely AA, et al. Racial differences in prescription of opioid analgesics for chronic noncancer pain in a national sample of veterans. J Pain. 2014;15(4):447-455.

14.   Hollingshead NA, Matthias MS, Bair MJ, Hirsh AT. Impact of race and sex on pain management by medical trainees: a mixed

methods pilot study of decision making and awareness of influence. Pain Med. 2015;16(2):280-290.

15.   Gu CN, Brinjikji W, El-Sayed AM, Cloft H, McDonald JS, Kallmes DF. Racial and health insurance disparities of inpatient spine augmentation for osteoporotic vertebral fractures from 2005 to 2010. AJNR Am J Neuroradiol. 2014;35(12):2397-2402.

16.   Carey TS, Garrett JM. The relation of race to outcomes and the use of health care services for acute low back pain. Spine (Phila Pa 1976). 2003;28(4):390-394.

17.   Jarvik JG, Comstock BA, Heagerty PJ, et al. Back pain in seniors: the Back pain Outcomes using Longitudinal Data (BOLD) cohort baseline data. BMC Musculoskelet Disord. 2014;15:134.

18.   Chibnall JT, Tait RC, Andresen EM, Hadler NM. Race differences in diagnosis and surgery for occupational low back injuries. Spine (Phila Pa 1976). 2006;31(11):1272-1275.

19.   Tait RC, Chibnall JT, Andresen EM, Hadler NM. Management of occupational back injuries: differences among African Americans and Caucasians. Pain. 2004;112(3):389-396.

17. Head Pain

A headache is pain felt within the skull, in the forehead, in the temples, or at the base of the skull. Most headaches are caused by emotional stress or fatigue, but some headaches are a symptom of a disease within the brain. Pain in your head can arise in your head or can be referred from your neck, too. Different types of headaches such as migraines, tension headaches, cluster headaches, head trauma headaches, and temporal arteritis headaches will be discussed.

Pain in your head can be divided into two divisions: Some pain receptors exist outside your skull, and other pain receptors exist within your skull. Structures outside of your skull that can cause pain in your head include the skin and scalp over the head, muscles about your head and neck, and the outer wrapper of the bone of your skull called the periosteum. Your sinuses can also cause you to have head pain. Within your skull, you have a lining that can become inflamed and irritated and cause pain. Your veins can cause pain as well if they become engorged.

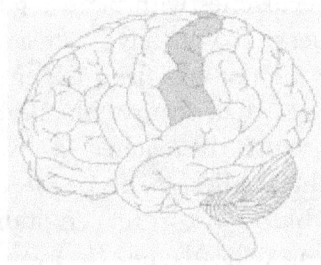

Figure 1. Headaches can originate from within the skull.

If you have tenderness around the arteries in your temples, you may have an inflammation of the temporal arteries. Your doctor will examine your pupils to see whether they are extremely small and will look at your upper eyelids for any drooping. Those with migraine headaches usually want to be left alone and usually seek a quiet, dark place. Those with cluster headaches find no relief in any position; they try many positions while attempting to eliminate their headaches and usually end up pacing the floor.

If your temperature is elevated, you may have an infection in your throat, sinuses, or even in your brain. Sometimes a CT scan is necessary to determine whether you have swelling in your brain or a brain abscess. An electroencephalogram (EEG) study is sometimes needed to determine whether you have a seizure disorder or a sleep problem. If you have had trauma to your head, your doctor may want a CT scan, which will show whether you have bleeding within your head. An MRI scan of your brain can be done to see whether you have loss of myelin, which is a substance in your brain. With loss of myelin, you may develop neurological symptoms that include memory loss and difficulty concentrating. Occasionally a spinal tap is done. This can investigate whether you have an infection. At the time that the spinal tap is done, a pressure monitor can be used to see whether you have increased pressure in your central nervous system.

Loss of consciousness could indicate seizures or a hemorrhage into your brain. If you have had no previous history of headaches, your doctor will need to run tests to see whether you have a bleed in your brain from a weakness in the arteries in your brain. A weakness in the blood vessel is called an aneurysm. If you have headaches accompanied by neurological abnormalities during and after your headache, your doctor will want to make sure that you don't have a bleed within your brain.

Tumors can cause headaches with neurological abnormalities such as forgetfulness and dizziness. If you have a headache that first begins after age 50, your pain may be coming from degeneration of the discs in your neck. Hormonal changes that occur with the decreased function of your thyroid gland can cause headaches as well. Remember that depression also can cause headaches. A headache that occurs when you have an increase in your blood pressure can indicate various medical diseases that may be causing a headache. Be aware that headaches can come from the soft tissues in your neck. An x-ray of your neck will not reveal soft tissue problems. An MRI can usually reveal problems in structures that could cause you to have a headache.

A common type of headache is the classic migraine headache. By definition a migraine headache is a headache that returns and varies widely in its intensity and frequency of the attacks and the duration. Usually the headaches occur on one side and are associated with nausea, vomiting, and a loss of appetite. Sometimes you may have visual problems associated with this headache. You can have a headache with sensations that forewarn you of an attack of an impending headache.

You may have a sensation of flickering lights or blurred vision or weakness in your arms or legs. These sensations are called an aura. Some migraines occur without an aura. If you have migraines with an aura, usually you have visual disturbances. In the United States, migraine prevalence is highest among Native Americans, then Whites, followed closely by Hispanics and Blacks. Asians have the lowest prevalence of severe, frequent headache or migraine of the major racial or ethnic groups.[1] In another study however, migraine prevalence was found to be higher in blacks and other unspecified minorities than in the white population.[2]

This type of visual disturbance is seen in 90 percent of patients who have migraine headaches with an aura. Migraine headaches can be triggered if you have abnormal response to stress. Migraine treatment utilization, diagnosis, and treatment are low for both African Americans and Caucasians.[3] However, this was especially true for African Americans, who also reported lower levels of trust and communication with doctors relative to Caucasians. The findings highlight the need for improved physician and patient education about migraine diagnosis and treatment. In the United States, migraine prevalence is highest among Native Americans, then Whites, followed closely by Hispanics and Blacks. Asians have the lowest prevalence of severe, frequent headache or migraine of the major racial or ethnic groups.[2,3]

More than 50 years ago, doctors thought that the source of migraine pain was related to decreased blood flow to the brain, which in turn decreased the oxygen in the brain, causing headaches. However, more recent studies have demonstrated that the migraine headaches occur in brain cells. Sometimes the blood flow in the brain can decrease and the thickness of the blood can increase. These events can release chemicals in your brain that activate the pain impulses in your brain. When you have one of these headaches, you may experience mood disturbances as well as pain. You may have nausea and vomiting, too.

Migraine headaches usually begin when you are a teenager. However, some migraine headaches can begin at age 40. Before you suffer a migraine headache, you may have changes in your vision or speech and balance. You may notice zigzag lines in front of your eyes or small specks in one eye. You may notice different lines that come and go in front of your eyes. You may have numbness in your hands. When the headache occurs following these visual disturbances, your headache is usually on one side of your head. If you are seeing lines only in front of your left eye, usually your headache will be on the right side of your brain.

Sometimes you can have headaches that occur several times a week followed by a long period of having no headaches. Sometimes your migraine headaches can be incapacitating. Movements such as bending over, coughing or sneezing can worsen your headache. You will want to lie down. Following your headache, it can take approximately 24 hours for you to feel normal again. It has been found that African-Americans and Whites reported significant reductions in headache frequency and disability and improvements in life quality over a 6-month treatment period.4 However, Africans-Americans had significantly more frequent and disabling headaches and lower quality of life after treatment relative to Whites.

Seventy percent of people inherit the tendency to have migraine headaches. If you have migraine headaches, you usually have less than two attacks per month. However, 10 percent of patients have attacks every week. Another type of migraine headache can occur that does not have changes in sensation that can forewarn you of an impending headache. This type of headache is called a migraine headache without an aura. Sometimes these headaches occur on both sides of the head.

The treatment of your migraines can be divided into acute treatment of the attack as well as treatment to prevent the onset of headaches. Whenever possible, the factors that cause your headaches should be avoided. Stay away from foods that could trigger your migraine headache. Cheese, chocolate, red wine, and some Chinese foods that contain the additive MSG are commonly considered migraine headache triggers.

If you have an onset of a headache, a mild attack can be treated with aspirin. Nonsteroidal anti-inflammatory drugs can also be used to treat your headache. Ibuprofen is commonly used to treat headaches and can be purchased without a prescription. If you have nausea and vomiting associated with your migraine headache, you may need to take a nonsteroidal anti-inflammatory drug by the rectal route. New drugs called triptans have been developed and can decrease your headache within a significant time after its onset. Sumatriptan was the first triptan drug to be used for the treatment of migraine headaches.

Triptans are much better tolerated than the older caffeine-ergotamine medications. Be aware that the triptans are expensive. When you first suspect that you are having a migraine, take your triptan immediately. Stronger drugs such as Percocet have been prescribed for the treatment of migraine headaches.

If you have frequent migraine attacks and if these attacks are disabling, you should consider prophylactic treatment. You may have to make life adjustments. If you are having too much stress at work, you may need to consider changing your job. Medications can be helpful in preventing your headaches, but you should not become dependent on these drugs to solve any emotional problems that you may have. Avoid an overly busy schedule. Have one hour per day of free time to relax from a busy workday. Attempt to take one afternoon off per week and even one day off from work per month. When you have this time free, do whatever you feel like doing.

If anxiety causes you to have migraine headaches, consider relaxation techniques such as yoga or hypnotherapy. If you have significant psychological problems, consider a consultation with a psychologist. Sometimes breathing into a plastic bag for 10 minutes can prevent the onset of a headache. You may benefit from the administration of nitroglycerin placed under your tongue, which can decrease the onset of migraine headaches.

Remember, however, that nitroglycerin can cause headaches if the dose taken is too high. Aspirin can prevent the onset of headaches. Benadryl has been used to prevent the onset of migraine headaches as well. Antihypertensive medications such as Nadolol and Verapamil have been used to prevent the onset of migraine headaches. Amitriptyline, an antidepressant, also has been demonstrated to prevent the onset of migraine headache.

Migraine headaches appear to be hormonally related. They are more common in women until age 60 when the incidence is about equal. Migraine headaches commonly occur with the onset of menses in women. These headaches may also occur in the first trimester of pregnancy. The headaches can disappear following a complete hysterectomy. After the onset of menopause, your migraine headaches may disappear or at least decrease in intensity and frequency. However, if you receive hormone therapy at the time of menopause, this can prolong your headache symptoms. Sometimes your migraine headaches can worsen when you begin using oral contraceptives. Concern exists about the use of oral contraceptives by those who suffer migraine headaches, because they run a higher risk of stroke. The risk of a stroke is further increased if you smoke.

Numerous studies have assessed the prevalence of migraines within the general population, college students, professional groups, industrial/work place settings, and overseas populations, but little has been done with athletes. It was found that the prevalence of migraines in National Collegiate Athletic Association Division I men's and women's basketball players was generally less than in the general population, that women showed an increased prevalence of migraines when compared with men, and that Caucasians and African Americans did not differ in prevalence of migraines.[5]

Another type of headache that you could experience is called a tension-type headache. This also is called a muscle contraction headache or a psychogenic headache. The term "tension type" is used to imply that muscle tension plays a role in the onset of the headache. If you have chronic tension-type headaches, you may have headaches 15 days a month. For your doctor to make a diagnosis of your tension-type headache, you should have at least 10 previous headache episodes. The headaches should last from 30 minutes to 7 days. You will usually have a headache on both sides of your head. Your headaches should not be aggravated by walking or routine physical activity. If you have a tension-type headache, you should not experience nausea or vomiting. You should not have visual disturbances that are associated with migraine headaches.

Be aware that some individuals have chronic daily tension-type headaches. Migraine headaches and tension-type headaches are experienced more in women than men. Studies have been done that indicated that tight muscles around the scalp and neck can cause tension-type headaches. Studies used to objectively identify muscle tension have been done and have validated muscle tension as a cause of tension-type headaches. Remember that if you have significant stress in your life that the muscles in your neck and scalp can have sustained contractions. When you have prolonged muscle contractions of your scalp and neck, the muscles have less blood flow and, therefore, less oxygen going to your muscles. This decrease in blood flow can result in the formation of lactic acid in your muscles, which can cause you to have significant pain.

Muscle tension-type headaches can start at any age. Tension-type headaches can begin in childhood if a child is physically and emotionally abused. When you have a tension-type headache, you will feel a tight band and pressure around your head in the form of a tight cap. Your neck muscles will feel as if they are in a knot. The location of your head is usually all around your head on both sides. Try to avoid stress to prevent this type of headache from occurring. Usually a tension-type headache is seen in tense or anxious people. A family history of tension-type headaches is not as common as with migraine headaches.

Treatment for this type of headache is the avoidance of stress. Biofeedback as administered by a psychologist can decrease your muscle tension and, therefore, decrease your headaches. If you have tension-type headaches, you must learn to relax. Aspirin and acetaminophen can be of some help. Heat also can cause your muscles to relax.

If depression perpetuates your headaches, you can take antidepressants at bedtime. Sometimes muscle relaxants can be used to decrease your pain. Anti-anxiety drugs such as Valium have sometimes been used preventatively to decrease the chance of one of these headaches developing. When your headache occurs, one of the nonsteroidal anti-inflammatory drugs may be helpful in decreasing your headache.

Another type of headache that you should be aware of is called a cluster headache. For your doctor to make a diagnosis of cluster headache, you should have had at least five attacks before seeing your doctor. Usually the headache is on one side of your head and can be above your eye or in your temple. The headache usually lasts 15 minutes to 3 hours if untreated. Usually you will have tearing of your eye as well as nasal congestion on the side of your cluster headache. You may have forehead sweating. Your pupil may be extremely small and your upper eyelid may droop.

You may have clustering of headaches for several weeks and then no headaches for two weeks. You may go for a year without having a headache. A cluster headache is different from a migraine headache. Usually there is no nausea and vomiting associated with a cluster headache. Usually if you have a cluster headache, you are agitated and have to pace the floor. This is different from your migraine headache, which causes you to lie down and rest during the attack. Cluster headaches can occur while you are asleep or at rest during the evening. The overall incidence of cluster headaches is extremely rare. Less than 10 percent of the population suffers from cluster headaches. You may have your first attack between the ages of 20 and 40 years. Cluster headaches are associated with cigarette smoking and trauma to your head. Also, if anyone in your family has a history of cluster headaches, you may be prone to these headaches.

The exact cause of these cluster headaches is unknown. The cluster headache occurs more frequently in men than in women. There is a 5:1 man-to-woman ratio of cluster headaches. If you suffer from a cluster headache, your doctor will want to make sure that you do not have a pituitary tumor. A pituitary tumor is an abnormal growth in your pituitary gland in your brain. Not only can it cause you to have a headache but sometimes it can decrease your vision. An MRI can help detect this tumor. If it is malignant not only may you need surgery but irradiation as well as drug therapy.

To treat a cluster headache attack, some doctors suggest inhalation of 100 percent oxygen using a face mask. Usually your headache will settle in 15 minutes. If this does not work, an injection of sumatriptan (Imitrex) may decrease your pain. Some studies have even recommended the use of local anesthetics on a cotton swab placed in the nose.

Steroids in high doses can sometimes be used to decrease the onset of cluster headaches. Medrol can be given in various doses and schedules as directed by your treating physician. This drug must be discontinued slowly after treatment for five to seven days. It may take up to three weeks to taper the drug. Nonsteroidal anti-inflammatory drugs may be effective to decrease the headaches. Sometimes sufferers need to see a neurosurgeon in consultation to see whether there is a surgical procedure that can be done to decrease the headache.

If you have had a history of trauma to your head, you may develop headaches associated with your head trauma. These headaches continue for more than eight weeks after trauma to your head. Your headache is often severe and is throbbing. You may have nausea and vomiting associated with this headache. You may be drowsy or you may become irritable. Your memory may be temporarily impaired.

A headache following trauma can be made worse with physical exercise. A post-traumatic headache differs from migraine symptoms in that a chronic post-traumatic headache is usually generalized and permanent. However, it can be made worse by physical or mental strain. Usually this type of headache subsides in 8 to 10 weeks. You may develop a post-traumatic headache with only a minor injury to your head. In fact, the more severe the injury, the less chance you have of developing one of these headaches. Post-traumatic headache is reported more often in women than men. The incidence of a post-traumatic headache can be 40 percent following a head injury.

Treatment of this headache is with anti-inflammatory drugs or mild pain relievers such as Darvon. Your doctor must help you deal with any loss of memory. If you have had mood changes, your doctor may have you see a psychologist to help you through this post-traumatic psychological period. You may have chronic headaches associated with trauma to the head if the injury occurred when you were older than 40. If you have a low educational level as well as a low intelligence, your headache could be chronic. Furthermore, a history of previous head trauma or a history of alcohol abuse can predispose you to have post-traumatic headaches for a long time.

If you are over 60 years old, you could develop a headache associated with temporal arteritis. This usually occurs after you have had a fever. You have a burning pain caused by inflammation of your temporal artery on the side of your head. It is usually accompanied by a throbbing headache about your temple. You may have a burning pain about your scalp. Temporal arteritis headaches are worsened by jaw movement such as chewing. This type of headache can be accompanied by loss of vision, which is a medical emergency. The diagnosis sometimes has to be made with a biopsy of the arterial tissue. Steroids are usually the treatment of choice for this pain.

Do you know what structure in your brain cause headaches? Pain in your head can come from direct pressure on structures such as muscles or blood vessels. Traction on your muscles and nerves can cause you pain. If your blood vessels become engorged and if the diameter of your vessels becomes enlarged, the enlarged vessel can compress your nerves in your brain and cause you pain. A prolonged muscle contraction in your neck can cause pain as well. On occasion, more than one mechanism can cause you to have a headache. If you have a migraine and tense your muscles, you can have two causes for your headaches.

Keep a diary of your headaches. Your history of your headaches is a most important part of your doctor's workup. Your doctor needs to know about your general medical health. The progression of your headaches over days to months to years is important. A history of any headaches in your family is important as well. You must know that migraine headaches tend to run in families. Muscle contraction headaches and brain tumors also run in families. You need to keep a daily diary. You should write down what factors cause your pain and how long your headaches last and what medications you took either before, during, or after your headaches have resolved. Your doctor will examine your diary to look for a consistent pattern in the occurrence of your headaches.

There are clear sexual differences in the incidence of headaches, with women being more likely than men to experience headaches. Women are two to three times more likely to suffer migraine headaches than men. Women experience more disabling daily muscle tension-type headaches. Tension-type headache is a highly prevalent condition. Episodic tension-type headache is a highly prevalent condition with a significant functional impact at work, home, and school.[6] The overall prevalence of episodic tension-type headache in the past year was 38.3%. Women had a higher 1-year prevalence than men in all age, race, and education groups. Whites had a higher prevalence than African Americans in men and women. The prevalence increased with increasing educational levels in both sexes, reaching a peak in subjects with graduate school educations of 48.5% for men and 48.9% for women.

Patients in previous sumatriptan studies for migraine headache treatment have been predominantly Caucasian and the effects of sumatriptan between different ethnic groups are unknown. Sumatriptan injection is effective and well tolerated in non-Caucasians and Caucasians for the treatment of acute migraine attacks. Only minor differences in efficacy or tolerability were observed between blacks, Hispanics, and others.[7]

Be aware that there are no gender differences in children prior to puberty. This suggests that reproductive hormones have an effect on the onset of headaches. However, men have more cluster headaches than women in a prevalence ratio of 5:1. It is estimated that more than 50 percent of women suffering from migraine headaches miss approximately one week of work per year, whereas approximately 40 percent of men miss one week of work per year.

Obesity can increase the risk of migraine headaches in females.[8] The odds of episodic migraine are increased in those with obesity, with the strongest relationships among those younger than 50 years, white individuals, and women. Women who suffer from headaches are more likely than men to seek treatment for their headaches. Women are more likely to receive a headache diagnosis than men. Further study reveals that women are more likely than men to receive prescription medications for their headaches. Women receive more prescriptions than men for all migraine headaches except for the nonsteroidal anti-inflammatory drug category.

Women are more likely to relate that weather changes, perfumes, and cigarette smoke can trigger their migraine headaches. The sex hormones estradiol and progestin are believed to cause the increased incidence of headaches in women. A significant fall of estrogen in the bloodstream that occurs just before the onset of menstruation can cause migraines in some women. However, exactly how estrogen triggers migraine headaches remains to be further.

Recent studies report that migraine headaches with an aura are occur more frequently in women, whereas migraine headaches without an aura occur more frequently in men. Cluster headaches and post-traumatic headaches occur more frequently in men. Chronic muscle tension headaches are more prevalent in women. Headaches arising from degeneration of the neck or muscle spasms of the neck are more common in women. Some people who have been administered a spinal anesthetic develop a headache. The spinal headaches are more common in women. The reason for this finding is unknown.

Sex hormones do affect pain, including headaches. If you are a woman and if your progesterone increases, your migraine headaches could go away. This is the reason why women have fewer migraine headaches during pregnancy. As progesterone increases during the menstrual cycle, headaches may be fewer. In men, when testosterone increases, cluster headaches become frequent. Cluster headaches are noted at the time of puberty. With the increase in progesterone, estrogen, and testosterone, there is an increase in migraine as well as tension headaches. Be aware that women produce testosterone as well as men. Pain increases in both men and women when progesterone, estrogen, and testosterone increase.

Post dural puncture headache is a known complication after lumbar puncture. A spinal headache can occur as a result of a procedure such as a spinal tap or epidural block. In these procedures, a needle is placed within the fluid-filled space surrounding the spinal cord. This creates a passage for the spinal fluid to leak out, changing the fluid pressure around the brain and spinal cord. If enough of the fluid leaks out, a spinal headache may develop. The elderly may also develop postdural puncture headache, and epidural blood patch is an effective and well-tolerated treatment of persistent and severe symptoms.[9,10]

During the menstrual cycle, a woman retains more fluid. This retention of fluid increases the water content of the woman's bloodstream and dilutes the effects of any medications. It is, therefore, believed that the mass of drug that needs to be administered at different times during a woman's menstrual cycle may vary. If this variation of fluid and drug responses is evident, your dose of drug will need to be changed periodically.

One of the opioids that can be used for the management of severe migraine headaches is butorphanol (Stadol). This drug is administered nasally. Some doctors advocate the use of this drug for the treatment of headaches. This drug is believed to work better in women than in men. Women show a greater analgesic response to kappa-stimulating opioids. The other types of opioids are mu-stimulating opioids and include morphine and Demerol.

These mu-stimulating opioids have been shown to work better in men than in women. For this reason, studies are being done and more studies need to be done that can evaluate the effects of these drugs for the treatment of severe headaches. African American subjects showed greater analgesic responses in general to both butorphanol and morphine for pain management medications compared with non-Hispanic whites.[11] For thermal pain threshold, butorphanol but not morphine analgesia was greater for African American vs non-Hispanic whites.

References

1.　　Stang P, Sternfeld B, Sidney S. Migraine headache in a prepaid health plan: ascertainment, demographics, physiological, and behavioral factors. Headache. 1996;36(2):69-76.

2.　　Loder S, Sheikh HU, Loder E. The prevalence, burden, and treatment of severe, frequent, and migraine headaches in US minority populations: statistics from National Survey studies. Headache. 2015;55(2):214-228.

3.　　Nicholson RA, Rooney M, Vo K, O'Laughlin E, Gordon M. Migraine care among different ethnicities: do disparities exist? Headache. 2006;46(5):754-765.

4.　　Heckman BD, Holroyd KA, Tietjen G, et al. Whites and African-Americans in headache specialty clinics respond equally well to treatment. Cephalalgia. 2009;29(6):650-661.

5.　　Kinart CM, Cuppett MM, Berg K. Prevalence of migraines in NCAA division I male and female basketball players. National Collegiate Athletic Association. Headache. 2002;42(7):620-629.

6.　　Schwartz BS, Stewart WF, Simon D, Lipton RB. Epidemiology of tension-type headache. JAMA. 1998;279(5):381-383.

7.　　Burke-Ramirez P, Asgharnejad M, Webster C, Davis R, Laurenza A. Efficacy and tolerability of subcutaneous sumatriptan for acute migraine: a comparison between ethnic groups. Headache. 2001;41(9):873-882.

8.　　Peterlin BL, Rosso AL, Williams MA, et al. Episodic migraine and obesity and the influence of age, race, and sex. Neurology. 2013;81(15):1314-1321.

9.　　Sjovall S, Kokki M, Turunen E, Laisalmi M, Alahuhta S, Kokki H. Postdural puncture headache and epidural blood patch use in elderly patients. J Clin Anesth. 2015;27(7):574-578.

10.　　Ohtonari T, Ota S, Sekihara Y, et al. [The Clinical Features of Cerebrospinal Fluid Leaks--Based on Our Experiences]. J UOEH. 2015;37(3):231-242.

11.　　Sibille KT, Kindler LL, Glover TL, et al. Individual differences in morphine and butorphanol analgesia: a laboratory pain study. Pain Med. 2011;12(7):1076-1085.

18. Nerve Pain

A neuropathy by definition is any disease of your peripheral nerves. These are the nerves that exist outside of your brain and spinal cord. A disease of these nerves can cause a weakness as well as numbness in the area where the nerve travels. If only one nerve is affected by a disease state, it is called a mononeuropathy. Your symptoms will depend upon the distribution of that nerve in your tissue. A polyneuropathy involves many nerves. With a polyneuropathy, your symptoms are more exaggerated as compared to a mononeuropathy. A polyneuropathy can involve more than one extremity and is usually related to a metabolic disease. A momoneuropathy is usually related to a nerve compression.

Basically the symptoms of your neuropathy can be divided into two groups, one of which occurs where your symptoms are spontaneous and another which involves maneuvers that can cause you to experience pain. Examples of the latter group are scratching your skin, putting pressure over the diseased nerves, or related to changes in temperature (usually cold).

Typically with the onset of your neuropathy you will feel a burning or stinging pain in the area of the affected nerve. Like neuralgias, you can also have shock-like stabbing pain. Neuralgia is "nerve pain" by definition. Sometimes the pain can radiate through your entire arm or leg. Sometimes a slight touch of the skin over your diseased nerve can cause incapacitating pain.

Basically any neuropathy may cause a burning, gnawing pain. You can have some decreased sensation about the painful nerve. Extreme pain from just a light touch can occur in tissues over the nerve. You can have increased sweating, cold sensations, or skin discoloration in the extremity associated with your neuropathy. The onset of your pain following an injury to your nerve can either be of an immediate onset or a delayed gradual onset. Your pain intensity can be affected by both emotion and fatigue. Not all neuropathies cause pain. Some neuropathies cause only numbness.

You may have tests done by placing a needle into your nerves, called a nerve conduction velocity test, and an electromyography (EMG). Nerve conduction testing examines your nerve while the EMG examines any effects on your muscles with respect to muscle pathology. The needles used for these tests are attached to an oscilloscope and can measure the speed of the transmission of impulses in your nerves or muscles. These tests are extremely helpful to your doctor in diagnosing your pain syndrome. Frequently a nerve biopsy is needed as well for your doctor to diagnose a neuropathy. Mononeuropathies occur more often in diabetic patients than in the normal population. Diabetes can affect the muscles around your eye. A diabetic mononeuropathy can affect the nerves in your arms as well as your legs. A nerve lesion is a traumatic event to a nerve such as compression which can cause a neuropathy. If you have a peripheral nerve lesion, you will probably experience pain. The pain usually comes and goes.

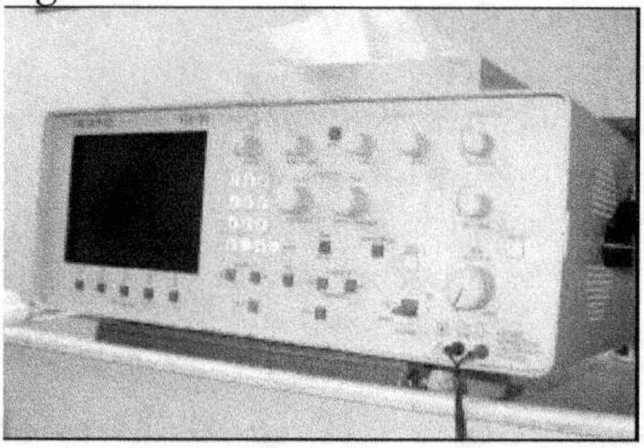

Figure 1. EMG/NCV oscilloscope.

It is important to diagnose diabetic neuropathies. However, half of all diabetes in the United States remains undiagnosed. It is unsurprising given only 60.9% of doctors would diagnose it when the condition is strongly suggested, and nearly one-quarter suspecting diabetes would not order tests necessary to confirm it. The diagnosis of diabetes is significantly influenced by a patient's race/ethnicity, and clinical management is influenced by patient socio-economic status and the doctor's gender.

Bone tissue is innervated and diabetes can adversely affect this innervation. Therefore peripheral nerve function may impact bone mass density.[1] Older Black and White men and women are equally affected. Poor peripheral nerve function may contribute to lower bone mass density and higher fracture risk, in those with diabetic neuropathy. Poor peripheral nerve function may directly be related to lower bone mass density. There appears to be a tendency for white individuals to have a higher prevalence of sensorimotor neuropathy than other ethnic groups with diabetes.[2]

Chronic pain conditions, such as neuropathic pain, are a common problem that poses a major challenge to pain management providers due to its complex natural history, unclear etiology and poor response towards therapy. Entrapment neuropathies such as the carpal tunnel syndrome are characterized by abnormal sensations in the area of the nerve as well as pain. Usually if your nerve is compressed, your blood supply to your nerve is also compromised.

Entrapment neuropathies occur when a nerve is compressed. For example, tissue at your wrist can compress a nerve going to your hand and fingers which can result in weakness and pain in your hand. The basic pathology of an entrapment neuropathy is that the compression over your nerve can destroy your larger fibers that have a fatty wrapper around them called myelin. As these nerves are destroyed, it leaves only your C-fibers in the affected nerve. With the preservation of your C-fibers, you will have pain as well as tenderness at the location of your nerve entrapment.

You can have a neuropathy that is not painful but it can cause you to have abnormal feelings in the tissue around your injured nerve. You have probably heard of a Morton's neuralgia. This can cause a severe entrapment of the small nerves that are around the bones that make up the foot. If you destroy your large nerve fibers, you will have mainly the smaller C-fibers left in the diseased nerve. These C-fibers will cause you to have significant burning pain. The exact causes of many neuropathies remain unknown.

If you suffer from rheumatoid arthritis, you may suffer from a neuropathy related to your rheumatoid arthritis. A degeneration that can occur in your joints can also occur in your nerves. Some neuropathies cause you to have a loss of sensation instead of causing you to feel pain. An example of a neuropathy with a loss of sensation is called congenital analgesia with anhydrous. This means that you have some degree of numbness of an extremity but that the extremity never sweats.

The drug Isonizid used for the treatment of tuberculosis can cause you to have pain in your nerves. You may develop a painful neuropathy related to chronic renal failure (kidney failure). This is one of the side effects of this drug. You feel some numbness but also some tingling and later significant pain that is both burning and aching. Muscles in your calves can also become painful. If you have this neuropathy, you may have difficulty walking.

You may be awakened at night by the onset of spontaneous pain. On examination you will have a decreased sensation in your legs. Other types of drugs can also cause you to have a neuropathy. For example, arsenic has been implicated as a cause of neuropathy. In addition, people who suffer with the HIV or AIDS can have extremely debilitating neuropathies associated with their disease.

Cancers can cause you to have a neuropathy. Your malignancy can cause you to have a progressive sensory neuropathy that usually is not painful. You may develop weakness or numbness in one or several of your nerves. If your cancer invades one of your nerves, you may develop pain that mimics reflex sympathetic dystrophy (RSD). RSD symptoms cause burning pain and swelling of your hand or foot.

A neuropathy as a child can cause permanent anesthesia to an arm or leg. For example, if you have numbness in an area of your hand and you place your hand on a hot stove, you run the risk of a heat injury to your hand. If you have a loss of sensation in the area of one of your nerves, the tissue that does not feel sensation can be prone to future injury.

If your thyroid glands do not produce enough thyroid hormone, you may develop pain related to a hypothyroid neuropathy. You may have pain or decreased or abnormal sensations in both your hands and feet. Compression of the nerves in your arms or legs for whatever reason can cause you to have pressure damage to these nerves. The neuropathy caused by this compression is called a compression neuropathy. Pressure over your nerve or nerves can come from a brace or cast or can come from tumors or muscle or connective tissue thickening. Compression of your nerves can occur at different points throughout your body. If you have neuropathies associated with disease states, your nerves can be more susceptible to injury with compression. You can have numbness as well as the pain in your extremities and can also have abnormal sensations.

Nerve conduction studies are helpful in diagnosing neuropathies. Nerve conduction studies are done by inserting a needle into your tissue and studying the conduction of the nerve impulses. Electromyography (EMG) can also be used to evaluate a compression neuropathy. This task can determine if the neuropathy has affected your muscles. A myeloma can cause you to have pain in the distribution of one or more of your nerves. A myeloma is a malignant disease that affects your bone marrow.

Carpal tunnel syndrome starts gradually with aching in your wrist that can extend to your forearm. You will develop pins and needles in your hand and fingers. This sensation can occur while you are driving, holding a phone, or reading this book. You may develop weakness in your hands and drop objects. The diagnosis of your carpal tunnel syndrome can be done by arthroscopy, which consists of putting a scope into your carpal tunnel. An MRI of your wrist and hand can be beneficial as well.

You may ask whether laboratory tests can help diagnose carpal tunnel syndrome. At present, however, there are no tests that can be done to definitively diagnose this condition.

The carpal tunnel is a narrow passage in your wrist about the diameter of your thumb. The purpose of this tunnel is to protect your median nerve as well as the tendons that go to your fingers. The problem is that excessive pressure on this nerve will cause you to have numbness and pain and can lead to hand weakness. With proper treatment, most people who develop carpal tunnel syndrome can have normal restoration of their hand function. Compared to whites, African-Americans had a lower percentage of costs due to carpal tunnel syndrome.[3]

Repetitive-motion injuries are being reported at an increasing rate. This is reported from newsrooms to meat-packing plants to occupations where employees have to do repetitive motion daily. If you are taking birth control pills or have a sudden weight gain, which causes fluid retention, you may develop carpal tunnel syndrome. Compression of the median nerve in the carpal tunnel is a common compression neuropathy. This entity affects women more than men. The average age of the onset of this ailment is between 40 and 60 years of age.

Your carpal tunnel is the space between your bones in your hand at your wrist and the connective tissue over your tendons. The carpal tunnel contains the tendons that flex your wrist (bend it downward) and your median nerve. A carpal tunnel syndrome can cause you to have pins and needles sensations and numbness in most of your hand except for the little finger. You can also have weakness of your thumb. This entity is caused by pressure on your median nerve as it passes through the carpal tunnel at your wrist.

This condition can be caused by any continuous repetitive movement of your hand, such as typing or working with a computer. If you are obese, pregnant, have a decrease in your thyroid function, or have Raynaud's disease or diabetes or renal failure, you are at a higher risk of developing a carpal tunnel syndrome than the population in general.

If you have this syndrome, you will probably have abnormal sensations as well as pain in your affected hand while you sleep. The pins and needles sensations are usually on the palm side of your hand. You can also have wrist and forearm pain. The feeling of pins and needles as well as pain can be caused by repeated wrist and finger flexion. Remember that flexion is a downward position of your fingers as well as your hand.

You may develop hand weakness. The symptoms begin in your dominant hand (the one that you use to write, to brush your teeth, comb your hair, etc.). However, your other hand can also be affected as well. If your doctor taps over the middle of your wrist on your palm side, you may have the production of pins and needles that go from your wrist to your fingers. This is called Tinel's sign.

The Phalen test is another test to diagnose carpal tunnel syndrome. A blood pressure cuff is applied to your arm. If you have carpal tunnel syndrome, you will develop pins and needles in your hand when the blood pressure cuff is inflated. Repetitive motion has been downplayed as a cause of carpal tunnel syndrome. However, some jurisdictions allow repetitive motion as a cause of carpal tunnel syndrome. Fluid retention during menses or pregnancy is a cause of carpal tunnel syndrome. It is important for you to know that carpal tunnel syndrome can be idiopathic. This means that the cause of your carpal tunnel syndrome is unknown.

If you have carpal tunnel syndrome, you run a 1 percent chance that you will develop permanent injury. When you are initially seen by your health-care provider, you probably will be treated with immobilization of your wrist with a splint. This will prevent pressure on your nerve. If this method fails, you will be given an anti-inflammatory drug or an injection of Cortisone into your carpal tunnel to decrease the swelling in your tendons and ligaments within the tunnel. If this method fails, you will be a candidate for surgery.

Surgery to release the tissue that is compressing your median nerve has been shown to be effective for the treatment of carpal tunnel syndrome. There have even been cases of gout or arthritis causing carpal tunnel syndrome that have been successfully treated by surgery. You may ask whether you should have a surgical versus nonsurgical treatment for your carpal tunnel syndrome. A follow-up study of one year after surgery revealed excellent results with open carpal tunnel surgery. Surgical treatment appears to have better results than splinting.

You need to know that there could be some post-operative complications associated with carpal tunnel surgery. This can include increased pain in your scar, probably related to where the nerve endings in your skin come together during the healing process. You can also have recurrent symptoms of your pain and weakness of your grip. The exact causes of these problems remain unclear. This can happen whether or not your surgery is done through an open incision or by an endoscopic approach. During endoscopy your surgeon places a scope into your carpal tunnel space to be able to operate without having to make an incision.

You may also develop reflex sympathetic dystrophy (RSD) for an unknown reason following carpal tunnel surgery.

Carpal tunnel syndrome is treated frequently in a primary care environment. Workplace task modification and wrist splints can defer a referral for surgical decompression. Nerve and tendon exercises can be of benefit. Steroid injections into the mouth of the carpal tunnel can be helpful in some patients, especially in women. If your doctor accidentally injects your median nerve, however, this can cause you disabling chronic pain. Only a small percentage of patients with carpel tunnel syndrome actually require surgery.

Your chances of recovering completely following treatment are excellent. You should avoid re-injury by changing the way that you do repetitive movements. The incidence of an occupational carpal tunnel syndrome is usually a combination of genetics, your physiology, and your lifestyle factors in addition to general biomechanics. Therefore, no general rule of thumb applies to occupations in general.

The anatomy of the carpal tunnel in Koreans is somewhat different, in part, from the results obtained from studies of whites.[4] This information can help obtain a better surgical outcome and complete decompression of the median nerve during operation while preventing inappropriate or inadvertent injury to the motor branch of the median nerve in Koreans.

Also be aware that your carpal tunnel syndrome can be due to a congenital predisposition. This means that your carpal tunnel is smaller than in other people. This can cause you to develop carpal tunnel syndrome, especially if you are doing repetitive-motion work or using vibrating hand tools. A smaller carpal tunnel noted in women may be the reason why they are three times more likely than men to develop carpal tunnel syndrome because their carpal tunnel syndrome

Occupations with the highest prevalence of the Carpal tunnel syndrome were mail service, health care, construction, and assembly and fabrication. Industries with the highest prevalence were food products, repair services, transportation, and construction. The risk factor most strongly associated with CTS was exposure to repetitive bending/twisting of the hands/wrists at work, followed by race (whites higher than nonwhites), gender (females higher than males), use of vibrating hand tools and age. This result is consistent with previous reports in that repeated bending/twisting of the hands and wrists during manual work is etiologically related to occupational carpal tunnel syndrome.[5] Awkward posture and psychological demand, and decreased skill variety and job control at work are all related to CTS.[6]

Diabetes can be associated with a polyneuropathy, which means that many nerves are involved in the disease process. If you develop polyneuropathy, it occurs usually on both sides of your body and usually in both lower extremities from the knees down to your feet.

Numbness and abnormal sensations are the most frequent complaints associated with this neuropathy. You can have complaints of burning pain ranging from mild to severe in both legs. On occasion you may have symptoms of pains that are described as sharp, bolting, shock-like pain. Because diabetes can cause you to have a decrease in blood flow to your feet, make sure that you wear proper fitting shoes. Poor fitting shoes can cause ulcers on the bottom of your feet.

Sometimes both of your upper extremities can be involved with your diabetic neuropathy. The nerves in your extremities that have a myelin sheath around them will lose the sheath if you develop a diabetic neuropathy. If you have a diabetic neuropathy, you can have both pain as well as a decrease in sensation in your legs.

It is interesting to note that if you have a painless diabetic neuropathy that you usually do not have reflexes in your lower extremities at your knees and ankles when your doctor taps you with a reflex hammer. However, if you have a painful diabetic neuropathy, usually your deep tendon reflexes are normal at your knee and ankle.

If you are diabetic and have an elevated blood sugar, for some reason this increased blood sugar can lower your pain threshold. This means that you will be more responsive to a certain pain stimulus than if you did not have a diabetic neuropathy. For example, if you do not have a diabetic neuropathy and prick yourself with a safety pin, you will complain of the pain that is gone within a reasonable time. However, if you have a diabetic neuropathy, a simple pin prick can cause you to have significant pain because your pain threshold has been decreased. Furthermore, if you have a diabetic neuropathy with an increase in your blood sugar, your tolerance to pain will be decreased.

It has furthermore been published in animal studies that an elevated blood sugar will reduce the analgesic effects of morphine in the animal model. In other words, glucose can affect your morphine pain receptors. If you have a diabetic neuropathy, you can have a decrease in tissue blood flow in your legs.

Your sympathetic nervous system can also be altered if you suffer from a diabetic neuropathy. In many instances, your sympathetic stimulation can be decreased. You can have a high blood flow in both extremities. However, this blood flow can be decreased by an increase in the activity of your sympathetic nervous system.

Blood flow to certain areas of your body can be decreased by sympathetic stimulation of your sympathetic nervous system if you have a painful neuropathy. This reduction in blood flow usually results in an improvement of your pain if your pain was caused by swelling of your tissue related to an increased blood flow to your tissue. Blood flow effect in a nonpainful diabetic neuropathy has just the opposite effect.

Be aware that diabetes can cause multiple nerve disorders in the nerves outside of your brain and spinal cord. However, some of the nerves coming off of your brain can transmit pain fibers and your diabetes can also adversely affect these nerves. Not only can you develop pain in your legs, you can also develop weakness in your legs as a result of your diabetic neuropathy. On occasion some individuals with a diabetic neuropathy can have constant pain. The type of diabetic neuropathy is the diabetic amyotrophy. This entity occurs on one side of your body. It occurs most often in the nerves that go to your muscles.

The nerves that go to your muscles are called motor nerves. The diabetic amyotrophy is a motor neuropathy. The diabetic amyotrophy neuropathy, as well as other diabetic neuropathies, can be seen if you have poor control over your diabetes. Diabetic neuropathies are found in middle-aged as well as elderly patients who suffer with diabetes. Careful attention to control over blood sugar in the long term is the best way to prevent diabetic neuropathy.

The treatment of painful diabetic neuropathy has included anticonvulsive medications such as Tegretol. Neurontin and Lyrica have become more popular over the past several years. Tricyclic antidepressant drugs such as Elavil can help to relieve your pain. A drug that has been used successfully for the treatment of a painful diabetic neuropathy is mexiletine. This drug is essentially a medication that is used if you have abnormal heartbeats. This drug has been shown to be effective for the treatment of your diabetic neuropathy. Lidocaine is not only a numbing medicine but it is also a drug used for irregular rhythms of your heart.

If you have significant pain relief with the administration of lidocaine administered intravenously the chances are that you will have excellent relief with the oral mexiletine. The problem with mexiletene is that you can get side effects such as nausea and vomiting. Tremors, dizziness, and blurred vision can also occur. If you have any heart problems that you know of, you must tell your doctor before starting mexiletine.

Another medication that can help you control your painful diabetic neuropathy is a topical capsaicin cream. Almost 75 percent of patients with diabetic neuropathy who used this cream reported significant pain relief. The problem with this cream is that you can have side effects that include a burning sensation at the sight of the cream on application. If you take a warm bath or shower, the pain about your skin can be magnified.

Alcoholic neuropathy is fairly common in the United States. Approximately 20 percent of chronic alcoholics develop peripheral neuropathy related to their alcoholism. The neuropathy affects not only sensation but can affect strength in your lower extremities. Alcoholics who develop this neuropathy complain of burning feet. As the neuropathy becomes more severe, the alcoholic will develop weakness in both legs.

Occasionally the arms can be affected as well. One important treatment for this neuropathy is to stop drinking. When alcohol consumption has been abolished, the neuropathy can recover, but the recovery is slow. The alcoholic neuropathy is believed to be due to a deficiency of thiamine as well as other B vitamins.

Alcoholics usually have an inadequate food intake. The alcohol can affect the absorption of vitamins through their gastrointestinal systems. Alcoholics have a greater need for thiamine but are not obtaining the thiamine in their diet. It is furthermore known that alcohol itself can exert a direct toxic effect on nerves in the arms and legs. Besides stopping alcohol consumption, alcoholics should take nutritional supplements containing both thiamine and a vitamin B complex.

Tegretol or Neurontin or a tricyclic antidepressant such as Elavil can also be used for the treatment of this disease. The radiological features of alcoholic ulcero-osteolytic neuropathy have been studied in Blacks. Infective and resorptive changes in the bones of the forefeet of the patients were noted and these features are related to chronic infection or to the toxic effects of the alcohol.7

If you or someone you know has kidney failure, a severe neuropathy can occur that is called a uremic neuropathy. This type of neuropathy is associated with chronic renal failure. Uremia is the presence of an excessive amount of urea as well as other nitrogen waste compounds that are in your bloodstream. Normally these waste products are excreted by your kidneys into your urine. However, if you have kidney failure, your urea is not eliminated from your bloodstream. This will cause your urea to accumulate in your blood. This will cause you to have drowsiness as well as nausea and vomiting and can progress to death.

If you have uremia, you have a 50 percent chance that you can develop a uremic neuropathy. This disease is becoming less prevalent because of the treatment of kidney failure with hemodialysis as well as kidney transplants. This disease progresses slowly. At first it affects your sensory nerves. It can progress to cause weakness in the muscles about your feet.

You can have cramps in your calves. With dialysis, this disease will stabilize. It can even improve with dialysis. If this disorder worsens during dialysis, the frequency and duration of your dialysis will be increased until your symptoms improve. After renal transplant, you can expect to have a significant improvement in your renal neuropathy.

There is another class of neuropathy called nutritional neuropathy. This class of neuropathy is seen not only in alcoholics but in individuals who are on restrictive diets. Thiamine deficiency can lead to heart failure. With this nutritional neuropathy, you may have hand, feet, and calf pain. You can have extreme pain just from light touch.

You may have some numbness and weakness in your extremities. The administration of thiamine can reduce your symptoms. Severe nutritional deficiency can cause you to develop significant pain related to your nutritional neuropathy. If you don't get enough thiamine, you can develop beriberi. This is a result of a deficiency of vitamin B1 (thiamine).

Beriberi is another nutritional neuropathy that is widespread in rice-eating countries. It is noted in individuals who eat polished rice from which the thiamine-rich seed coat is removed. Two types of beriberi exist. One form is called wet beriberi. In this type of beriberi, there is an accumulation of tissue fluid in your body.

With dry beriberi, there are signs of starvation. If you starve yourself, you will become too thin. The nervous system can degenerate if you are not obtaining a proper amount of thiamine. Also, nutritional deficiencies in a woman at the time of conception can cause abnormalities in a fetus, which can cause significant harm. Pellegra is another neuropathy caused by nutritional deficiency. It is characterized by weakness, tingling, and even pain. This neuropathy is caused by niacin deficiency. Niacin is also a B vitamin. Pellegra is a result of a poor diet that does not have enough niacin or doesn't have sufficient tryptophane. Tryptophane is an amino acid from which niacin can be synthesized in your body. Pellegra is more common in corn-eating communities.

Chemicals also can cause you to develop a neuropathy. Cisplatin is an agent used in chemotherapy to treat tumors. This chemical can cause you to develop a painful peripheral neuropathy as well. The neuropathy associated with this drug can cause you to have severe pain in your extremities. However, this neuropathy is reversible at the end of your chemotherapy. Arsenic is another chemical associated with a painful neuropathy. It can also cause you to have renal failure.

Arsenic can be toxic to your heart and can cause your heart to stop. It takes one to two weeks for you to develop a neuropathy associated with arsenic ingestion. You will have burning pain as well as tingling and numbness in your extremities associated with this neuropathy. If you have a severe neuropathy from arsenic poisoning, you may not have a good prognosis on your recovery.

Thallium is an insecticide as well as a rodenticide (kills rats and mice). It can also be used to image your heart by your cardiologist when examining you for heart disease. If you suffer from thallium poisoning, you will now develop the pain in your gut including nausea and vomiting. Your symptoms can progress through a stoppage of your heart. You can develop a psychosis as well as confusion, which can lead to a coma.

You can develop a neuropathy within 48 hours of adjusting to this chemical. You can develop pain in both your arms and legs. In severe cases, the nerves coming off of your brain can be affected as well. This chemical can affect your nerves that are involved in your breathing. If you recover from this poisoning, your recovery may never be complete. One of the hallmarks of this disease is loss of hair.

The prevalence, predictors, and consequences of peripheral neuropathy in the elderly have not been well defined. Neurologic deficits in one study were associated with numbness, pain, restless legs, trouble walking, trouble with balance, and reduced quality of life.[8] Peripheral sensory deficits are common in the elderly. In most cases, a medical cause is not obvious. Mechanisms related to neuropathic or microvascular factors, inflammation, or hyperglycemia may be mediating the association of diabetes and hearing impairment.[9] The diagnosis of diabetes is significantly influenced by a patient's race/ethnicity, and clinical management (specifically for foot neuropathy) and is influenced by a patient socio-economic status and the doctor's gender.[10]

Genetic predisposition, particularly specific mitochondrial DNA (mtDNA) backgrounds, has been proposed as a contributing factor in the expression of an epidemic of bilateral optic neuropathy that has affected residents of Cuba since 1991. Approximately 50% of Cuban mtDNAs originated from Europeans, 46% from Africans, and 4% from Native Americans.

These findings demonstrate that mutations arising in specific mtDNAs are unlikely to play a role in the epidemic neuropathy.[11] The risks of diabetes and cardiovascular disease are elevated worldwide in Indian Asians. However, risks of other diabetes-related complications, i.e., foot ulceration and amputation, also with a vascular basis, are substantially lower in Asians than in white Europeans. Asians with diabetes have substantially less large and small fiber neuropathy than Europeans, despite comparable traditional risk factors. Independent from smoking, the lower risk of neuropathy in Asians is due to better skin microvascularization.[12]

References

1.   Strotmeyer ES, Cauley JA, Schwartz AV, et al. Reduced peripheral nerve function is related to lower hip BMD and calcaneal QUS in older white and black adults: the Health, Aging, and Body Composition Study. J Bone Miner Res. 2006;21(11):1803-1810.

2.   Sosenko JM. The prevalence of diabetic neuropathy according to ethnicity. Curr Diab Rep. 2009;9(6):435-439.

3.   Leigh JP, Waehrer G, Miller TR, McCurdy SA. Costs differences across demographic groups and types of occupational injuries and illnesses. Am J Ind Med. 2006;49(10):845-853.

4.   Ahn DS, Yoon ES, Koo SH, Park SH. A prospective study of the anatomic variations of the median nerve in the carpal tunnel in Asians. Ann Plast Surg. 2000;44(3):282-287.

5.   Tanaka S, Wild DK, Seligman PJ, Halperin WE, Behrens VJ, Putz-Anderson V. Prevalence and work-relatedness of self-reported carpal tunnel syndrome among U.S. workers: analysis of the Occupational Health Supplement data of 1988 National Health Interview Survey. Am J Ind Med. 1995;27(4):451-470.

6.   Arcury TA, Cartwright MS, Chen H, et al. Musculoskeletal and neurological injuries associated with work organization among immigrant Latino women manual workers in North Carolina. Am J Ind Med. 2014;57(4):468-475.

7.   Miller RM, Hunt JA. The radiological features of alcoholic ulcero-osteolytic neuropathy in Blacks. S Afr Med J. 1978;54(4):159-161.

8.   Mold JW, Vesely SK, Keyl BA, Schenk JB, Roberts M. The prevalence, predictors, and consequences of peripheral sensory neuropathy in older patients. J Am Board Fam Pract. 2004;17(5):309-318.

9.   Bainbridge KE, Cheng YJ, Cowie CC. Potential mediators of diabetes-related hearing impairment in the U.S. population: National

Health and Nutrition Examination Survey 1999-2004. Diabetes Care. 2010;33(4):811-816.

10. McKinlay J, Piccolo R, Marceau L. An additional cause of health care disparities: the variable clinical decisions of primary care doctors. J Eval Clin Pract. 2013;19(4):664-673.

11. Torroni A, Brown MD, Lott MT, Newman NJ, Wallace DC. African, Native American, and European mitochondrial DNAs in Cubans from Pinar del Rio Province and implications for the recent epidemic neuropathy in Cuba. Cuba Neuropathy Field Investigation Team. Hum Mutat. 1995;5(4):310-317.

12. Abbott CA, Chaturvedi N, Malik RA, et al. Explanations for the lower rates of diabetic neuropathy in Indian Asians versus Europeans. Diabetes Care. 2010;33(6):1325-1330.

19. Arthritic Pain

Arthritis is the painful inflammation of the joints in your body. Approximately one out of seven people has some form of arthritis, and there are many different types you can have. And if you know someone who has arthritis, you know that arthritis can be devastating. More than 35 million people in the United States suffer from this disease.

Inflammation that occurs in your joints can cause you to have pain as well as swelling of your joints. For you to understand why you develop pain in arthritis, you must have some knowledge of joint anatomy. Joints in your arms and legs permit movement of your arms and legs. The bones of your joints are held together by a capsule that consists of a dense strong tissue; further, your joints are held by ligaments, which connect bones to each other. Your joint is supported by muscles or tendons that lie over your joints. Tendons connect muscles to bones.

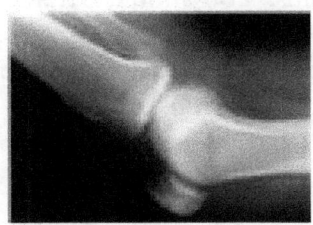

Figure 1. Arthritis can cause joint deterioration.

On the inside of your joint, the surface of your joint is covered with a tissue called a synovium. This tissue has special cells that exist within the lining of your synovial tissue. Some of these cells help to form some of the components that make the fluid in your synovial tissue thick. This thick fluid is like motor oil. A thick fluid will provide your joints with better lubricating properties than a watery fluid. The fluid that exists in your synovium lubricates the surfaces of the bones and cartilage that make up your joint. Cartilage is a tough, slippery layer of tissue that covers the surfaces where bones contact each other in joints.

Synovial tissues contain many blood vessels. Your synovium also contains sympathetic fibers. This anatomical feature can be important if one develops an entity called reflex sympathetic dystrophy. There is also a joint in your body where your back bone meets your hip bone. This is called your sacroiliac joint. This joint is only slightly movable. Even though this joint does not move freely, it can cause you significant pain. Other sites or cells exist in your joint that secretes chemicals that rebuild and degrade your joint. This process of rebuilding and degrading your joint keeps your joint anatomy in balance. If your joint becomes degraded, it will degenerate and you will develop arthritis in the degenerating joint.

Your health-care provider will want to know whether your pain is localized to one joint or many of your joints. If you have arthritis, you may realize that you have stiffness of your joints in the morning but that the stiffness progressively decreases as you become more active. If you have the rapid onset of joint pain that involves one joint such as the joint in your great toe, this usually signifies a gouty arthritis, known more simply as gout. You may know a young man who complains of pain in his buttocks and the back of his thigh along with morning stiffness. These symptoms can be associated with an arthritic condition called ankylosing spondylitis.

If you have any nodules under your skin, you may have rheumatoid arthritis. You should be able to feel these nodules over your elbows. If you have a relative who has a history of rheumatoid arthritis, you run the risk of developing this type of arthritis. If you have had weight loss as well as chronic fatigue, you must include this in your pain diary. Weight loss and fatigue can be associated with rheumatoid arthritis. Your health-care provider will examine your joints for normal range of motion. Any limitation in your range of motion about your joints will be recorded. If you have pain on passive range of motion of your joints usually indicates that you have inflammation of your joints.

Your joints will be examined for warmth as well as tenderness, and your muscles will be evaluated for strength as well as size. If you have significant pain, sometimes you will not use certain muscles in your arms or legs. This can cause your muscles to shrink in size and cause you to have weakness. Your shoulders will be examined for tenderness as well as range of motion. Your wrist joints, finger joints, elbow joints, hip joints, knee joints, and the joints in your feet will be examined.

If you suffer from one of the arthritic diseases, you may notice on occasion that your joints are swollen and red. When you go to your doctor, they may not be swollen and red at that time. This is why it is important for you to keep a pain diary. If you are seeing a doctor for pain in your joints, your doctor may want to get some laboratory tests. Your doctor may use a needle and syringe to extract fluid from your joints.

Your doctor will look at the fluid to see whether it is clear. Normal joint fluid should be clear and straw colored.

If you have osteoarthritis, the fluid can be straw colored. Other types of arthritis that you may have include rheumatoid arthritis or gout. Your fluid may be yellow. Your doctor will examine your fluids for cells. Your doctor also will obtain blood from you. Your blood will be examined for any elevation in your white cells (a sign of inflammation) and a test for rheumatoid arthritis can be done at the same time.

Your doctor may also order x-rays or even a CT scan or MRI of your painful area. Furthermore, it is not unusual for your doctor to eventually order a bone scan if your pain persists in spite of conservative treatment. A bone scan consists of injecting a very small dose of radioactive dye into your vein. After this has been done, a special camera takes a picture. If you have arthritis, there will be an increased uptake of the radioactive material into your painful joint, showing that the joint is inflamed. Inflammation is the responses of your body's tissues to irritation or injury. Your affected tissue can become warm swollen and/or red. The severity of inflammation depends on the cause and the area affected.

Osteoarthritis is the most common arthritic disease. It also is called degenerative joint disease. Most of us will eventually develop osteoarthritis as we experience wear and tear on the joints in our body. Osteoarthritis occurs in the joints of your body when your cartilage is worn down and damaged by overuse, sometimes allowing the rigid and brittle bone ends to come into direct contact with each other. Your bones that compose your joint can then break down and develop irregular growths called osteophytes that can interfere with the proper movement of the joint and cause pain. Your joints provide you with range of motion and do support your body as well. To have normal and painless range of motion, your joints must have cartilage in between your bones.

Cartilage is a tissue that coats the ends of your bones. The synovium surrounds your bones as well as the cartilage. Your cartilage does not have its own blood supply. This synovium is, therefore, filled with a liquid, and the synovial fluid supplies sugar and other nutrients as well as oxygen to your cartilage. When you are young, your cartilage contains approximately 85 percent water and it decreases to 70 percent as you age. Molecules called proteoglycans are in your synovial joint. Your cartilage is also composed of collagen. Collagen gives your joint support as well as flexibility.

When the cartilage in your joint deteriorates, you have the beginnings of osteoarthritis in your joints. Osteoarthritis does not cause you to have immediate pain in your joints. Your pain appears gradually. In the early phases of this disease, your cartilage swells. The cartilage will lose water. As the cartilage loses its hydration, cracks appear in the cartilage. Your synovium can become inflamed and swollen.

If the disease progresses, more tissue is subsequently lost and your cartilage then loses its elasticity. Over time the cartilage in your joint can be completely destroyed. This will leave the ends of your bones without a protective cartilage. As a result, the two bones that form the joint can rub against each other, causing you to have significant pain.

Osteoarthritis does not spread throughout your entire body and cause problems outside of your joints as may happen in other arthritic diseases such as rheumatoid arthritis. It is confined to your joints. Other arthritic diseases such as rheumatoid arthritis can affect you lungs and your heart. Pain in a joint in your arm or leg or your back or neck is usually your major symptom if you suffer from osteoarthritis. Pain is the reason why you will seek medical care. Pain also is the major reason why you may suffer functional loss of your arms or legs. Osteoarthritis can cause not only pain in your arms and legs, but also in your spine.

Osteoarthritis can affect the elastic cartilage in your discs between your bones. These discs between your bones in your back act as cushions between the bones. You also have joints where each in your back stacks on top of one another. These bones stack on top of each other and fit like Lego blocks. These joints can degenerate, which will cause you to become stiff and will decrease your range of motion.

In addition to pain and decreased range of motion, you may have muscle spasms. If the holes where the nerves from your spinal cord come out of your vertebral bodies, the hole can decrease in size and compress the nerves going to your extremities. This can cause you to have pain, weakness, and numbness. Osteoarthritis of your spine can occur in your neck, lower back, or even your mid back.

Degenerative arthritis can become evident in your hips. Pain usually develops in your hips slowly. The pain in your hips can be referred to your buttocks or to your groin. If you have osteoarthritis that affects your hips, you will probably walk with a limp. As you walk with a limp, the excessive stress on your knees, ankles, and back can cause you pain as well.

Osteoarthritis also can become evident in your knees. Your knee may become warm as well as swollen. You may have decreased range of motion in your knees over time. This decreased range of knee motion can make it painful for you to walk through a shopping center or go up and down steps. Osteoarthritis also can affect the joints in your hands. You may notice a bony growth about the joints in your fingers. Osteoarthritis can cause painful range of motion around your fingers.

In all of these boney structures affected by osteoarthritis, be aware that osteophytes can form in your joints. The osteophytes that form at the margins of your joints can be a source of pain. Your joint pain originates from nerves that transmit pain impulses located in the tendons, ligaments, periosteum of your bones, and the synovium of your joints.

You also need to be aware that the periosteum, which wraps your bone, contains many nerve endings that can cause you to have significant pain if one bone of your joint rubs on the other bone of your joint. Various chemicals in your nerve endings in your joint can be released. One chemical, substance P, is frequently released in joints. Capsaicin cream that depletes substance P from the nerve endings can be used to manage your joint pain.

Your joint pain associated with osteoarthritis usually begins gradually and progresses slowly over years. Originally you may have the condition but not experience any pain. With the passage of time, symptoms may begin. You will be become stiff and the stiffness will probably cause you to decrease your activity.

You will notice an increase in your pain when it rains or when the weather becomes cold. Your pain may become severe to the point that it keeps you up at night. Osteoarthritis usually occurs in older people. Approximately 85 percent of people over 65 develop osteoarthritis. However, only half of these people experience any symptoms.

Studies have shown that perceived racial discrimination is a significant predictor of clinical pain severity among African Americans.[1] African Americans were more sensitive to heat pain and reported greater perceived racial discrimination as well as greater mistrust of medical researchers compared with non-Hispanic Whites.

Caucasians have a higher incidence of osteoarthritis than other ethnic groups. Osteoarthritis is not common in people younger than the age of 45. Before age 45, this disease occurs more frequently in men. After age 55, osteoarthritis is seen more often in women. Osteoarthritis involving the knee is more prevalent in women than in men, perhaps a result of wearing high-heeled shoes.

Obesity puts an increased pressure and stress on your joints in your legs. Obesity is an abnormal increase in your body fat resulting in excessive weight. There must be a 20 percent weight gain greater than the ideal for your height and body build. If you are obese, you have an increased chance of developing osteoarthritis. Any excess weight that you carry may cause deterioration of the joints in your hips, knees, and ankles.

If you have morning stiffness and pain in your joints, you are more likely to report your pain to a health-care provider. You should know that women tend to report joint pain more often than men. Age does not affect the incidence of pain reporting. If you have weakness in your thigh muscles, called the quadriceps, you may be prone to develop osteoarthritis of your knees. Any type of chronic pain syndrome can cause you to suffer from depression. If you are depressed, tell your doctor so that your doctor could prescribe antidepressant medications for you.

Osteoarthritis can occur after trauma to a joint. Repetitive motions required in your job can also cause the onset of osteoarthritis. The management of your osteoarthritic pain first involves correction of any abnormal biomechanics. One way of changing an abnormal biomechanical factor is weight reduction. Obesity increases the incidence of osteoarthritis of the knees more in women than men. A cane or shoes that fit right and provide a cushion can decrease symptoms associated with osteoarthritis.

Fatigue is common among persons with osteoarthritis (OA), but little is known about racial/ethnic differences in the prevalence, correlates, or dynamics of fatigue in OA. African Americans and non-Hispanic Whites with OA demonstrated that fatigue is a significant factor for both African Americans and non-Hispanic Whites with OA, and is negatively related to quality of life.2 Pain symptoms, at both the momentary level and across individuals, were predictors of fatigue. Although overall levels of reported symptoms were similar across these 2 groups, the pattern of fatigue symptoms across the day differed.

Nonsteroidal anti-inflammatory medications are commonly used to treat osteoarthritis (for example, Celebrex, Mobic, and Day Pro). Be aware that nonsteroidal anti-inflammatory drugs may cause gastrointestinal complications. Steroids injections into your joints can also decrease the inflammation of your joints, which will decrease your pain. Your doctor can also inject hyaluronic acid into your joints for pain modification. Glucosamine, which is available without a prescription, has been demonstrated to decrease pain associated with osteoarthritis. If you persist with chronic pain and disability, consultation with a surgeon may be indicated to see whether you quality for and would benefit from a total joint replacement.

Celecoxib is an effective treatment for osteoarthritis. However, information on its efficacy and safety profile in different racial/ethnic groups is limited. Noticeable differences among racial groups are found in other disease states, but a thorough investigation of OA is lacking. Celecoxib 200 mg once daily was compared to naproxen 500 mg twice daily in the treatment of OA of the knee in Hispanic patients. Celecoxib 200 mg once daily was as effective as naproxen 500 mg twice daily in the treatment of signs and symptoms of knee OA in Hispanic patients. Celecoxib was shown to be safe and well tolerated in this patient population.[3]

Prior investigations have suggested that physician-related factors may contribute to differential use of TKA among women and ethnic minorities.4 Patient race and sex were not associated with a different likelihood of a surgical recommendation.

Another form of arthritis is rheumatic arthritis. Rheumatic arthritis is characterized by redness, warmth, swelling, and painful joints. If you have rheumatoid arthritis, you will have decreased range of motion of some of your joints in your body. You also may complain of stiffness. This disease attacks the synovial linings of your joints as well as the tendons about your joints. If you develop rheumatoid arthritis, you may suffer generalized weakness and weight loss.

The exact cause of rheumatoid arthritis is unknown. Rheumatoid arthritis affects men and women, all races, and all ages. However, rheumatoid arthritis is three times more common in women than in men. Family history plays an important role in the development of rheumatoid arthritis. Rheumatoid arthritis may result from an abnormality in the immune system. Your antibodies may attack your joints to cause significant degeneration within your joints. It can usually have a slow onset. However, be aware that it can have an acute onset as well. The onset of rheumatoid arthritis occurs more often in the winter. If you are between the ages of 30 and 50, your chance of developing rheumatoid arthritis are increased.

You probably have rheumatoid arthritis if you have four of the following seven criteria: morning stiffness around your joints, arthritis of three or more joints, arthritis of your hands, arthritis that occurs on both sides of your body, nodules over your bony joints, an elevated rheumatoid factor in your bloodstream can aid in the diagnosis as well as X-ray changes of your joints. The treatment of rheumatoid arthritis is to relieve your pain and decrease your joint inflammation. In addition, your health-care provider will want to maintain as much range of motion about your joints as possible. Splinting, range of motion exercises and strengthening exercises can be extremely beneficial to you. Occasionally, you may need a brace on one of your extremities.

Usually nonsteroidal anti-inflammatory drugs are prescribed for the management of your arthritic pain. As mentioned with regard to osteoarthritis, the COX-2 inhibitors are safer for your gastrointestinal system than the older nonsteroidal anti-inflammatory drugs. Some doctors prescribe medications such as gold compounds, antimalarial drugs, and sulfasalazine. However, each of these drugs has the potential to cause serious side effects. Steroids also may be necessary to decrease the inflammation of your joints. Steroids typically decrease pain and swelling.

If these methods do not relieve your pain, you may be a candidate for immunosuppressive therapy. Immunosuppressive therapy is the administration of a drug which eliminates or lessens an immune response. Methotrexate is used frequently for the treatment of your rheumatoid arthritis. Methotrexate can cause liver pathology.

Surgery is the last resort for the treatment of rheumatoid arthritis and consists of total joint replacement. If your pain becomes intolerable and if you have significant limitations in joint function, surgery can provide you with relief. Joint replacements are now available for hips, knees, shoulders, elbows, and ankles.

Be aware that sex hormones may play a role in the development of rheumatoid arthritis. Sex hormones can block some of the mechanisms involved in the development of rheumatoid arthritis. If you are a premenopausal woman, you could develop rheumatoid arthritis if you have low levels of DHEA as well as testosterone. Postmenopausal women have high levels of both testosterone and DHEA. Both of these chemicals are called androgens. Apparently androgens are of some benefit to you in preventing progression of this disease. On the other hand, men who have rheumatoid arthritis usually have low testosterone levels. Some medical scientists think that testosterone may decrease the incidence of rheumatoid arthritis. In addition, a history of smoking is associated with an increased risk for the development of rheumatoid arthritis in men but not in women.

Despite the high prevalence of depression among vulnerable Hispanics with rheumatoid arthritis many do not disclose it or seek treatment.[5] Use, duration, and goals of antidepressant therapy should be clarified to patients.. Providers should strive to establish trust and conduct in-person depression screening to facilitate disclosure. Interventions with an interpersonal component, such as support groups or patient navigators, were preferred. Themes emphasizing coping strategies, stress reduction, positive thinking, self-efficacy, and resiliency are likely to be most acceptable.

Ankylosing spondylitis is a disease that predominantly affects men. Pain usually begins in the back and sacroiliac joint (the joint where the back and hip bones meet) early in life. An x-ray of the spine of a male with ankylosing spondylitis appears as bamboo and is called a bamboo spine. This pattern is also seen on MRI imaging studies. Ankylosing spondylitis usually affects men before the age of 40. If you have ankylosing spondylitis, you may develop arthritis of your spine as well as the large joints in your body.

Ankylosing spondylitis is present in 8 percent of Caucasians and 3 percent of African American men. A marker in the bloodstream called HLA-B27 is present in 90 percent of patients who have ankylosing spondylitis. Ankylosing spondylitis has been observed in rats when the HLA-B27 gene is expressed.

Usually ankylosing spondylitis will become manifest in a male around age 20. This arthritic disease does occur in women, but the symptoms are more prominent in men. If you do suffer from ankylosing spondylitis, your primary symptoms may be symptoms in your hip joints. You may have progressive decrease of your back range of motion. You may have some pain in the joints of your arms and legs as well. X-rays have shown arthritis in sacroiliac joints. Over time, your spine will continue to stiffen. The onset of ankylosing spondylitis is gradual. If your disease progresses further, your symptoms will usually go upward toward your neck. You have a normal curve in your lower back that will become straight. You may have difficulty expanding your chest to take a breath.

If your ankylosing spondylitis advances, your entire spine may become fused, which restricts your motion about your spine in all directions. The earliest x-ray changes usually occur in your sacroiliac joints. Erosion of these joints becomes evident. The outer rings of your discs in your spine become calcified. Furthermore, calcification of the vertical ligaments that run in front and back of your vertebral bones occurs. When this happens, if you have an x-ray of your spine, it will appear as a bamboo stick. Remember that rheumatoid arthritis affects mostly small joints. Ankylosing spondylitis affects large joints. Osteoarthritis does not usually affect your sacroiliac joints.

If you have ankylosing spondylitis, physical therapy and nonsteroidal anti-inflammatory drugs are important for the treatment of the pain associated with this disease. No treatment is currently available that will eradicate ankylosing splondylitis. Occasionally stronger analgesics such as opioids are needed to control your pain. Sulfasalazine is sometimes useful for pain in arthritis in your arms and legs. The problem with ankylosing spondylitis is that you can have pain that is severe over decades of your life. The severity of the pain associated with this disease varies greatly. Approximately 10 percent of patients have disability so severe that they are unable to return to work after 10 years.

Gout is one of the most painful arthritic diseases. Gout results from crystals of uric acid that are deposited into joint spaces between your bones. These uric acid crystals deposited into your joints cause inflammation with swelling, redness, and warmth about your joint. Gouty arthritis is noted in 5 percent of all cases of arthritis.

Uric acid is formed from the breakdown of chemicals called purines that are found in many foods. You should avoid foods that will elevate your uric acid blood level. If you have an onset of gout, avoid meat and seafood. Avoid yeast products, including beer and other alcoholic beverages. You must also avoid oatmeal, asparagus, cauliflower, and mushrooms.

Gout has a significant impact on a patient's quality of life. Important differences in the impact of gout by gender and race were noted as well.[6] Compared with Caucasians, African-Americans ranked the following concerns high more often: dietary restrictions, severe pain, effect on emotional health and the need for canes/crutches during flares.

In most people, uric acid is dissolved in the bloodstream and excreted through the kidneys. If your kidneys do not eliminate enough uric acid from your bloodstream, the uric acid will increase in your bloodstream. If the uric acid forms crystals and deposits these crystals into your joints, gout will develop. In many people, the uric acid deposits affect the joints in their great toes. The big toe is affected in approximately 75 percent of people suffering gout. The ankles, heels, knees, wrists, and fingers may also be affected by gouty arthritis.

Gout is more common in men than in women and is more common in adults than in children. Obesity increases the risk of developing gout. An excess consumption of alcohol also interferes with the excretion of uric acid from your body. The increased uric acid that occurs can form crystals and deposit these crystals into your joints. Adult men between the ages of 40 and 50 are most likely to develop gout. It is occasionally seen in women. It rarely occurs before menopause. For some reason, people who have had organ transplants are more susceptible to gout.

A diagnosis of gout can be made by withdrawing fluid from your painful joints and analyzing the fluid for uric acid. When your gout attack is severe, you may be totally incapacitated. African American ethnicity is associated with a significantly lower risk for gout and hyperuricemia compared with Caucasian ethnicity.[7] Estrogen hormones noted in women can help the body eliminate uric acid. For this reason, gout is rarely seen in premenopausal women.[8] Be aware that if you have gout, you have an increased risk of developing kidney stones. These stones are usually composed of uric acid. If you have gout, you also have a higher risk of developing a kidney disease.

Sometimes overproduction of uric acid is related to a genetic disorder. Excessive exercise can also increase uric acid, as can obesity. Starvation or dehydration can increase uric acid, too. Thyroid disease can also increase uric acid. Diuretics (medications that make you urinate, such as furosemide and hydrochlorthiazide, and cyclosporine A (an immunosuppressive medicine) can increase the uric acid concentration in your bloodstream. The diagnosis of gout is made by finding uric acid crystals in the fluid of your joints.

If you develop an acute attack of gout, you need in most instances to be treated for your pain. Your doctor may give you nonsteroidal anti-inflammatory medications or steroids or colchicine. The use of COX-2 inhibitors is under investigation. Remember other nonsteroidal anti-inflammatory drugs could cause you to develop ulcers. Steroids can be used to treat gout and can be given orally or by injection into your muscle. The steroid can be given over approximately two weeks. Sometimes your doctor will inject your painful joint with a steroid.

Colchicine is the medication that has been used extensively over the past two decades for the treatment of gout. It is most effective during the first 24 hours of an acute attack. Colchicine can cause you to have vomiting and nausea. If you have liver problems, you should not take colchicine. Allopurinol is another drug that can decrease your uric acid levels. Allopurinol is usually used in people who produce excessive uric acid. Allopurinol should not be used during an acute gouty arthritis episode because Allopurinol can prolong the attack.

Probenecid is used by some rheumatologists because it has fewer side effects than Allopurinol. If you have developed tophi (nodules under your skin) that are painful, you may need to have these uric acid crystals removed surgically. The foundation for designing interventions to improve urate-lowering therapy adherence in racial minorities must be implemented. [9]

Avascular necrosis (AVN) is the death of bone tissue due to a lack of blood supply and can lead to tiny breaks in the bone and the bone's eventual collapse. The blood flow to a section of bone can be interrupted if the bone is fractured or the joint becomes dislocated. Anyone can be affected by avascular necrosis. However, it's most common in people between the ages of 30 and 60. Patients with allograft rejection, African American race, peritoneal dialysis and earlier date of transplant were at the highest risk of AVN, while diabetic recipients are at a decreased risk.

Many patients have no symptoms in the early stages of avascular necrosis. As the AVN condition worsens, a patient's affected joint may hurt only when weight is placed on it. Eventually, the joint may hurt even when lying down. Avascular necrosis primarily affects the joints at the shoulder, knee, and hip. Avascular necrosis may be caused by steroid use and most commonly affects the femoral head, humeral head, and tibial plateau.

Early joint changes can be demonstrated by bone scan or magnetic resonance imaging. Although osteonecrosis affects both men and women, it mainly affects men. However, in cases related to SLE, the disease mostly affects women. It can occur in people of any age, from children to the elderly. However, it is more common in people in their thirties, forties, and fifties.

Risks of developing AVN include diabetes, steroid use, alcoholism, gouty arthritis, sickle cell anemia, renal disease, trauma, Systemic Lupus Erythematosus, rheumatoid arthritis, air or fat embolism, Caissons disease, tumor or hematological malignancy. Avascular necrosis of bone is also an important complication of systemic lupus erythematosus. Traumatic osteonecrosis occurs when a fracture, dislocation, or joint injury damages surrounding blood vessels, disrupting blood circulation to the bone. For 20% of osteonecrosis patients, the cause is unknown and the condition is known as idiopathic osteonecrosis.

Reduced weight bearing is typically essential for healing and can be achieved by limiting activities or by using crutches or other mobility aids. Electrical stimulation is sometimes used to promote bone growth. Core decompression is a surgery in which the inner layer of bone is removed, theoretically allowing for better blood flow to the area of concern.

This surgery is most effective for people in the earliest stages of the disease. Osteotomy surgery reshapes either the affected bone or surrounding bones in order to decrease stress on the afflicted area. The surgery is most effective for patients with advanced forms of the disease and for when avascular necrosis affects a large area of bone.

Depending on how advanced the disease state is this surgery can be very effective with the right indications. In bone graft surgery, healthy bone is transplanted from one part of the patient to the area affected by avascular necrosis. Total joint replacement is used in late-stage avascular necrosis and when the joint is destroyed. The diseased joint is replaced with artificial parts, to recreate the mechanics of a human joint.

Anti-inflammatory medications such as ibuprofen will help reduce the swelling and pain sensations you are experiencing. Physical therapy can help relieve the pain associated with your arthritis. Massage therapy can relax your muscles and often relieve swelling in your muscles and help your arthritis pain. Acupuncture can stimulate nerve fibers and help decrease your pain.

Because of sex differences with respect to the effect of estrogen as well as progesterone on the absorption, metabolism and elimination of medications, drug dosing may fluctuate in the female patient depending on whether or not the female is pre- or post-menopausal. The physiological changes that occur during the menstrual cycle can affect the response of a drug in the female body. You must discuss the effects of your drug with your doctor because the effect of your drug may decrease during menses.

References

1.   Goodin BR, Pham QT, Glover TL, et al. Perceived racial discrimination, but not mistrust of medical researchers, predicts the heat pain tolerance of African Americans with symptomatic knee osteoarthritis. Health Psychol. 2013;32(11):1117-1126.

2.   Smith DM, Parmelee PA. Within-Day Variability of Fatigue and Pain Among African Americans and Non-Hispanic Whites With Osteoarthritis of the Knee. Arthritis Care Res (Hoboken). 2016;68(1):115-122.

3.   Essex MN, Behar R, O'Connell MA, Brown PB. Efficacy and tolerability of celecoxib and naproxen versus placebo in Hispanic patients with knee osteoarthritis. Int J Gen Med. 2014;7:227-235.

4.   Dy CJ, Lyman S, Boutin-Foster C, Felix K, Kang Y, Parks ML. Do patient race and sex change surgeon recommendations for TKA? Clinical orthopaedics and related research. 2015;473(2):410-417.

5.   Withers M, Moran R, Nicassio P, Weisman MH, Karpouzas GA. Perspectives of vulnerable U.S Hispanics with

rheumatoid arthritis on depression: awareness, barriers to disclosure, and treatment options. Arthritis Care Res (Hoboken). 2015;67(4):484-492.

6.   Singh JA. The impact of gout on patient's lives: a study of African-American and Caucasian men and women with gout. Arthritis Res Ther. 2014;16(3):R132.

7.   Krishnan E. Gout in African Americans. Am J Med. 2014;127(9):858-864.

8.   Bruderer SG, Bodmer M, Jick SS, Meier CR. Association of hormone therapy and incident gout: population-based case-control study. Menopause. 2015;22(12):1335-1342.

9.   Singh JA. Facilitators and barriers to adherence to urate-lowering therapy in African-Americans with gout: a qualitative study. Arthritis Res Ther. 2014;16(2):R82.

20. Osteoporosis

Osteoporosis is the most common type of bone disease that is related to the breakdown of substances that exist in your bones. If you suffer from osteoporosis, you will have a progressive reduction in your bone minerals as well as the structural components of your bones, but the normal composition of bone is preserved. Osteoporosis affects 20 million Americans and results in more than 1.3 million bone fractures in the United States every year. In a lifetime, women lose more than half of their spongy bone, which comprises the center of bones, and approximately 30 percent of the nonspongy (compact) bone, which composes the outer aspect of bones. The prevalence of osteoporosis and the incidence of fractures are substantially lower in black than in white subjects, a finding generally attributed to racial differences in adult bone mass.[1]

Differences in bone mineral density (BMD) as assessed with dual-energy x-ray absorptiometry are observed between geographic and ethnic groups, with important implications in clinical practice. Economic adversity was associated with higher bone turnover in men, and minority race status was associated with higher bone turnover in women, consistent with the hypothesis that higher levels of social stresses cause increased bone turnover.[2]

Osteoporosis can be a significant bone disease because it is potentially disabling. Approximately 30 percent of all postmenopausal Caucasian women will suffer from fractures related to osteoporosis. More than one third of all women and one sixth of all men over 65 years of age will sustain a hip fracture. This is a frightening statistic because hip fracture complications can be fatal. It is estimated that the annual cost of health care for those with osteoporosis in lost national productivity as well as medical costs exceeds $10 billion in the United States alone. Osteoporosis could be primarily a manifestation of normal aging, including the postmenopausal estrogen deficiency in women, regardless of gender or race.[3]

During your lifetime, bone is constantly being made and is constantly being lost. In normal circumstances, the production and reduction of your bone is balanced. Osteoporosis can result if you do not make enough bone or if you have an accelerated decrease in your bone minerals and the matrix structure (the components of your bone which make your bones hard) of your bone or both.

Your bone density increases significantly during puberty. This increase in bone density is the result of your response to sex steroids. Sex steroids increase your bone density. When you are a young adult, your bone density is twice what is when you were a child. If you have had a delay in the onset of puberty, you may have a decrease in your bone density.

Factors that can affect your bone mass include exercise or lack of exercise, calcium intake, growth hormones, sex hormones, genetics, race, and gender. If you have a relative who has a history of osteoporosis, tell your primary care doctor. Genetics play an important role in the development of osteoporosis. Studies have demonstrated that bone density is lower in the daughters of women who have osteoporosis than in those women who do not have osteoporosis.

Bone density tests in identical twins have been done indicating that genetics is an important factor in the development of osteoporosis. These studies have suggested that most of the genetic differences in bone density are the result of a gene that is linked to your vitamin D receptor gene. Further study has revealed that variations of the vitamin D receptor gene result in differences in bone density changes of 10 percent to 12 percent in osteoporosis-prone individuals. Further study is being done on the effect of the vitamin D receptor gene and the severity of osteoporosis in both men and women.

Men in general have been shown to have higher bone densities than women. Furthermore, African American men have higher bone density than Caucasian men. The same is true with African American and Caucasian women. Even though osteoporosis is a disease that mostly affects women, osteoporosis can be seen in a small percentage of men. If you are a woman and if you have had a delay in the onset of your menstrual periods by several years, you may be susceptible to osteoporosis.

A woman's first menstruation occurs when her reproductive organs become active and can take place at any time between the ages of 10 and 18. Studies have revealed that calcium supplementation can enhance prepuberty bone accumulation. An increase in physical activity can also increase bone density around the time of puberty. Osteoporosis is highly prevalent in severe COPD, and affects males and African Americans to a similar degree as females and Whites.[4] Osteoporosis should be considered in severe COPD regardless of race or gender.

Your bone density will continue to increase throughout your life until you reach an age where your bone density becomes stable. When you approach 40, your bone density can begin to decline. Bone density decreases are noted in women before menopause. In men, a decrease in their bone density occurs somewhere between 20 to 40 years of age. In women, after menopause has occurred, the rate of bone loss accelerates. During the first 10 years of menopause, the women's spongy bone is lost faster than the outer bone. Hip fracture rates among persons of Japanese ancestry were approximately half that of Caucasians for both sexes.[5]

Osteoporosis is usually without symptoms until a fracture occurs. Usually the fracture is in one of the bones of the back. However, your wrists, hips, ribs, pelvic bone, and your leg bones can sustain fractures. The bones in your spine can have a loss of height, which is called a compression fracture. If you have osteoporosis, you can sustain a fracture in one of the bones in your back with minimal stress. It usually takes significant stress to fracture a normal bone. Even bending over to pick up an object off the floor can cause a compression fracture. You will most likely notice the immediate onset of pain in your mid or lower back at the time of the compression fracture. Usually your pain decreases over several weeks.

If you have multiple fractures in your back, your pain may become chronic. Usually your back pain is worse with standing vertically. The increased weight on the bones in your back will cause you to have pain. Lying down will decrease your spine pain. Bone is lost with advancing age in men as in women, leading to an increased incidence of osteoporotic fractures of the fore-arm, vertebral body and femoral neck.[6]

You will also lose height as the bones in your back compress. If you fall, you may sustain a hip fracture. Hip fractures are dangerous for elderly patients. Usually a hip fracture will cause you to need hospitalization. On occasion your total hip has to be replaced surgically. If you are elderly, you may need nursing home care following a hip replacement. Medical complications, such as pulmonary embolus, that can be associated with hip surgery in elderly patients can be fatal.

If you have osteoporosis, your bones become more porous. This means that the bones in your body develop holes, which in turn weaken the structure of your bones. All of your bones can be affected, and each of your bones can be at an increased risk for a fracture. If you have a low calcium intake and are not physically active, you are also at risk of developing osteoporosis.

There is a type of osteoporosis that is called idiopathic osteoporosis. The cause of this type of osteoporosis is unknown, but it does affect middle-aged men and premenopausal women. Did you know that being weightless in space can contribute to the onset of osteoporosis? Individuals who suffer from anorexia nervosa also develop osteoporosis. Despite lower levels of activity, blacks and Hispanics were not more likely to have osteoporosis, and high levels of activity were significantly associated with higher bone density.[7]

There are other causes of osteoporosis besides the ones just mentioned. Hyperthyroidism and hyperparathyroidism in addition to your body's overproduction of cortisone (a steroid) are causes of osteoporosis. As previously mentioned, if you have a decrease in your growth hormone, you are prone to develop osteoporosis. It is important for your body to absorb calcium through your gastrointestinal system.

If you have a history of a gastrectomy (removal of a portion of your stomach), cirrhosis of the liver, or any other gastrointestinal malabsorption syndrome, you are more prone to develop osteoporosis. If you have a history of multiple myeloma or leukemia, you may develop osteoporosis. The exact cause of this finding is presently unknown. If you have been immobilized for any reason, you may develop osteoporosis. If you are unable to walk or exercise for whatever reason due to your immobilization, you may develop osteoporosis. Alcohol can contribute to your development of osteoporosis. Chemotherapy can also cause osteoporosis. Steroid use has been implicated in the development of osteoporosis.

Other diseases have a link to osteoporosis. An autoimmune disease is a disorder in which your body attacks its own tissue. Your joints can become damaged by your own antibodies. Systemic lupus erythematous is an autoimmune disease commonly known as lupus. If you have lupus, you will become fatigued and have painful joints in addition to developing skin rashes. Ninety percent of individuals diagnosed with lupus are women. If you have lupus, you are at an increased risk for developing osteoporosis.

Steroids are prescribed for the treatment of lupus. However, remember that steroids can trigger osteoporosis. The fatigue caused by lupus results in a decrease in exercise and activity. These factors increase your risk of developing osteoporosis. Furthermore, the disease itself can decrease your bone mass. Individuals who are HIV positive can also develop osteoporosis. The reason for the increase in osteoporosis in patients with HIV infection is not known. It is possible that the virus may infect the cells that produce bone.

In addition to Caucasian women being more prone to developing osteoporosis, Asian American women are also at a high risk for developing osteoporosis. African American and Hispanic women are at a lower risk for developing osteoporosis. The reason for the effect of race on the development of osteoporosis remains to be seen.

A diagnosis of osteoporosis can be made by a plain X-ray. If you have a vertebral bone compression in your mid back, for example, there will usually be a decrease in the height of your affected (compressed) bone that can be seen on X-ray. Sometimes a bone scan is needed to diagnosis osteoporosis. If you have a bone scan, a doctor will inject a radioactive material into your vein. You will have a picture of your body taken by a special camera. Compression fractures, which were not diagnosed by other means, can be detected on a bone scan.

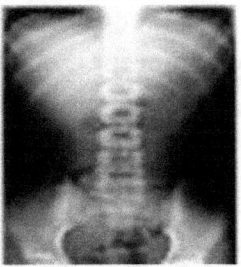

Figure 1. X rays may help to diagnose osteoporosis

Osteoporosis can also be diagnosed by measuring your bone mineral density. Your bone density value will be compared to a normal value that is noted for young adults of your same sex. A bone density test can predict the probability of you developing a fracture related to your bone density value. Quantitative computed tomography can also be used and is effective for diagnosing osteoporosis because it will not only measure your bone mineral density, this test can also measure the density of your spongy bone within your back and hip bones.

However, this test is expensive and will expose you to radiation. Different types of tests are being used and being developed to diagnosis osteoporosis. Bone scanning can be useful for the diagnosis of compression fractures. If you have a decreased bone density, your doctor should attempt to determine the cause of your osteoporosis.

Sometimes your doctor needs to obtain blood from you for further testing. Your doctor may take some blood from you to be sent to a lab to measure the calcium, organic phosphate, and alkaline phosphatase in your bloodstream. These minerals are usually normal if you have osteoporosis. However, your alkaline phosphate may be higher if you have a fracture.

Not all fractures associated with osteoporosis are painful. You may have a fracture and not know it. Your doctor will probably measure the level of your parathyroid hormone in your blood if you develop nonpainful bone fractures, which are not associated with bone trauma such as a fall. This is important because an elevation of parathyroid hormone can decrease your bone mass. Because a decrease in testosterone may be associated with osteoporosis in men, male patients should have their testosterone blood levels measured when they have their yearly physical examinations.

Bone density testing is important early in the development of osteoporosis because there is no cure for osteoporosis. In other words, there is no way to reverse osteoporosis after it has become established. However, early treatment can prevent the progression of osteoporosis. If it has been determined that alcohol is a cause of your osteoporosis, you must stop consuming alcohol. If your thyroid levels are elevated, this disease should be treated early to decrease the progression of your osteoporosis. Physical therapy and mild aerobic exercise may be important in retarding the early development of osteoporosis. If you have a compression fracture of one of your bones in your spine, a back brace can provide you with pain relief. Your physical therapist may want to strengthen your stomach muscles as well as the muscles in your back.

Orthopedic surgeons are frequently the first health-care providers to evaluate patients with fractures. This study reported that orthopedic surgeons, however, have been slow to develop awareness for identifying individuals who have osteoporosis who could benefit from drug therapies. Doctors need to realize that a patient who sustained a hip fracture is identified as an individual who has a high probability of developing osteoporosis. This individual is at a high risk for having a future bone fracture.

If you have had a hip fracture, you are a probable candidate for bone density testing. Communication between a patient's orthopedic surgeon and primary care doctor is essential. This communication could facilitate the diagnosis of decreased bone density in individuals who have suffered hip fractures.

Cortical bone is a compact form of bone that makes up the outer shell of your bones. It consists of a hard, solid mass made up of bony tissue that is arranged in concentric layers. This is similar to the layers noted in a tree. Your compact bone will surround your spongy bone. Bone is composed of collagen fibers that contain bone salts, which are mainly calcium carbonate salts as well as calcium phosphate salts. As previously stated, during the first 5 to 10 years of menopause, women can lose 10 to 15 percent of their compact bone and 25 percent of your spongy bone. It is important for you to know that this bone loss can be prevented by estrogen-replacement therapy. However, estrogen therapy can be associated with an increased risk of a stroke and heart disease.

The amount of bone loss varies among women, which has led medical investigators to derive a classification of osteoporosis. If your osteoporosis is more severe than is expected for your age, you have type I postmenopausal osteoporosis. If you have type I osteoporosis, you are at a higher risk to have compression or crush fractures of the bones in your spine. You may also be prone to a fracture at the bone above your wrist on the side of your thumb. This type of fracture is called a Colles fracture.

If your bones are weak and fragile, you can easily sustain a bone fracture. These types of fractures are related to bone density loss. If you have a decrease in your estrogen, you may have the production of chemicals that may decrease your bone mass. The prevalence and severity of disc space narrowing are higher in elderly women than in elderly men. With increasing age, disc space narrowing progresses at a greater rate in women than in men.[8]

An initially rapid rate of bone loss in the post-menopausal period is followed by a slower loss of bone throughout the rest of life. Your loss of bone mass does result from normal aging and occurs in both men and women. This type of bone loss is called type II osteoporosis. Fractures can occur in type II osteoporosis as well as in type I osteoporosis. Fractures can occur in your hip, pelvis, wrist, the bones in your legs, and the bones in your back. Sometimes type II osteoporosis is associated with a defect in the absorption of calcium through the gastrointestinal system. As you age, your calcium absorption through your stomach and intestine can decrease. A decreased absorption of this important substance will decrease the amount of calcium in your bloodstream.

In your body you have various chemicals stimulated by growth factor. Growth factor tells your body to make new cells and to maintain the cells that are already present in your body. These chemicals sit on the outer surface of your cells. Growth factor is needed in wound healing if you have had an injury to one of your tissues (bone, muscle, nerve). Estrogen, a female sex hormone, increases the production of this growth factor. Be aware that growth factor stimulates bone formation. If you have a decrease in estrogen, you can diminish your formation of bone. As a result, a decrease in estrogen will decrease your ability to form bone.

In your body you have two parathyroid glands. These glands are around your thyroid gland at the base of your neck above your breastbone (your sternum). Your parathyroid glands stimulate the production of parathyroid hormone, which is produced if you have a decrease in calcium in your bloodstream. Parathyroid glands produce parathyroid hormone. This hormone produced by your parathyroid gland is released into your bloodstream. The parathyroid hormone controls the distribution of both calcium and phosphate throughout your body.

A high level of parathyroid hormone will cause transfer of calcium from your bones to your bloodstream. If your parathyroid hormone level decreases in your bloodstream, it will lower your blood calcium level. If you have a decrease in your estrogen hormone, you will have a decrease in your blood calcium levels as well. If your estrogen goes down, your bone sensitivity to the transfer of calcium from your bones to your bloodstream is increased. Therefore, you will lose your bone density as your blood level of estrogen decreases.

If your calcium in your bloodstream increases, you will decrease your parathyroid hormone secretion. Estrogen deficiency can decrease your bone matrix formation in your body. You should now be aware that sex hormones play an important role in the maintenance of your bone structure. You should now realize that when your sex hormones decrease as you age, this decreased hormone level could adversely affect your skeletal system.

As previously stated, osteoporosis occurs more often in women as in men. However, it is also seen in men. It is estimated that more than 2 million men in the United States suffer from osteoporosis. Approximately 20 percent of all hip fractures in the United States occur in men. Compression fractures in the bones of the spine can occur in men as well. This observation demonstrates that osteoporosis is not solely a "woman's disease." Osteoporosis develops less often in men than in women because men have more bone mass and larger skeletons. Therefore, the bone loss in men starts later and progresses more slowly.

The development of osteoporosis in men has been recently recognized as an important public health issue. Men suffering from osteoporosis are a long-neglected group of individuals. The National Institutes of Health are currently studying osteoporosis in men. The results of this study should help doctors understand how to prevent and treat osteoporosis in men. Remember that when bone is lost, it cannot be replaced. Middle-aged and elderly men should have their testosterone levels measured periodically.

As previously stated, a reduced level of testosterone in men can cause osteoporosis. Thirty percent of men with osteoporotic fractures of the bones in their spine have low testosterone levels. Testosterone therapy may retard the development of osteoporosis in men. The research has shown that a decrease in estrogen in men can be a cause of osteoporosis. Be aware of the fact that men also have estrogen secreted in their bodies.

The prevention and treatment of osteoporosis includes synthetic estrogen or progesterone therapy if you are postmenopausal. However, you must take calcium in addition to the hormone therapy. A synthetic estrogen called raloxifene has been approved for the treatment of osteoporosis. This drug will increase your bone density. It has fewer side effects than other types of estrogen drugs.

Postmenopausal women who exercise for 60 minutes 3 times a week and take calcium supplements can stop bone loss. It is recommended that individuals over 50 use calcium supplements. If you do not want to use a calcium supplement, calcium-rich foods such as milk, yogurt, and cooked dry beans will provide you with calcium. Furthermore, some cheeses can increase the calcium in your bloodstream. Most individuals have trouble getting enough calcium in their diet and end up needing calcium supplements.

Remember that vitamin D is also an important vitamin that is necessary for strong bones. If you are not out in the sun, you should drink vitamin D-fortified milk or eat vitamin D fortified foods. Remember that vitamin D is important because it helps your body to absorb calcium. Vitamin D can help you increase your calcium absorption through your gastrointestinal tract by up to 65 percent.

Be aware that drugs used to treat asthma can increase your risk of fractures if you are prone to osteoporosis. Inhaled steroids can be used for the treatment of asthma. This drug increases your risk of sustaining a bone fracture. Steroids are used not only for the treatment of asthma but also for the treatment of rheumatoid arthritis and some bowel disease. If you are taking steroids for longer than three months, you may need to discuss this with your doctor and you and your doctor should consider a prescription for Fosamax, which is used to treat osteoporosis.

Smoking also increases bone loss. Hip and spinal bone fractures are higher in men and women who smoke. Research is being done to determine how nicotine damages bone. Preliminary investigations reveal that nicotine can inhibit absorption of calcium that is needed for bone health. Just like women, men need to take calcium. Men can inherit osteoporosis from their fathers.

Caucasian men are at a higher risk of developing osteoporosis than other races. Osteoporosis in men can be diagnosis by a bone mass measurement. This is a special type of x-ray that emits a trace amount of radiation. Middle-aged men who have complaints of back or hip pain may be candidates for a bone mass measurement as well as a measurement of the testosterone in their bloodstream.

Research has demonstrated that there is gender bias with respect to men who have suffered hip fractures. Doctors in the past have felt osteoporosis was a woman's disease. We now realize that osteoporosis affects both women and men. Medications to prevent bone loss are for the most part ignored for middle-aged and older men who have sustained hip fractures. Hip fracture complications are a cause of death in approximately 17 percent of women and 6 percent of men in the United States. By the age of 70, bone loss is equal in both men and women.

The absorption of calcium from your gastrointestinal system decreases with age. The United Stated recommended dietary allowance of calcium is up to 1,000 milligrams per day. Calcium can retard your osteoporosis but cannot completely stop it. An increase in calcium in your bloodstream may not protect you from compression fractures of the bones in your spine. Calcium therapy can help you if you are a woman and postmenopausal. Some endocrinologists have recommended that if you are postmenopausal that you should consume 1,500 milligrams per day of calcium.

As stated earlier in this chapter, sex steroids are important for the maintenance of proper bone density. Oral estrogen as well as estrogen in the form of a patch worn on the skin can prevent bone loss if you are estrogen deficient. Bone loss is rapid in the first years of menopause, so estrogen therapy is of great benefit if it is administered before you begin to lose a significant amount of bone mass. Studies have demonstrated that estrogen therapy decreases the risk of bone fractures in postmenopausal women. It is recommended that if you are taking estrogen supplements that you also take calcium supplements.

Estrogen supplements are not without side effects. If estrogen is not administered along with progestin, you run the risk of cancer. Estrogen replacement can be related to breast cancer as well as heart disease. These studies with respect to cancer are controversial, however. Other studies have noted that estrogen therapy can decrease the chance of you having a heart attack by up to 50 percent. However, routine use of estrogens is not recommended by most physicians because of potential side effects. Consult your doctor about the risks and benefits of estrogen therapy and make your own decision before using estrogen therapy.

Calcitonin is another drug that you could take to prevent bone loss in your vertebral bodies throughout your spine. Calcitonin is most effective in early and late menopause. Calcitonin is available for intranasal use. Calcitonin has been shown to produce pain-relieving effects. Calcitonin is most useful if you have a history of osteoporosis and have chronic pain related to fractures related to your osteoporosis.

Elderly individuals appear to be prone to vitamin D deficiency. Decreased vitamin D and decreased calcium in elderly patients' bloodstreams can lead to accelerated bone loss. It has been shown that vitamin D plus calcium can reduce the incidence of fractures in elderly women.

Falls can cause significant injury to your hips or the bones in your legs if you have osteoporosis. The rationale for this device is that the nervous system in elderly individuals, women and men, decreases touch and position sense. Touch and position sense are needed to maintain balance. It is thought that if you can stimulate the nervous system in the soles of the feet, improvement will be seen in the balance and posture control of elderly individuals. Improvement in the balance of elderly individuals is extremely important because bone fractures can be potentially lethal for them.

Elderly individuals who have suffered a hip or wrist fracture because of osteoporosis received the treatment that they need to prevent future fractures of their bones. Only 22 percent of elderly women and elderly men received a prescription drug for one of the drugs used to treat osteoporosis. It is important that elderly individuals who have sustained a fracture receive osteoporosis treatment medications because they are five times more likely to suffer another fracture.

By using osteoporosis drugs, they can reduce the risk of a future fracture by as much as 60 percent. Be aware that more than 550,000 hip and wrist fractures occur in elderly individuals suffering from osteoporosis every year. An initial fracture in an elderly individual should signal a red flag to a doctor that this individual probably has osteoporosis and needs prescription medications.

If you have had a fracture of one of the bones in your spine, treatment that puts bone cement into your bone can be used to treat any compression fracture that you may have. Be aware that leakage of this bone cement, called polymethylmethacrylate, can be associated with an embolus to your lungs, heart and lung failure, and death. The techniques that use this cement are called vertebroplasty and kyphoplasty.

Value and safety of these procedures continues to be studied. Vertebroplasty involves the injection of the bone cement into your vertebral bones. Kyphyplasty introduces a surgical instrument into one of the bones in your spine with intent to elevate the compressed bone. When this instrument is withdrawn, the space left is filled with bone cement. Each of these procedures remains to be studied.

Fluorides may be used to possibly strengthen bone. A small dose of sodium fluoride can increase your spinal bone density. As a result, you can have a reduced incidence of vertebral body fractures. Parathyroid hormone can prevent bone loss in young women who are estrogen deficient. Be aware that a new drug recently developed for the treatment of osteoporosis, Forteo, has been shown to cause bone cancer in laboratory rats. No cancers were seen in humans to date.

If you have decreased bone density, you must take the medicines prescribed for you. Studies have shown that compliance is sometimes as low as 66 percent. This means that only 66 percent of individuals in a study actually took the medications prescribed for them. Women who did not take their osteoporosis medications developed significant further decrease in their bone densities. On the other hand, a study of postmenopausal women who had a history of a fractures related to osteoporosis did not receive drug treatment for the osteoporosis within a year following their fracture. Improved adherence to osteoporosis treatment can be done if women are educated regarding their bone densities and the effects of drugs on their bone density.

Bisphosphonates are an important class of drug for osteoporosis. These drugs can increase the minerals in the bones in your back. Furthermore, the chance of you having a vertebral fracture is decreased if you are in late menopause. These drugs can also prevent bone loss in early menopause. Examples of these drugs include etidronate and alendronate. Further research is being done with respect to these drugs in the prevention of bone fractures. However, these drugs will not reverse osteoporosis.

There are other drugs available for women who have osteoporosis. Fosamax and Actonel are two of the drugs commonly used to decrease the progression of osteoporosis. This new drug is called ibandronate. This drug can cause generalized body aches. Actonel , Binosto, Boniva, and Fosamax (also available as generic) work by inhibiting cells that break down bone and slowing bone loss. Actonel,

Binosto, and Fosamax are usually taken once a week, while Boniva is taken once a month. Evista is an osteoporosis drug that has some actions similar to estrogen, such as the ability to maintain bone mass. Forteo is a medication used for the treatment of osteoporosis in postmenopausal women and men who are at high risk for a fracture. Red meats, soft drinks, and foods with phosphate food additives as well as excessive amounts of alcohol and caffeine should be avoided as well.

During the acute stage of fractures, attention is directed toward relieving your pain with pain pills, including narcotics and muscle relaxants for spasm that occurs related to the fracture. Heat, massage, and rest can also be of benefit to you. Physical therapy in many instances can help you with your pain. If you have a fracture of one of the vertebral bodies in your spine, a corset or a back brace can decrease your pain. Exercise can be useful if it strengthens your abdominal and back muscles.

Prevention is the best treatment.[9] A calcium supplement that contains Vitamin D, such as OsCal-D, will strengthen your bones and help prevent osteoporosis. Prescription medications such as Fosamax will keep you from losing more bone mass. Perform weight-bearing exercises to help maintain and build your bone mass. Be sure to follow all of your doctor's recommendations for exercises and medications.

Economic adversity was associated with higher bone turnover in men, and minority race status was associated with higher bone turnover in women, consistent with the hypothesis that higher levels of social stresses cause increased bone turnover. The magnitude of these associations was comparable to the effects of some osteoporosis medications on levels of turnover.2 A study examined the effect of low intensity exercise on bone density by conducting trunk stabilization exercise on females after menopause.[10] In females, trunk stability exercise could not change bone density meaningfully, but it could maintain bone density. There is a risk of osteoporosis and fracture risk in men with prostate cancer.[11]

Important differences exist in the metabolism of bone and mineral and the vitamin D endocrine system between whites and African Americans and include rate of skeletal remodeling, bone mass, and vitamin D metabolism.[12] A higher bone mineral density (BMD) in African Americans is associated with a diminished incidence of osteoporosis and fractures.

Vitamin D insufficiency is more prevalent among African Americans than other Americans and, in North America, most young, healthy Backs do not achieve optimal vitamin D concentrations at any time of year. This is primarily due to the fact that pigmentation reduces vitamin D production in the skin.[13] Lower-weight, older African-American men and women are at significantly increased risk for low bone mineral density and are likely to be at greater risk for osteoporotic fracture.[14] Vitamin D deficiency in older African Americans is associated with lower bone mineral density of the hips.[15]

Diabetes is also associated with an increased risk of bone fractures. However, bone mineral density, falls, diabetes complications nor other risk factors can explain why these fractures occur in this population. Among patients with diabetes, hyperglycaemia may have detrimental effects on bone, but also use of anti-diabetic treatment may have an impact on fracture risk.[16]

References

1.   Gilsanz V, Skaggs DL, Kovanlikaya A, et al. Differential effect of race on the axial and appendicular skeletons of children. J Clin Endocrinol Metab. 1998;83(5):1420-1427.

2.   Crandall CJ, Miller-Martinez D, Greendale GA, Binkley N, Seeman TE, Karlamangla AS. Socioeconomic status, race, and bone turnover in the Midlife in the US Study. Osteoporos Int. 2012;23(5):1503-1512.

3.   Kimura K. Aging of bone density in the second metacarpal. Okajimas Folia Anat Jpn. 1991;68(4):251-257.

4.   Li L, Brennan KJ, Gaughan JP, Ciccolella DE, Kuzma AM, Criner GJ. African Americans and men with severe COPD have a high prevalence of osteoporosis. COPD. 2008;5(5):291-297.

5.   Ross PD, Norimatsu H, Davis JW, et al. A comparison of hip fracture incidence among native Japanese, Japanese Americans, and American Caucasians. Am J Epidemiol. 1991;133(8):801-809.

6.   Scane AC, Sutcliffe AM, Francis RM. Osteoporosis in men. Baillieres Clin Rheumatol. 1993;7(3):589-601.

7.   Vasquez E, Shaw BA, Gensburg L, Okorodudu D, Corsino L. Racial and ethnic differences in physical activity and bone density: National Health and Nutrition Examination Survey, 2007-2008. Prev Chronic Dis. 2013;10:E216.

8.   Wang YX, Griffith JF, Zeng XJ, et al. Prevalence and sex difference of lumbar disc space narrowing in elderly chinese men and women: osteoporotic fractures in men (Hong Kong) and osteoporotic fractures in women (Hong Kong) studies. Arthritis Rheum. 2013;65(4):1004-1010.

9.   Riggs BL, Melton LJ, 3rd. The prevention and treatment of osteoporosis. N Engl J Med. 1992;327(9):620-627.

10.   Kang JI, Jeong DK, Choi H. The effects of trunk stabilization exercise on bone density after menopause. J Phys Ther Sci. 2015;27(12):3869-3872.

11.   Grey A. Osteoporosis and Fracture Risk in Men with Prostate Cancer. Eur Urol. 2015.

12.   Bell NH. Bone and mineral metabolism in African Americans. Trends Endocrinol Metab. 1997;8(6):240-245.

13.   Harris SS. Vitamin D and African Americans. J Nutr. 2006;136(4):1126-1129.

14.   Robbins J, Hirsch C, Cauley J. Associates of bone mineral density in older African Americans. Journal of the National Medical Association. 2004;96(12):1609-1615.

15.   Wilkins CH, Birge SJ, Sheline YI, Morris JC. Vitamin D deficiency is associated with worse cognitive performance and lower bone density in older African Americans. Journal of the National Medical Association. 2009;101(4):349-354.

16.   Starup-Linde J, Karahasanovic A, Vestergaard P, Eiken P. [Diabetes increases the risk of fractures]. Ugeskr Laeger. 2015;177(49):V08150663.

21. Irritable Bowel Syndrome

Pain in your abdomen can be disabling and can be severe. Abdominal pain in general occurs more often in women than in men. However, the incidence of abdominal pain decreases with age. Stress, diet, and the work environment are potential causes of abdominal pain in general. Your gastrointestinal pain will decline after age 40. The pattern of declining abdominal pain is consistent in both sexes. However, overall, the incidence of abdominal pain is higher in women than in men from childhood years to old age. These findings of various abdominal pains include pain in your upper, mid, or lower abdomen. Cramping and intermittent pain is easily caused by disorders of your bowel, gallbladder, ureter, or fallopian tubes. Age, education and urban/rural type of living were not related to the prevalence of IBS. IBS in females was higher in females than in males.

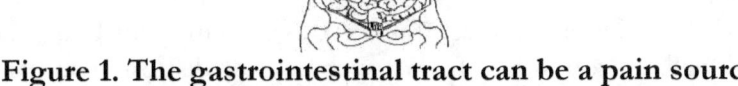

Figure 1. The gastrointestinal tract can be a pain source.

A common syndrome in adults is the irritable bowel syndrome (IBS), which is frequently diagnosed in the general population. Approximately 30 percent of patients seen by gastroenterologists suffer from IBS. It is more common in women and may even be seen in adolescents. If you have IBS, this disease can impair your quality of life. This disease has begun to become more closely studied and the pharmaceutical industry has begun marketing new drugs to decrease the symptoms of IBS.

The exact cause of IBS remains to be defined. IBS has become a defined clinical entity. IBS can be caused by physiological, psychological, and behavioral factors. Sometimes you may have severe symptoms without any physical findings. A diagnosis of IBS is determined by your symptoms. If you have IBS, you will frequently report pain or discomfort in your stomach area. Age, education and urban/rural type of living were not related to the prevalence of IBS but the female gender is related.[1]

Non-white IBS patients experience impairment in vitality, role limitations and bodily pain similar to white patients. [2]

The frequency of irritable bowel syndrome-type symptoms is greater in females than in males and is less in Hispanics than non-Hispanic whites. Additionally, females report more alternating bowel pattern and constipation than males and non-Hispanic white females more abdominal pain than the other subgroups. Ethnic differences in dietary factors that may be relevant to bowel function in ethnic groups.[3] Substantial similarities as well as differences in IBS patients of the two races support the concept that, while there is an important role for a biological component to the pathogenesis of IBS, it by itself may not be an exclusive determinant.[4]

This pain is not confined to one area of your gut but it is global over your stomach. Usually this abdominal pain is relieved followed a bowel movement. You may suffer diarrhea alternating with constipation. You can suffer bloating or the feeling of incomplete evacuation of your stool. Some investigators believe that your colon is the cause of IBS. You can have symptoms daily or you may have symptoms once a week or once a month. If you have IBS, you may also have heartburn and nausea. If you have IBS, you can suffer from fibromyalgia or other muscle pains. You can have headaches or bladder symptoms. In addition to other body disturbances, you may also suffer from chronic fatigue and significant depression.

IBS can involve the central nervous system (your brain and spinal cord) as well. If you suffer from psychological distress, you can have a negative effect on your central nervous system that may send signals to your peripheral nervous system and cause you to have hypersensitivity with respect to your gastrointestinal (mouth to rectum) system. IBS can coexist with ulcerative colitis or Crohn's disease. If you suffer from IBS, the underlying causes may be psychological.

Pain associated with IBS can be a result of depression or other illness. If you have psychosocial factors, these factors can influence the frequency of your symptoms as well as the severity of your symptoms. If you suffer from IBS, you may have a history of physical, sexual, or emotional abuse. Usually extensive diagnostic tests are not utilized for your doctor to diagnose your IBS because there are no definitive tests for this disease.

A diagnostic criterion for the diagnosis of IBS is hard to establish because of the variety of physical complaints associated with IBS. In other words, the pattern of the pain as well as the location and severity differs among patients. To be diagnosed with IBS, you need to have abdominal pain first of all. Your pain must be relieved with a bowel movement. The onset of your pain must be associated with a change in the frequency of your stool habits. The onset of your pain must be associated with a change in the appearance of your stool. You may possibly have IBS if you have an abnormal stool (in which it differs in appearance from usual stool appearance) one out of every four defecations.

Be aware that just because you have continuation of your symptoms, this does not justify expensive diagnostic testing. You do not have a severe life-threatening medical disease if you have IBS. Your doctor will reassure you that you do not have a dangerous disease. If you do notice blood in your stool, notify your doctor so that your doctor can determine whether or not you need further diagnostic tests. If you develop weight loss, symptoms that are worse at night, blood in your stools or have a family history of colon cancer, follow up with your doctor.

If you have feelings of having to strain or have a feeling of incomplete evacuation of your stool in one out of four defecations, you may possibly have IBS. If you have bloating or abdominal distention in one out of four days or passage of mucus in one out of four defecations, there is a high probability that you have IBS. You should have symptoms for at least 12 weeks or more over the previous 12 months. Your symptoms do not have to be consecutive.

Approximately 70 percent of individuals with IBS have only mild symptoms. On the other hand, 25 percent of patients have symptoms that can interfere with work, school, or social functions. Approximately 5 percent of individuals have severe symptoms that severely limit their activities of daily living and their quality of life. If you have mild or moderate symptoms, these symptoms can be managed by your primary care doctor. You may only need a dietary or lifestyle change.

Be aware that upper abdominal pain not associated with ulcers can be present in 50 percent of the IBS population and nausea and vomiting can also be present in 50 percent of the IBS population. Increased urination among women is also associated with IBS. Women who have IBS can also have chronic pelvic pain and other gynecological symptoms. If you have a history of physical or sexual abuse or have suffered the loss of a parent or other important person during childhood, you are more prone to develop IBS. You can have sexual dysfunction if you have IBS. Decreased sexual drive has been seen in both men and women who suffer from IBS. If you are a female, you may suffer significant stomach pains premenstrually. Stomach pain as well as pelvic cramping was noted to be higher in individuals with IBS during menses.

At one time, doctors thought that IBS was a psychosomatic (mental) entity. If you suffer from IBS, you are not "crazy." It is now known that nerves in your gastrointestinal system can become oversensitive, causing them to overreact to both gas as well as food passing by these nerves. The stimulation of your nerves in your gastrointestinal tract will cause you to have pain as well as cramping. Current studies reveal that symptoms associated with IBS are not imagined but are real and have a neurological basis.

If you have moderate symptoms, you may require psychological treatment and occasionally pharmacologic management. If you have severe and constant symptoms, you may require antidepressants as well as psychological testing and treatment and you may need to be referred to a gastroenterologist. As previously stated, your doctor may want to test for parasites in your blood. A general consensus among treating doctors in general is that you do not need extensive testing when you initially present to your doctor. You will be re-evaluated over time and any additional diagnostic tests will be done depending on your clinical status and your response to treatment.

More than 50 percent of patients with IBS who were seen in gastroenterologist clinics had psychiatric problems. The possibility of developing IBS is extremely high in individuals who suffer panic disorders. If you have depression, you are also prone to IBS. Greater sympathetic nervous system responses to abdominal pain have been reported in men when compared to women. Studies have demonstrated that men have heightened sympathetic nervous system activation. In other words, women have lower sympathetic nervous system activation when compared to men.

IBS occurs less frequently among older adults than among younger patients. While IBS affects the quality of life at all ages, social functioning was actually better on average among older compared to younger IBS patients.[5] The IBS symptoms have equal applicability to both genders and to African-Americans as well as to Caucasians.[6]

In 1917, a German scientist determined that in the wall of the gut was a self-contained nervous system that could function on its own without impulses from either the brain or the spinal cord. In other words, your gut has a brain of its own. Small nerves are in the lining of your esophagus, stomach, small intestine, and your colon. Because of new findings associated with IBS, a pharmaceutical company has developed a drug called Lotronex. This drug can help manage your symptoms associated with IBS.

Your brain can affect the nerves in your stomach, on the other hand. For example, if you are anxious or have to give a speech in front of a large crowd, you may develop "butterflies" in your stomach. In other words, you feel the effect of your stress within your gastrointestinal system. If you are facing a stressful situation, your brain can influence specialized cells in your gastrointestinal system called mast cells to release histamine. Histamine makes the nerves in your gastrointestinal system to contract the smooth muscle in your gut. This will cause you to have cramps. It can also cause you to have diarrhea. Be aware that medications that affect your brain can also affect your gut.

There was a significant sex difference in mean number of stools per week with Hispanic males greater than Hispanic females and non-Hispanic white males greater than non-Hispanic white females. The frequency of irritable bowel syndrome-type symptoms was greater in females than in males and was less in Hispanics than non-Hispanic whites. Hispanic females reported more alternating bowel pattern and constipation than males, and non-Hispanic white females reported more abdominal pain.[3]

Prozac can work on serotonin in your brain and spinal cord but also cause you to have abdominal cramping and diarrhea. Anti-anxiety drugs are currently being studied to determine whether they can decrease your symptoms associated with your IBS. Imitrex, which is used to treat migraine headaches, is being studied for the treatment of your IBS symptoms. Lotronex is an anxiety type of drug. This drug is becoming increasingly popular for the treatment of IBS.

IBS has become the most diagnosed but the least understood medical ailment. Lotronex is used to treat abdominal pain and discomfort in female patients. Be aware that more individuals suffer from IBS than asthma or diabetes. Lotronex is the first drug approved by the FDA to be used for IBS treatment. At one time, you did not hear much information about IBS in the lay press. The reason for this was that subjects about the bowels and defecation were considered taboo by the press. Now you may note that there are television advertisements touting the use of medications for the treatment of IBS. It is important for you to be able to talk to your doctor openly about your IBS. You must talk openly and not suffer any embarrassment when you talk to your health-care provider about your symptoms. As people age, the incidences of women suffering from IBS outnumber men by three to one.

A new drug that was available in 2006 is called Zelnorm. However, The FDA announced that this irritable bowel syndrome drug was voluntarily taken off the market because of possible cardiovascular risks by the drug manufacturer. It was a drug that is in a class of medications called gastrointestinal serotonin agonists. This drug was used for the treatment of constipation, bloating, and abdominal pain. In the United Kingdom, another drug called renzapride was studied for the treatment of IBS. Preliminary studies that were done with respect to this drug for the treatment of IBS symptoms were extremely promising.

Renzapride was not shown to be superior to placebo in relieving IBS symptoms and caused significant incidences of diarrhea and drop-outs due to adverse effects in treated patients. Thus, this medicine might be a cost burden to patients without providing good effectiveness.[7] Research however, continues into the development of new drugs for the treatment of IBS because this disease costs the health-care system approximately $30 billion per year.

Sometimes anti-anxiety drugs can be used for the treatment of your IBS. Anti-anxiety drugs can be effective if you get abdominal cramps when you become stressed. In addition to the utilization of drugs for the treatment of your IBS, also consider meditation, exercise, yoga, and getting enough sleep. All of these methods can decrease your stress, which ultimately could decrease your symptoms associates with IBS. Another method that you may want to consider for the treatment of your IBS is hypnosis. Hypnosis has been shown to be effective for the treatment of symptoms associated with IBS.

Sex steroids may work to modulate abdominal pain associated with IBS. They can have direct effects on your gastrointestinal motility and inhibit the emptying of your stomach. Studies have shown that premenopausal and postmenopausal women who are taking hormones had slower stomach-emptying times with solids when compared with men and when compared with postmenopausal women who were not taking hormones. Testosterone has no influence on the gastric emptying in men. However, estrogen and progesterone will slow down the gastric emptying time in men. A study has demonstrated that a male's complaint of discomfort with distention of a balloon in the male's rectum was higher if the male had a low testosterone level.

Non-white IBS patients experience impairment in vitality, physical limitations, and bodily pain. Yet overall, non-white IBS patients report similar quality of life limitations to white IBS patients.[2]

When considering your treatment for your IBS, your doctor will assure you that your symptoms are not from a serious illness. Your doctor will recommend a change in your diet with an emphasis on a high-fiber diet and low fat. You will be prescribed medications for constipation, diarrhea, and pain. You may require antidepressant medication as well as psychological intervention. Because of the differences in gender with the prevalence of IBS, pharmaceutical companies are now looking at gender as they search for new IBS gender-specific medications. One drug company has asked for approval to study the drug for the treatment of IBS in women only. Early studies have revealed that Alosetron may demonstrate gender specificity for the treatment of IBS in women.

If you have severe IBS, you may have had stomach and bowel problems all of your life. If you have IBS, you will be fearful that your symptoms can occur at any moment. As a result, you will always attempt to know where the closest restroom is. As a result, this can influence your social interaction. Traveling can become a problem for you. In addition to the medication mentioned, dietary fiber and biofeedback as well as occasional antidepressants can alleviate your symptoms.

If you suffer from IBS, you may want to minimize your fat intake. Many foods inhibit your intestinal gas transit. By decreasing the passage of gas through your gastrointestinal system, bloating and the expansion of your bowel can cause you to have pain. Fructose is another food substance that can worsen your IBS symptoms. Fructose is found in honey, fruit, and in some soft drinks. Fructose can cause you to have bloating, cramps, and diarrhea. Bacteria in your colon may use fructose as their food source. In the process of utilizing fructose, hydrogen gas is liberated in your colon from the breakdown of sugars.

Inflammatory (as opposed to irritable) bowel disease is another entity that can also cause you to have significant pain. Both IBS and inflammatory bowel diseases have similar symptoms. Your IBS is characterized by pathology within your intestine. Both IBS as well as inflammatory bowel disease can be affected by stress. They both can be affected by your central nervous system as well as your immune system within your gastrointestinal system. Antibiotics and anti-inflammatory agents are used in inflammatory bowel syndromes. There has been some suggestion that these pharmacologic methods can be useful also in IBS.

Inflammatory bowel disease is believed to be a disease of your immune system. IBS can respond to diet. However, the inflammatory bowel disease rarely responds to changes in diet. Inflammatory bowel disease includes ulcerative colitis and Crohn's disease. Ulcerative colitis is a chronic disease and a recurrent disease. It involves inflammation of the lining of the colon. It can also involve your rectum. Crohn's disease can involve any part of your gastrointestinal tract, including your mouth all the way to your anus. The cause of Crohn's disease and ulcerative colitis are unknown.

Inflammatory bowel disease is more common in Caucasians and more common in Jewish men and women. The incidence is almost equal in men and women. The incidence of ulcerative colitis and Crohn's disease is similar. Usually inflammatory bowel disease begins in early adult life. However, there are cases reported in the elderly. Genetic factors can make you prone to inflammatory bowel disease. If you have a disorder of your immune system, you are again prone to develop irritable bowel disease. It is possible that your immune system may attack the lining of your gastrointestinal system. Emotional stress can worsen your symptoms of inflammatory bowel disease.

Crohn's disease usually involves the lower ileum (the lowest part of the small intestine). Your rectum can be involved. Approximately one third of Crohn's disease patients have their pathology in the colon, whereas one third of patients have their pathology in the ileum and one third have their pathology in both the ilem and colon. The inflammation of your gastrointestinal system can go from the inside of your bowel to the outside. The inner lining of your gastrointestinal system can develop ulcers. An ulcer is a break in the lining of the wall of your gut. This break in your gut lining can fail to heal and can be accompanied by inflammation. A fistula from the inside of your bowel to the outside can develop. A fistula is an abnormal communication between a hollow organ and the exterior.

With Crohn's disease, you can have fever, diarrhea, pain, and tenderness in the right lower part of your abdomen. You can also develop an abscess around your anus. The inner aspect of your intestine or colon can decrease in diameter, which is called a stricture. If you have Crohn's disease, you can have an increased incidence of gallstones. The bile salts are not absorbed properly through your ileum. You can also develop kidney stones. You can have a history of frequent liquid bowel movements.

Because of absorption problems of nutrients, you may have a poor nutritional status. You can feel fatigued and suffer from a loss of energy. If your bowel becomes swollen, you can feel the inflamed bowel, which feels like a mass. This thickened loop of inflamed bowel can be tender to deep palpation. If you develop a tract from the inside of your bowel to the outside, this fistula can cause you to develop an abscess behind the lining of your bowel. You will have fever, chills, and tenderness to deep palpation about your abdomen. Your health-care provider will obtain a complete blood count from you.

A chronic inflammation of your gastrointestinal system can cause you to have anemia. You may suffer from iron deficiency or a vitamin B12 deficiency. Your gastrointestinal system may not be able to absorb protein. Your doctor may want to obtain a stool sample from you and have it examined for parasites. Your doctor will want to do an x-ray series involving your upper gastrointestinal system. A barium enema and a colonoscopy may be necessary as well.

A barium enema is an enema with opaque contrast liquid that outlines your intestines on x-ray images. This test helps your doctor look for abnormalities in your bowel. To examine your lower bowel, your doctor may also use air with the barium to distend your bowel. Through the colonoscope (a flexible fiberoptic instrument), your doctor can obtain biopsies of your colon and ilium. White blood cells protect your body against foreign substances. If your white cells are elevated and your abdomen is tender, this will necessitate a CT of your abdomen (because you might have a serious infection). You will be given antibiotics and will be given nutritional supplements. Occasionally surgery is required to drain the abscess.

If your gastrointestinal system develops an obstruction somewhere in your system, your food cannot pass through this obstruction. You will be treated with fluids through your veins, and a tube will be placed through your nose to suction out substances that are unable to pass through your bowel. Steroids can be necessary to treat the inflammation caused by Crohn's disease. Be aware that chronic cramping, abdominal pain, and diarrhea are noted in both IBS and Crohn's disease.

The problem with Crohn's disease is that it is a lifelong illness. You must eat a well-balanced diet. If you have Crohn's disease, you may have intolerance to milk products. You may need B12 shots monthly. Steroids are usually indicated as part of your treatment. Your diarrhea will be treated pharmacologically. Your doctor will treat your pain with the appropriate pain medication.

Medicines for Crohn's disease include: aminosalicylates (sulfasalazine). These medicines help manage symptoms, Antibiotics (such as ciprofloxacin or metronidazole) may help. These may be tried if aminosalicylates aren't helping. They are also used to treat fistulas and abscesses. Corticosteroids (prednisone) may be given for a few weeks or months to control swelling. These steroid medicines usually stop symptoms and put the disease in remission. But they are not used as long-term treatment to keep symptoms from coming back. Medicines that suppress the immune system (methotrexate) may be used as well. Cyclosporine and intravenous corticosteroids, may be needed for severe cases.

If you smoke, stop smoking; smoking can cause you to have a recurrence of Crohn's symptoms. If conservative treatments fail, you may require surgery. As previously stated, there is no cure for the disease. However with proper medical and surgical treatment, you should be able to cope with this disease as well as its complications and lead a productive life. Ulcerative colitis is another form of inflammatory bowel disease.

Ulcerative colitis involves the inner lining of your colon. You remember that Crohn's disease can go through the entire lining of your gastrointestinal system. You will have bloody diarrhea if you have ulcerative colitis. You will have pain in your abdomen. You will develop anemia and the protein in your bloodstream, albumin, will be decreased. A scope in your colon is the key to the diagnosis of your disease.

With respect to children and ethnicity, the incidence of Ulcerative Colitis revealed that Hispanic and Asian children had development of Ulcerative Colitis (UC) more often than Crohn's disease (CD), suggesting possible etiologic differences across racial and ethnic groups.[8] There are significant differences in Irritable Bowel Disease subtypes and serologic markers among racial/ ethnic groups with IBD in the United States. However, African Americans and whites predominantly had CD, whereas Mexican Americans predominantly had UC. There was no difference between African Americans and Mexican Americans when separately compared to whites in terms of intestinal manifestations of CD and UC. IBS occurs less frequently among African Americans. Although IBS affects quality of life among both ethnicities, the degree of impairment is similar however.[9]

Be aware that other structures in your abdomen can cause you to have abdominal pain. If you have a problem in one of the major arteries, for instance, you can have abdominal pain. It is difficult for your health-care provider to diagnose and treat your pain without a detailed history of your symptoms as well as with an examination. For this reason, you must keep an accurate pain diary. You may need x-rays or an MRI. Your examination by your doctor will be important. Your kidneys and ureters (as well as your ovaries and uterus if you are a female) can cause you to have abdominal pain on occasion.

With respect to race, appendicitis and diverticular disease were comparatively low in most non-White groups, while ulcerative colitis and Crohn's disease were mostly higher in South Asians.[10]

Endometriosis is a common and painful disorder in women where tissue that normally lines the inside of the uterus becomes implanted on tissue outside the uterus. This can cause women to have pain in their abdomen. However, organs that are part of your gastrointestinal system are usually the cause of your abdominal pain. If you have pain in your upper abdomen on the right side, you may have an inflamed gallbladder or an ulcer. Hepatitis can cause you to have pain. Pancreatitis, a painful inflammation of the pancreas, can cause pain in your mid abdomen that radiates to your back. Renal stones and kidney stones on occasion can cause abdominal pain in addition to pain in your flanks.

Interstitial cystitis is an inflammatory disease of your bladder that can cause you to have lower abdominal pain. If your abdominal pain is associated with your menstrual cycle, keep a diary of how the pain is affected. Ovarian cysts can cause you to have pain in your lower abdomen. Abdominal pain is the pain that you feel in your abdominal area which is between your chest and groin. Another term for abdomen is your stomach or "belly." Always be aware that pain in your abdomen can originate from your chest or your pelvis (the area below your abdomen).

There are many organs in your body. You can have pain in any one of these organs. For example, you can have pain in your stomach, your large and small intestines, your liver, gallbladder, and pancreas, for instance. Your aorta, which is a major blood vessel that comes off of your heart, runs down through your abdomen. If you have an aneurysm, which is a defect in the wall of this great vessel, you can have pain in your abdomen. An aneurysm needs to be evaluated by your doctor. An aneurysm is a weakness in the wall of your aorta. This weak area could rupture, which could be fatal.

Your appendix, if it is inflamed, can cause you to have abdominal pain as well. Your appendix is part of your gastrointestinal system. A viral infection in your intestine or gas can cause you to have significant abdominal pain. As you probably know, this pain can be severe.

This should alert you that the severity of the pain does not correlate with the severity of the disease. In other words, you can have cancer of your colon and have only mild pain. Causes of abdominal pain include gas, constipation, milk intolerance, stomach flu, an irritable bowel syndrome, indigestion, esophageal reflux, ulcers, gallstones, and diverticular disease.

If you have an obstruction of your bowel, you can have significant disabling pain. A food allergy can cause you to have gastrointestinal pain. Kidney stones and urinary tract infections can also cause you to have pain. If you have a sickle cell crisis, you can also experience abdominal pain. Crohn's disease and ulcerative colitis are two types of inflammatory bowel disease that can cause you to suffer significant pain. If one of your inflamed organs ruptures, you will have excruciating pain and your stomach will be as hard as a board. You will probably have a fever associated with this pain. These symptoms are usually seen in peritonitis. Peritonitis is an inflammation of the membrane which lines your abdominal cavity.

If you have abdominal pain that occurs during your period, your pain may be from menstrual cramps. Pneumonia can cause you to have referred abdominal pain, and even a heart attack can occasionally cause you to experience abdominal pain. Cancer of the stomach, colon, and pancreas can also cause abdominal pain. Emotional upset can also cause you to have abdominal pain.

Parasites as well as helicobacter pylori can cause you to have abdominal pain. This bacterium is called in microbiological terms gram-negative bacteria and can be found in the moist membrane lining of your stomach. It can cause you to develop a progressive gastritis (an inflammation of the lining of your stomach) as well as stomach cancer, heart disease, and gastric and duodenal ulcers. Your doctor will help your body eradicate this bacterium with antibiotics and other drugs.

Keep a diary of your stool frequency and note the amount of rectal bleeding, cramps, and abdominal pain that you have. If you have frequent diarrhea, the fluid volume of your body can become depleted. You may have up to 10 bloody bowel movements a day, which can cause you to develop severe anemia. If you have ulcerative colitis, you may also have ankylosing spondylitis, which is an arthritic type of disease that can affect your joints. Plain x-rays of your abdomen can be helpful for the diagnosis of ulcerative colitis. There may be increases in the diameter of your colon in certain areas of your abdomen.

Sometimes children can have abdominal pain. The ratio of girls to boys with abdominal pain is four to three. There can be a psychological origin of their abdominal pain in a significant number of these children. Chronic abdominal pain in children without obvious pathology such as a diseased appendix is psychogenic in approximately 90 percent of cases. Psycogenic means that the origin is in your mind as opposed to your body. The etiology of this abdominal pain arises from stress, anxiety, and/or depression. Sometimes this entity can be caused by inflammatory bowel disease or an ulcer.

You need to keep a diary as to whether or not your pain is severe, cramping, persistent, or constant. Does your pain only awaken you at night? Have you ever had a similar pain pattern previously? How often do you have the pain? In other words, does it occur daily, weekly, or monthly? Does it occur after meals? Is the pain referred to your back, shoulder blades, or legs?

Is it worse after lying down or after drinking or eating greasy foods? Is the pain worse with stress? Is your pain relieved after eating or after drinking milk? What medicines are you taking? If you are taking over-the-counter nonsteroidal anti-inflammatory drugs, you need to tell your doctor. Have you had a recent injury to your stomach? As you can see, your history is important factors in helping your doctor diagnose what is causing your abdominal pain.

Sometimes your doctor will obtain laboratory values, including blood samples, stool samples, and a urinalysis. An x-ray of your abdomen may be necessary to diagnose the cause of your pain. A barium enema or an upper GI and small bowel series are sometimes done as well. A scope can be placed into your gastrointestinal tract to attempt to diagnose the cause of your pain as well.

The treatment goal of any gastrointestinal disease is twofold. The first is your doctor will terminate your acute symptoms (symptoms of recent onset and not necessarily of great severity), and then your doctor will attempt to prevent a recurrence of your symptoms. If you have mild symptoms, eat a regular balanced diet but decrease your intake of caffeine and any vegetables that can produce gas. Fiber supplements decrease diarrhea. Your doctor may prescribe medications for you to take for your diarrhea. If your disease is confined to your rectum, your doctor may prescribe topical medications only. Topical steroids and steroid suppositories can also be used.

If you have mild to moderate symptoms, you will be given oral medications. Taking fiber supplements, such as psyllium (Metamucil) or methylcellulose (Citrucel), with fluids may help control constipation. Fiber obtained from food may cause much more bloating compared with a fiber supplement. Over-the-counter medications, such as loperamide (Imodium), can help control diarrhea. Some people will benefit from medications called bile acid binders, such as cholestyramine (Prevalite), colestipol (Colestid) or colesevelam (Welchol), but these can lead to bloating. medications, such as hyoscyamine (Levsin) and dicyclomine (Bentyl), can help relieve painful bowel spasms.

If your symptoms include pain or depression, your doctor may recommend a tricyclic antidepressant or a selective serotonin reuptake inhibitor (SSRI). These medications help relieve depression as well as inhibit the activity of neurons that control the intestines. Some people whose symptoms are due to an overgrowth of bacteria in their intestines may benefit from antibiotic treatment. Some people with symptoms of diarrhea have benefited from rifaximin (Xifaxan), but more research is needed.

Sulfasalazine can be prescribed to treat your symptoms. Mesalamine can also be used. For some reason, the use of a nicotine patch has been shown to be effective in some patients suffering from this disease. The reason for this finding remains unknown. Steroid enemas can be used to treat your symptoms. Oral steroids can be used as well. If you develop severe symptoms, you may require hospitalization. Approximately 15 percent of individuals with ulcerative colitis develop symptoms that are severe. You must stop all oral intakes. You will require fluids. Stop all opioid drugs. If your disease progresses, your fluid volume can decrease and this can make you dehydrated. You may require blood transfusions if you are hemorrhaging.

If your abdomen distends and becomes increasingly tender, you run the risk of perforation of your bowel (the creation of a hole in your tissue). Your colon can become excessively dilated. This finding is in less than two percent of cases of ulcerative colitis. This expansion of your bowel can cause a decrease in the blood flow to the bowel tissue. This is called toxic megacolon. If you have this disease, you run the risk of developing colon cancer. If your symptoms remain severe, you may require surgery.

Severe bleeding as well as the perforation of your bowel are indications for surgery. You may want to try to avoid surgery because of your self-image as you will probably require placement of an external pouch to evacuate your feces. However, if your colon is removed, your surgeon may be able to do a surgical procedure where you don't need an ostomy (opening into a tissue). Be aware that ulcerative colitis is a lifelong disease. In most instances, your symptoms will be controlled by medical therapy. You probably will not need surgery. You may never need hospitalization. Be aware that if you do need surgery, however, this could result in a complete cure of your disease. If you do suffer from ulcerative colitis, you have a better overall prognosis than if you suffer from Crohn's disease.

Nonwhite patients who presented to an emergency room in 2011 for abdominal pain were less likely than whites to receive analgesia and waited longer for their opiate medication.[11]   Numerous studies have shown differences in pain perception between men and women, which may affect pain management strategies. Younger patients received less potent analgesic treatment.[12] There is no reason for certain groups to receive suboptimal treatment, and greater efforts should be made to offer consistent treatment to all patients.

Prior studies have suggested gender-based differences in the care of elderly patients with acute medical conditions such as myocardial infarction and stroke, but it is unknown whether these differences are seen in the care of abdominal pain. Unlike prior research in younger patients with abdominal pain and among elders with other acute conditions, we noted no difference in management and diagnoses between older men and women who presented with abdominal pain.[13]

References

1.   Baretic M, Bilic A, Jurcic D, et al. Epidemiology of irritable bowel syndrome in Croatia. Coll Antropol. 2002;26 Suppl:85-91.

2.   Gralnek IM, Hays RD, Kilbourne AM, Chang L, Mayer EA. Racial differences in the impact of irritable bowel syndrome on health-related quality of life. J Clin Gastroenterol. 2004;38(9):782-789.

3.   Zuckerman MJ, Guerra LG, Drossman DA, Foland JA, Gregory GG. Comparison of bowel patterns in Hispanics and non-Hispanic whites. Dig Dis Sci. 1995;40(8):1763-1769.

4.   Minocha A, Bollineni D, Johnson WD, Wigington WC. Racial differences in general health, suicidal thoughts, physical and sexual abuse in African-Americans and Caucasians with irritable bowel syndrome. South Med J. 2010;103(8):764-770.

5.   Minocha A, Johnson WD, Abell TL, Wigington WC. Prevalence, sociodemography, and quality of life of older versus younger patients with irritable bowel syndrome: a population-based study. Dig Dis Sci. 2006;51(3):446-453.

6.   Taub E, Cuevas JL, Cook EW, 3rd, Crowell M, Whitehead WE. Irritable bowel syndrome defined by factor analysis. Gender and race comparisons. Dig Dis Sci. 1995;40(12):2647-2655.

7.   Mozaffari S, Nikfar S, Abdollahi M. Efficacy and tolerability of renzapride in irritable bowel syndrome: a meta-analysis of

randomized, controlled clinical trials including 2528 patients. Arch Med Sci. 2014;10(1):10-18.

8.   Abramson O, Durant M, Mow W, et al. Incidence, prevalence, and time trends of pediatric inflammatory bowel disease in Northern California, 1996 to 2006. J Pediatr. 2010;157(2):233-239 e231.

9.   Wigington WC, Johnson WD, Minocha A. Epidemiology of irritable bowel syndrome among African Americans as compared with whites: a population-based study. Clin Gastroenterol Hepatol. 2005;3(7):647-653.

10.   Bhopal RS, Cezard G, Bansal N, Ward HJ, Bhala N, researchers S. Ethnic variations in five lower gastrointestinal diseases: Scottish health and ethnicity linkage study. BMJ Open. 2014;4(10):e006120.

11.   Mills AM, Shofer FS, Boulis AK, Holena DN, Abbuhl SB. Racial disparity in analgesic treatment for ED patients with abdominal or back pain. Am J Emerg Med. 2011;29(7):752-756.

12.   Banz VM, Christen B, Paul K, et al. Gender, age and ethnic aspects of analgesia in acute abdominal pain: is analgesia even across the groups? Intern Med J. 2012;42(3):281-288.

13.   Gardner RL, Almeida R, Maselli JH, Auerbach A. Does gender influence emergency department management and outcomes in geriatric abdominal pain? J Emerg Med. 2010;39(3):275-281.

22. Fibromyalgia

Fibromyalgia is a chronic pain syndrome that affects soft tissue, tendons, and fascia. Fibromyalgia can be a debilitating, chronic pain disorder.[1] Also referred to as fibromyositis, it affects about 5 percent of the population, 90 percent of which are women of childbearing age. Chronic means that your doctor does not have an immediate fix for your pain. You must choose a physician who you feel comfortable with because you will probably see this person every month. You and your doctor must take control of your pain and not let your pain control your life. Changes in diet and exercise or lack of exercise must be addressed by you and your physician. You and your physician must function together as a team.

Fibromyalgia (FM) has been described and studied in various sociocultural settings in both developed and developing countries. For example, FM is relatively common in the unique setting of Muslim Bedouin women and has a very significant impact on their quality of life as well as on their dependents.[2] FM exists in Latin America as well.[3]

Fibromyalgia causes you to have muscle pain throughout the body, joint stiffness, and fatigue. You also may experience sleep disturbances and depression. It can cause many places on your body to become extremely tender. You are only diagnosed with fibromyalgia after other pain-causing conditions have been eliminated as the reason for your pain. Fibromyalgia is a condition that can be painful, but it is benign and will rarely cause you to be totally disabled. Only you can let it become disabling.

The reasons for diagnosing fibromyalgia vary and are based on the complaints that you have mentioned to your doctor. Right now no laboratory tests lead to a specific diagnosis of fibromyalgia, so your doctors must rely on you to explain the specific complications you are having. Your doctor also will test you by taking a small amount of blood from your vein to make sure that you do not have arthritis or another condition that could be causing your pain. You must tell your doctor if you have been bitten by tics or mosquitoes in the past six months, because West Nile virus symptoms and Lyme disease symptoms may mimic the symptoms of fibromyalgia.

The criteria for the diagnosis fibromyalgia are as follows: aches, pains, and stiffness involving three or more places on your body for at least three months. No traumatic injury to your body. Your symptoms of pain either get better or get worse when you do a lot of physical activity. Your pain gets worse when the weather changes. Your pain gets worse when you are under a lot of stress. You have a history of anxiety. You have a history of a lot of headaches. You have a history of irritable bowel syndrome. Your doctor finds tender spots on your body in at least 12 of 14 specific places. You have a history of being extremely sluggish and tired in the morning. This disturbance is reflected by an overall deficit in a positive affect and an inability to sustain a positive effect in the face of pain and a negative effect.[4]

People without fibromyalgia also may have similar tender points on their body like you do. Their tenderness could be caused by diseases such as rheumatoid arthritis, or they may be experiencing tenderness after a traumatic event such as a whiplash injury or a lifting injury. The difference is that your tender areas will be more sensitive to pressure than the surrounding areas of muscle. In other words, there will be one small extremely tender area of the muscle that is surrounded by a nontender area of the same muscle. It is common for these tender "trigger points" on your body to be extremely sensitive. This is because the fibromyalgia causes you to have a less of a pain tolerance in all the muscles throughout your body.

If you are like other people with fibromyalgia, the muscle pain that you experience is probably most common in your neck and lower back. However, it can affect any muscle part of your body. Your pain can range from sharp or cramping to a burning sensation. Your pain may be worse in one specific area, even though the pain can be felt all over your body. You also will notice that fibromyalgia pain affects tender areas on your body that are symmetrical, or located in the same places on the opposite side of your body.

Tenderness and swelling of the hands or feet is common. Other common places where you may notice tenderness include the areas under the base of the skull; above the shoulder blade, elbows, the buttocks (gluteal muscle); the front of the neck midway from the chin to the collar bone; the chest; the sides of the body over the hip regions; and the inner aspects of the knees.

It is more common for women to have fibromyalgia than men. Because of this, researchers are trying to find gender-specific causes of fibromyalgia. In general the amount of pain that women can withstand is lower than the amount of pain that men can withstand. Some researchers think that the differences in hormones between men and women can cause the differences in the amount of pain they can each withstand. Fibromyalgia is seen mostly in women between 20 and 50 years of age. However, it can affect children and elderly people as well.

FM and FM-like manifestations correlate best with the presence of Caucasian ethnicity, concomitant anxiety or an affective disorder, and to a lesser extent with poorer self-reported physical functioning.5 African American ethnicity is negatively associated with the combination of FM There is no difference noted between those with and without FM with respect to gender, education level, income below poverty level, disease activity or damage.

Caucasian ethnicity was strongly associated with FM and African American ethnicity was negatively associated with FM.[6] Widespread pain and tenderness is highly prevalent in these young women. Racial differences seem to exist; Caucasian women had significantly increased tenderness while African American women had more widespread pain.7 The association of depressive symptoms and pain was stronger in African American women. Education, rather than ethnic identity, has been found to be an important factor in clinical features of FM.[6]

The exact cause of fibromyalgia remains unknown. Studies of muscle tissue in people with fibromyalgia have shown changes that are similar to muscle tissues that have not been used very much. As a fibromyalgia sufferer, you may not be getting enough deep sleep. Even in normal people, not getting enough sleep can produce symptoms of fibromyalgia. It is not known if the lack of deep sleep is a cause of the beginnings of fibromyalgia. Some doctors think the loss of this deep sleep pattern can speed up the symptoms of fibromyalgia once they show up, but they do not think this explains what causes the syndrome.

You may have either an increase or a decrease in blood flow to your muscle tissues. This may be the direct result of an abnormal nervous system. As a result of either an increased blood flow or a decreased blood flow, your blood vessels can become a filter for blood to leak into your muscle tissues. The blood or plasma that is leaking into your muscles is the reason why you may sometimes notice that individual tissues, such as your hands or feet, are swelling up on your body.

If you have a decreased flow of blood to your muscle tissues, the tissue then does not have enough oxygen. This causes a type of pain called ischemic pain (meaning a decrease or loss of oxygen supply to a tissue). This is the type of pain someone having a heart attack may experience. In much the same way, your feeling of pain results when your muscle has a sudden loss of its oxygen supply. In a group of Puerto

Ricans with FM, the number of trigger points was associated with several FM symptoms and comorbidities.[8]

Not having enough oxygen going to your muscle cells lowers the levels of some chemicals in your muscles, causing you to feel pain. Your specific muscle groups that are affected by the fibromyalgia pain will usually become weaker than your other muscles. The rest of your muscle groups should continue to show their normal strength. This weakness in your muscles is what lessens your ability to function normally. On occasion, you may feel overly fatigued.

Hormones and other chemicals released by your body also affect symptoms of pain. Serotonin and norepinepherine are two chemicals in your central nervous system (brain and spinal cord) that calm down pain signals traveling to your brain. Not having enough serotonin going to your brain and spinal cord can cause you to not get enough deep sleep, which can cause symptoms of depression as well as fibromyalgia pain.

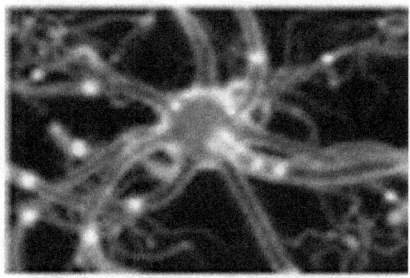

Figure 1. Hyper excitable nerve

Fibromyalgia also affects your levels of norepinepherine, which is a chemical in the central nervous system that functions in response to your short-term stress (such as work-related or spousal problems). Urine studies in people diagnosed with fibromyalgia have shown above normal urinary norepinephrine levels. These same high urinary norepinepherine levels also are seen in patients with anxiety. Just the opposite, people who don't have fibromyalgia, but who have a history of depression, do not show high urinary norepinepherine levels.

Another chemical in your body that causes pain is substance P. Substance P is found basically in all neurons of your central nervous system as well as nerves that go to your muscles. After your muscle tissues have been hurt, substance P is released. This can trigger burning pain sensations in your body. High substance P levels have been noted in the spinal fluid of people with fibromyalgia. Endorphins, substances produced by your body and deposited in the spinal cord to decrease pain transmission to your brain, are known to slow down the pain-causing effects of substance P. The low levels of endorphins in your brain and spinal cord may be another cause of pain associated with this condition. Substance P receptor modulates stress, depression, anxiety and pain. Substance P is increased in the spinal fluid of fibromyalgia patients.[9]

It is well known that vigorous exercise can produce endorphins that are then released in your body. Along with decreasing the pain signals that are sent to your brain, endorphins can affect your mood. It is thought that a lower than normal blood level of endorphins may be another cause of fibromyalgia. People with and without fibromyalgia who do physical exercise have noted a decrease in their pain following aerobic exercise. Normal people usually have an increase in endorphins in their bloodstream following exercise. However, you may show no increase in endorphin levels after you exercise.

Another theory of the cause of fibromyalgia is related to the increase in substance P in the spinal fluid of people with fibromyalgia. An increase in substance P in your spinal fluid can cause the nerves that go to your muscles to become excited. After these nerve endings are stimulated, your muscles will become excited and they will tense up and contract. After they have been contracted for a period of time, your muscles will not get enough blood to them. This causes your muscles to become injured. Incorrect posture also can cause your muscles unnecessary contraction. This can be an additional cause of fibromyalgia.

Researchers have discovered a higher lifetime rate of anxiety and depression among people suffering from fibromyalgia. Your complaints also may be the same as complaints from people who have hormone deficiencies. Growth hormone helps your body to heal muscle trauma. Their production in your body depends on certain sleep patterns. If you do not get enough sleep or you are fatigued a lot, your body may not produce as many growth hormones. If your growth hormone level is decreased, your muscles will not heal as well as they should.

In some studies, injections of growth hormones have decreased the symptoms of fibromyalgia, but many people are unhappy with the overall effects of the growth hormone and the extremely expensive cost of regular injections of growth hormone. You also may have symptoms similar to someone with low thyroid hormone production. This low blood level of thyroid hormone can cause you to have symptoms that include fatigue, weakness, and muscle aches. It is possible that the lower levels of serotonin in your bloodstream and central nervous system cause these symptoms.

Some doctors and researchers think that mental illness also could be a cause of fibromyalgia. Other doctors think that fibromyalgia is a made up expression from people with depression or anxiety. However, in some people with chronic pain, depression and anxiety can be a result of their chronic pain symptoms. About 40 percent of people with fibromyalgia are depressed, whereas 10 percent of the healthy population suffers from depression as well. The common thinking among current is that depression does not cause fibromyalgia, but that it occurs after the fibromyalgia itself sets in.

Your sex hormones interact with the nerves that go out to your arms and legs as well as with the nerves going to and from your spinal cord. They also can affect the nerve pathways in your brain and spinal cord, which are involved in determining how sensitive you are to pain. The sex hormones in your spinal cord can reduce the pain signals that are ultimately going to your brain.

Related to women's hormones, 72 percent of women with fibromyalgia had more pain during the premenstrual phase of their menstrual cycle. This means that right before the beginning of their menstrual cycle, levels of certain hormones are changing that cause women to experience more pain. Women with fibromyalgia have a decrease in a body chemical called nociceptin.10 This is similar to morphine-like chemicals that reduce pain.

Women suffering from fibromyalgia have a lower blood level of nociceptin than do normal women throughout the entire menstrual cycle. This could be a cause for their increase in pain sensitivity during that time. However, women suffering from fibromyalgia do not appear to have a decrease in their symptoms following menopause when their hormone levels are decreasing.

There is increased evidence that fibromyalgia can be genetically inherited. You may even know of a relative who has symptoms similar to yours. The exact gene that causes fibromyalgia has not been isolated, but several genes have been proposed as a possible explanation for the genetic inheritance of fibromyalgia and they are being studied. Research into the causes of fibromyalgia must continue. Continued research may ultimately lead to the answer of why men and women respond to pain differently.

Your understanding of fibromyalgia will diminish some of the fears associated with this disorder that you may have and help you to understand why certain methods of treatment have been prescribed by your doctor. This will help you to become more involved in your own treatment. It is important that you see only one doctor for your treatment of fibromyalgia. This will ensure that your condition is closely and consistently monitored. If you have any concerns about your treatment, tell your doctor.

Always stay away from things that cause you to become stressed or depressed. Stress and depression cause the hormones and other chemicals in your body to become unbalanced and could lead to more symptoms of pain. If you live in a cold environment, it is important that you keep warm to keep your blood flowing properly. Otherwise, your muscles will not get enough oxygen, causing you more muscle injury and pain.

It is a good idea for you to keep a daily diary of your activities and pain levels. When you visit your doctor, be sure to take your diary with you so your doctor can see your daily activities such as exercise, sleep, and eating habits. Also be sure to write down any medications you have taken and what their effects were. This will help your doctor determine what areas you need help in the most, and can help the doctor prescribe an effective treatment to relieve your pain symptoms.

It is important that you do exercise or any type of low-impact aerobic activity. Aerobic exercise is extremely helpful in decreasing your pain and improving your sleep pattern. Swimming and water aerobics are excellent ways for you to accomplish this goal. They are some of the best exercise activities for patients with fibromyalgia. These types of nonimpact activities will help strengthen and condition your muscles, unlike high-impact exercise that can actually do more damage to your muscles. A study published in 1996 said that following physical exercise, almost 50 percent of people had a significant decrease in their signs and symptoms of fibromyalgia. Exercise will improve your muscle range of motion.

Taking steroids to treat your fibromyalgia will not improve your symptoms of pain. People with other muscle or bone conditions such as rheumatoid arthritis do respond well to steroids. However, nonsteroidal anti-inflammatory medications such as ibuprofen may relieve or at least decrease your muscle pain.Most pain medicine physicians who treat fibromyalgia agree that you should not use morphine-like drugs.

Tramadol (Ultram or Ultracet) may be extremely helpful to people suffering from fibromyalgia. It has two mechanisms of action that can effectively reduce your pain. First, Tramadol exerts its pain-relieving effects by stimulating receptors in your brain and spinal cord. Activation of these receptors can significantly block the amount of pain impulses that ultimately reach the pain center in your brain. Second, the added advantage of using this drug to treat your pain is that it increases the levels of serotonin and norepinephrine in your spinal cord and brain. These two substances in turn can decrease the amount of pain signals that reach your brain. This drug should no cause you to become addicted to it.

The main goal in treating your fibromyalgia is to attempt to break the pain cycle. One way of accomplishing this goal is to correct any disturbance in your sleep pattern. Amitriptyline (Elavil) can be an important drug in restoring your sleep. Numerous studies have shown that getting enough sleep can significantly reduce your pain. If you are allergic to Amitriptyline, cyclobenzaprine (Flexeril) can be used. In some people, nonsteroidal anti-inflammatory medications such as ibuprofen can be successfully used.

Amantadine hydrochloride (Symmetrel) also may be used. This medication is an antiviral as well as an anti-Parkinson medication. Serotonin reuptake inhibitors (Paxil) may also have a positive effect on reducing your pain.

As stated previously, avoid any narcotic types of pain-relieving medications. These narcotic medications could cause you to feel depressed. They also can reduce your hormone production. A reduction in the levels of the hormone testosterone can occur in both men and women. In men, a large decrease of testosterone in the blood can cause depression and osteoporosis. It also is possible that you could become addicted to narcotic-type medications. In many cases, people with a lot of pain request narcotic therapy because they think it is the only thing that could possibly take care of relieving their pain. However, there is rarely a need for you to use these types of medications for the management of your fibromyalgia pain. If they are prescribed to you at all, only take them for three to five days.

Pain-relieving creams that can be applied directly to your skin also are an effective way to reduce your pain symptoms. Capsaicin cream contains chemicals that are obtained from red peppers. These substances lessen the amount of substance P in the nerve endings around your muscle tissue. Zostrix or a similar cream also may effective for you. This cream is expected to be more effective for managing pain than creams such as Ben-Gay that contain menthol.

Be aware of the fact that capsaicin-containing creams can cause your skin to feel like it is burning. This is a normal occurrence and will lessen with repetitive applications. Ben-Gay is most useful in managing inflammatory pain such as arthritis. You may even find it helpful to have an injection of a local anesthetic and a steroid directly into your most sensitive areas of pain.

Nerve stimulation is another method of relieving pain that you may find helpful. A TENS unit (Transcutaneous Electrical Nerve Stimulator) is useful in managing fibromyalgia pain in many patients. This small battery-powered instrument has two to four patches that are placed over your painful muscle areas. Electrical impulses will stimulate the nerves around your areas of pain. This stimulation will cause the production of the pain-relieving chemical enkephalin into your spinal cord.

Enkephalin will diminish the intensity of your pain signals which ultimately reach your brain. Another useful machine that is gaining in popularity is a muscle stimulator. These devices have six to eight patches that are placed over your painful muscle areas. The muscle stimulator machine will stimulate and work your muscles until they are fatigued and weakened. It is possible for your muscles that have been weakened by the fibromyalgia to be strengthened this way.

Your muscles are not the only entity that needs to be treated in order to manage your pain. You may have psychological needs related to coping with your fibromyalgia that should be addressed. Fibromyalgia support groups exist in many communities. In these groups you will share with each other what treatments work best for you. You may discover a new treatment you would like to try, and you may even find a friend to exercise with or just talk to about your experiences with fibromyalgia. Psychological counseling can be another useful way to cope with your pain. A psychologist can help you deal with the suffering aspect of your pain. Your psychologist also may want to teach you biofeedback. This is a good way for you to learn relaxing techniques that can significantly reduce your pain. Aromatherapy also could be effective for helping you manage your pain. This method is more effective in women because their scent perception is better than a man's. You may also find that hypnosis can decrease your pain intensity. You may want to try self-hypnosis as another modality for the management of your chronic pain.

You can see that there are many proposed causes of fibromyalgia and there are as many treatments recommend for the control of fibromyalgia pain. Empower yourself by becoming involved in your treatment. No matter what treatment method your doctor prescribes, make sure you understand why it is being suggested and that you can correctly follow the treatment guidelines. Always be honest with your doctor and let him or her know how you feel during your treatment. With good communication, you and your doctor together can find the causes of your pain and learn how to manage them effectively with the treatment modality or modalities that works best for you.

The symptoms of fibromyalgia in men are generally fewer and milder than those of women. However, the conditions caused by this syndrome can be just as painful. It is important that you discuss treatment with your doctor and follow your doctor's advice carefully. It is equally as important to educate yourself on the condition and pay attention to actions that may be aggravating your symptoms.   Change   your lifestyle habits. Keep a diary of your daily activities. Try to pinpoint actions that could be causing your fibromyalgia symptoms to worsen and eliminate them.

Assess your posture. If you slouch while sitting or standing, learn and follow proper posture techniques. This will keep your muscles from being unnecessarily contracted, which can cause you pain. Get more sleep. The more sleep and rest you accumulate, the more your muscles will be allowed to rest. Begin an exercise program. Exercising your muscles can help reduce some of the symptoms of fibromyalgia.

Water aerobics and swimming are good, nonimpact types of exercise that are beneficial. Exercising also will produce serotonin, which will in turn help you sleep better. If maneuvers that you do at work worsen your pain, notify your supervisor. If you continue to work with pain you could ultimately injure yourself or a co-worker. If you frequently use a computer, do not keep your neck in a bent position.

Take nonsteroidal anti-inflammatory medications such as ibuprofen to decrease your muscle pain. Applying topical pain-relieving creams such as capsaicin or Zostrix over your area of pain will help reduce your muscle pain. If your pain is keeping you awake at night, take a sleep-inducing medication such as Elavil to help you sleep. Getting enough sleep is important in helping your bodies heal. Tricyclic anti-depressant medications will help stabilize chemicals in your brain that respond to pain and reduce some of that pain. Taking pain medications such as Tramadol can provide you with some relief of your pain symptoms.

If you are depressed or need psychological help to deal with your pain, psychological therapy or support groups can help you cope with the suffering aspect of your pain. Biofeedback with a psychologist can teach you techniques that will help you relax and deal with your pain. If maneuvers that you do at work worsen your pain, notify your supervisor. If you continue to work with pain you could ultimately injure yourself or a co-worker. If you frequently use a computer, do not keep your neck in a bent position.

Outcomes show the needed to design different treatments for men and women with fibromyalgia.[11] Compared with placebo, pregabalin (Lyrica) significantly improved FM pain and other symptoms in patients taking antidepressant medication for comorbid depression.[12,13] Extended release gabapentin relieved FM pain symptoms and improved quality-of-life for FM subjects as well.[13] Acupuncture has proven effective in the immediate pain reduction in patients with fibromyalgia.[14] An evaluation of the effect of 1 year of a gluten-free diet was performed previously in patients with irritable bowel syndrome and fibromyalgia syndrome. Gluten withdrawal produced a significant improvement of the functional symptoms, suggesting that gluten might be partly responsible for FM.[15]

References

1. Chopra K, Kuhad A, Arora V. Neoteric pharmacotherapeutic targets in fibromyalgia. Expert Opin Ther Targets. 2011;15(11):1267-1281.

2. Peleg R, Ablin JN, Peleg A, Neumann L, Rabia RA, Buskila D. Characteristics of fibromyalgia in Muslim Bedouin women in a primary care clinic. Semin Arthritis Rheum. 2008;37(6):398-402.

3. Caballero-Uribe CV. The fibromyalgia problem. A Latin American point of view. Rheumatology (Oxford). 2004;43(10):1311-1313; author reply 1313-1314.

4. Finan PH, Zautra AJ, Davis MC. Daily affect relations in fibromyalgia patients reveal positive affective disturbance. Psychosom Med. 2009;71(4):474-482.

5. Friedman AW, Tewi MB, Ahn C, et al. Systemic lupus erythematosus in three ethnic groups: XV. Prevalence and correlates of fibromyalgia. Lupus. 2003;12(4):274-279.

6. Neumann L, Buskila D. Ethnocultural and educational differences in Israeli women correlate with pain perception in fibromyalgia. J Rheumatol. 1998;25(7):1369-1373.

7. Gansky SA, Plesh O. Widespread pain and fibromyalgia in a biracial cohort of young women. J Rheumatol. 2007;34(4):810-817.

8. Rios G, Estrada M, Mayor AM, Vila LM. Factors associated with tender point count in Puerto Ricans with fibromyalgia syndrome. P R Health Sci J. 2014;33(3):112-116.

9. Ablin JN, Bar-Shira A, Yaron M, Orr-Urtreger A. Candidate-gene approach in fibromyalgia syndrome: association analysis of the genes encoding substance P receptor, dopamine transporter and alpha1-antitrypsin. Clin Exp Rheumatol. 2009;27(5 Suppl 56):S33-38.

10. Anderberg UM, Liu Z, Berglund L, Nyberg F. Plasma levels on nociceptin in female fibromyalgia syndrome patients. Z Rheumatol. 1998;57 Suppl 2:77-80.

11. Lami MJ, Martinez MP, Sanchez AI, et al. Gender Differences in Patients with Fibromyalgia Undergoing Cognitive-Behavioral Therapy for Insomnia: Preliminary Data. Pain Pract. 2016;16(2):E23-34.

12. Arnold LM, Sarzi-Puttini P, Arsenault P, et al. Efficacy and Safety of Pregabalin in Patients with Fibromyalgia and Comorbid Depression Taking Concurrent Antidepressant Medication: A Randomized, Placebo-controlled Study. J Rheumatol. 2015;42(7):1237-1244.

13. North JM, Hong KJ, Rauck RL. The Effect of a Novel form of Extended-Release Gabapentin on Pain and Sleep in Fibromyalgia Subjects: An Open-Label Pilot Study. Pain Pract. 2015.

14. Stival RS, Cavalheiro PR, Stasiak CE, Galdino DT, Hoekstra BE, Schafranski MD. [Acupuncture in fibromyalgia: a randomized, controlled study addressing the immediate pain response]. Rev Bras Reumatol. 2014;54(6):431-436.

15. Volta U. Gluten-free diet in the management of patients with irritable bowel syndrome, fibromyalgia and lymphocytic enteritis. Arthritis Res Ther. 2014;16(6):505.

23. Myofascial Pain

A myofascial pain syndrome is a soft tissue disorder of your muscles that can cause you not only to have pain for a long time, but it can also cause you to have some disability. Your overall activities of daily living, including work, can be significantly decreased. Myofascial pain is pain related to muscle injury or overuse resulting in taut bands and palpable areas of pain which is referred to other areas of your body.

The problem with a myofascial pain syndrome is it can present with your pain symptoms that are similar to other muscle-causing pain syndromes such as fibromyalgia. Fibromyalgia is a disorder characterized by pain in the fibrous tissue of muscle. Muscle strains and ligament sprains can cause pain in your muscles and can contribute to the onset of the myofascial pain syndrome. Be aware that your myofascial pain syndrome is a distinct entity. Myofascial pain may develop from a muscle injury or from excessive strain on a particular muscle or muscle group, ligament or tendon. Myofascial pain syndrome (MPS) prevalence among chronic back pain patients was significantly high, with female gender being a significant risk factor.[1]

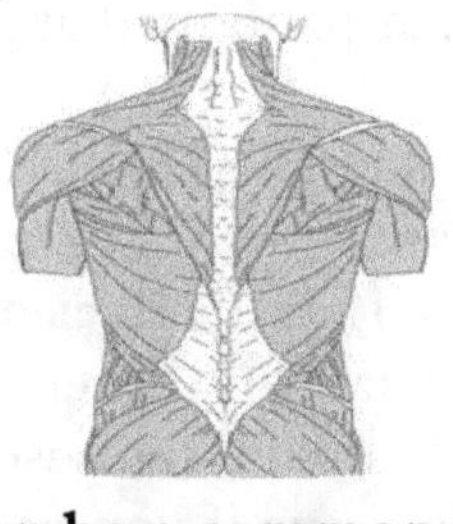

Figure 1. Muscles can be a common pain source.

Chronic myofascial pain is a painful condition that affects the muscles and the sheath of the tissue called the fascia that surrounds the muscles. Myofascial pain involves trigger points. Trigger points are highly sensitive areas within the muscle that are painful to touch and cause pain that can be felt in another area of the body, called referred pain

The pain intensity of myofascial disorders can vary from painless decreases in range of motion about your arms, legs, neck, and lower back, which are common in older individuals, to pain that is agonizing and incapacitating. This latter type of pain is seen if you are young and are extremely active. If you have a severe attack of myofascial pain, the pain may be so severe that it can cause you to fall to the floor. Pain related to myofascial pain syndrome can be as severe as that caused by a heart attack or by kidney stones. On the other hand, you need to realize that myofascial pain is not life threatening. Myofascial pain can decrease your activities of daily living and if it becomes chronic, can be a major cause of time lost at work.

In 1843, painful areas around muscles called "muscle callouses" were described. The doctor who identified these tender spots reported that the areas felt like a rope cord or a wide band. In the latter 1800s, it was thought that this muscle pain was associated with rheumatism. In 1904, fibrositis was a term used to describe inflammation of muscles. The muscles were noted to be hard to touch, and by the scientist who reported these findings thought that the pain was due to inflammation of the muscle tissue. Some health-care providers still use the different term fibromyositis.

In 1938, a doctor reported that pressing on the tender spots in a patient's muscle(s) could cause the individual to experience pain in other areas that were remote from the tender points. Before 1938, medical investigators did not realize that the pain was referred to areas distant from the tender spots. To define areas of the referred pain, the scientist injected saline or saltwater into areas that were painful (the volume of fluid induced pain). He then observed an individual's complaints of pain and established referred pain patterns that were related to an individual's trigger points.

In 1942, Dr. Travell emphasized that referred pain to areas away from the trigger point was evident if a patient had a myofascial pain syndrome. It was not until 1973 that scientists took biopsies of muscle tissues from areas of myofascial trigger points. Researchers reported abnormalities in the muscle tissue. Because it is known that there is an abnormality in your muscle tissue if you have muscle pain syndrome and that palpation of these areas causes you to have referred pain, the term "myofascial trigger points" is now used to define your painful areas throughout your body.

Myofascial trigger points occur when there is trauma to your muscle or prolonged tension to your muscle from slouching over a desk or slouching over a work table. This slouching results in disruption of the muscle cell. When your muscle cell becomes disrupted, your cell releases calcium. Calcium released inside of the muscle cell stimulates another contraction of your muscle. The prolonged contraction will exceed the available oxygen, glucose, and other nutrients that are needed for the energy to allow your muscle to continue to contract. With a sustained contraction, you run out of oxygen as well as other nutrients. This allows your muscle cell to build up a substance called lactic acid.

Lactic acid is seen when your body does not have sufficient oxygen. This substance then causes your body to produce pain-causing substances such as prostaglandins. These pain transmitters then stimulate nerve endings around your muscle cells. These nerve endings go to other structures in your body. This is why you notice a referred pain pattern when you have a myofascial pain syndrome. You will notice nodular, ropelike bands under your painful muscles when you have myofascial pain syndrome. The lack of oxygen in your muscle tissue will cause some of your muscle cells to die. This will cause scar tissue to form about your muscles. This scar tissue gives you the nodular feeling when you press over these painful areas. Rocky Mountain Spotted Fever or Lyme disease can also cause you to have muscle pain.

No laboratory tests are useful for the diagnosis of the myofascial pain syndrome. If you have the myofascial pain syndrome, you will complain of localized muscle pain and tenderness as well as the referred pain. If you have myofascial trigger points around your head and neck, you may complain of headaches as well as problems with your vision. Remember that you can have myofascial trigger points in one muscle or many muscles.

To make a diagnosis of myofascial trigger points, you must have the presence of painful areas on examination. These painful areas must be nodular and must be reproducible. Different amounts of pressure from your examining health-care provider will give you trigger point referred pain. Your doctor will record whether you have a "jump sign." This means that when your doctor applies pressure on your trigger point, you jump away from the pressure. Your health-care provider will usually notice a twitch about the area that has had pressure applied to it. At the time of your examination, your health care provided will notice that your pain diminishes with stretching or injection of your muscle with local anesthetics.

Your trigger points are classified as either active or latent. Your active trigger point causes you to have pain at the time of palpation. The latent trigger point on the other hand does not cause you to have pain at rest but can cause you to have restriction of movement about a certain part of your body and will cause weakness of the muscle that has the trigger point.

Remember that we described a latent trigger point that can persist for years after recovery from an injury. However, this latent trigger point will predispose you to have attacks of pain with overuse of your muscle. Sometimes in cold weather, your muscle will contract and cause you to have pain. Remember, only the active trigger points cause you pain. The latent trigger points, if they do become active, will then cause you to suffer some degree of pain.

Normal muscles do not have trigger points that can be felt. You should feel your normal muscles. Normal muscles have no ropelike, nodular areas or tender areas to pressure and exhibit no observable twitch when the muscle is palpated by your health-care provider. Furthermore, you will not have referred pain with this applied pressure. You can have different degrees of severity of myofascial pain. Some trigger points are much more sensitive than others. An extremely sensitive trigger point can cause you to have greater referred nerve pain than a less-severe or -intense trigger point. Myofascial pain is usually not symmetrical on either side of your body. However, medical conditions that cause muscle pain such as fibromyalgia are symmetrical.

Usually, patients come to their doctor with complaints due to the most recent active trigger point. When this trigger point has been eliminated, you may have other active or latent trigger points. These trigger points must also be inactivated. Usually the most severe trigger point is manifest. In other words, you can have three trigger points but the most severe trigger point is the one that actives the pain processing center in your brain. After this trigger point has been eliminated, the next most severe trigger point will be appreciated value. The three trigger points were always there but you concentrated on the more severe trigger point. This is why you have "movement" of your trigger points. Usually when your trigger point returns, it will return to the same areas that have been treated.

Trigger points are usually activated by overuse of your muscle. You stretch your muscle beyond its normal capability, which will cause your muscle to become injured. Bleeding can occur within your muscle tissue, which will cause scar formation in your muscle. Active trigger points can develop in your muscles following excessive, repetitive, or sustained motions. For example, if you work in a warehouse and load heavy boxes all day over months, you can begin to develop active trigger points.

Be aware that emotional stress can cause the formation of trigger points. Remember that stress causes your muscles to stay in a contracted state. When your muscles are contracted for a length of time as previously stated, you lose oxygen and other nutrients to your muscle tissues. This is the reason that you must attempt to relax and do the breathing exercises and range-of-motion exercises. You must take control of your myofascial pain. Use heat if you develop myofascial pain. The application of cold can also decrease your active myofascial trigger points. However, you should not use cold packs more than one than two days because chilling can contract your muscles and cause you to have worsening of your myofascial pain.

Your active trigger points can vary in pain severity from hour by hour or from day by day. The stress required to produce pain is variable. Again, if you are under much stress, it does not take much muscle stress to produce myofascial pain. The amount of stress that is needed to make your latent trigger become an active trigger point depends on your degree of conditioning of your muscles and your exercise tolerance as well. If you do not exercise and do aerobic activity and are under a lot of stress, you have susceptibility to develop active trigger points. If your muscle is stiff, avoid placing cold packs on a muscle that may already be contracted. Viral illnesses can cause muscle pain. If you have a virus, do not put cold packs on your muscles.

Your myofascial pain will outlast any precipitating traumatic event. The pain duration is longer in duration than the muscle strain duration. The problem exists that when you were injured; your muscles have developed a way of trying to prevent further pain. In doing so, these other muscles will cause your injured muscle to be protected. Eventually your active trigger points will become latent. If you rest your muscle and use a splint or an elastic bandage, your active trigger point may revert to become a latent trigger point. Occasionally you may do an activity that will activate your latent trigger point.

You should remember that your pain is frequently caused by pressure over your muscles. When you are lying in bed, you may have some pressure on your body in the area of the trigger points from your mattress. This pressure from your bed can cause you to have pain. On the other hand, be aware that sleep disturbances can cause your muscles to contract and become stiff and can worsen your myofascial pain syndrome. When this happens, consult your doctor as to whether you should be prescribed sleep aids. At times, melatonin before retiring at night can enhance your sleep.

You should attempt to avoid allowing your painful muscles to become stiff while you are at work or doing recreational activities. To decrease the change of stiffness, you must do range of motion lightly using the muscle. For example, if you have myofascial pain in your shoulder, do range of motion about your shoulder without a weight in your hand. Your muscle stiffness can increase in the painful muscle with inactivity. Therefore, when you wake up in the morning, do range-of-motion exercises.

Stretch the contracted muscle. If you pain is in your arm, neck, or shoulder, be aware that this extremity can become weak. Also be aware that you could unexpectedly drop an object from your hand. If you are picking up an expensive vase, for example, use both hands. When you have an injured muscle and if you go to pick up an object, your brain through the spinal cord has developed a protective mechanism to keep you from injuring your muscle further. This is the reason why you will occasionally drop an object.

No blood tests show any abnormalities attributed to a myofascial pain syndrome. X-rays, MRI images, and CT scans have not demonstrated any changes that can be associated with myofascial trigger points either active or latent. There have been no reported electromyographic (EMG) changes when you have a myofascial pain syndrome. However, the needle tip can touch a trigger point that can elicit a twitch which will be manifest on the EMG screen.

There is conflicting information on temperature changes associated with myofascial trigger points. Some investigators have noted that your temperature can be decreased over the area of the trigger point. However, for some reason, other investigators have noted increased temperature in the area of your trigger points. The reason for the discrepancy in these findings remains unknown at present.

The muscles of your skeleton are collectively the largest organ of your body. These muscles account for approximately 40 percent of your total body weight. You have approximately 696 muscles in your body. The problem is that any one of these muscles can develop pain. What is even worse is that any of these muscles can cause you to have referred pain. Your muscles receive minimal attention in medical textbooks. Your muscles collectively are the largest organ in your body; and if any part of this muscular organ can cause you to have pain, be aware that myofascial pain is a common occurrence.

Injection at myofascial trigger points in patients with nocturnal calf cramps not only alleviated pain and reduced the frequency of cramps but also lessened the severity of insomnia in a previous study.[2] Myofascial trigger point areas are common and can significantly increase your activity of daily living. Myofascial pain can even cause you to miss work if it is severe. The first part of this chapter mentioned that a previous injury could cause you to have current manifestations of myofascial pain. The areas of pain that are now manifest from a previous injury are called latent myofascial trigger points. Be aware that latent trigger points are more common than more recent active trigger points.

The greatest number of trigger points occurs between ages 31 and 50. When you are over 50, maximum activity will cause you to suffer from myofascial pain. As you continue to age and reduce your activity as a result of pain, your range of motion as a result of latent trigger points will become manifest. Many health-care providers are aware of myofascial trigger points. Chiropractors treat myofascial trigger points, as do physical therapists. Acupuncturists, anesthesiologists, dentists, pediatricians, rheumatologists, and specialists in physical medicine and rehabilitation all treat myofascial pain syndrome. The manner in which each of these health-care providers treats myofascial pain will vary from each of the health-care provider specialties.

As stated previously, a myofascial pain syndrome is a distinct entity from fibromyalgia and other pain syndromes. President John F. Kennedy sustained muscle injuries as well as other injuries as a result of a war related accident. Dr. Travell, his treating physician noted that President Kennedy had areas throughout his body that when touched or when pressed upon caused him to have significant pain. She first reported that he was suffering from "tender points" throughout his body. However, as time progressed, she noted that his condition was chronic. She also noted that if she pressed deeply into his muscle tissue that he would have pain that was referred to other areas about his body. Eventually the term "tender points" was changed to "trigger points" because palpation of the muscle would elicit referred pain elsewhere in the body.

For example, if you suffer from a myofascial pain syndrome, if your doctor presses on one of your painful areas in your shoulder for example, you may have referred pain that actually goes to your neck. Dr. Travell would do trigger point injections on President Kennedy. Trigger point injections with lidocaine have been reported to be effective for relief of painful trigger points.[3] However clinical results support the use of 5% lidocaine patches for treating patients with myofascial trigger points.[4]

If you suffer from the myofascial pain syndrome and if you are receiving adequate treatment for this syndrome, you will know that the diagnosis of myofascial pain syndrome needs to be accurate for you to receive the appropriate treatment. For example, traction on your spine could increase your myofascial pain but improve your pain if you have a disc herniation. Your chiropractor, doctor, or physical therapist may make the diagnosis of a myofascial pain syndrome.

You may note that you have areas in your body that are nodular like a rope and painful and if you press on these nodular areas it causes you to have pain. Your diagnosis is made by your health-care provider following a detailed medical history of your pain as well as an examination of your body.

Because other painful syndromes such as fibromyalgia can cause muscle pain, you must keep a pain diary of how your pain occurred, where your pain is located, and how severe your pain is. You must keep your diary information as to whether your pain stays in an isolated area or whether your pain moves in areas throughout your body. If you have had a motor vehicle injury at some time in your life, you must tell your doctor. For example, you may have had a whiplash injury 2 to 10 years ago. You may not have noticed significant muscle pain following the injury. However, with a muscle stretching, injury can become evident and can now cause you daily pain.

You must remember that in myofascial pain you will have a history of a sudden onset of pain following a stressful event to your muscles. You can have a gradual onset if you are doing chronic manual lifting. On the other hand, with fibromyalgia, the pain will be gradual and will be on both sides of your body, whereas your pain from your myofascial pain syndrome will be on one side. Remember that you will have tight ropelike bands in your muscles if you have myofascial pain but will have normal muscle tone if you have fibromyalgia.

Different types of treatment can be used to treat your myofascial pain syndrome. As with other tissues in your body, the muscles in your injured area go through different changes. If your muscle has direct trauma to it, it can develop some scar tissue around your injured muscle. These developing scars will limit your muscle's ability to either contract further or relax. These phenomena can result in shortened, weakened muscles. If you sustained a sprained ankle, you may have been placed in a brace. You will then have disuse of your muscles, which can cause your muscles to shrink in size, called atrophy.

If you had a fracture of one of your bones, you may have been placed in a cast by your doctor for six to eight weeks. The muscles about the injured joint under the cast will become weak. As you attempt to regain strength in the muscles, you may experience the onset of trigger points. Therefore, your therapist will need to do stretching exercises and conditioning exercises to help you regain strength and eliminate any active or latent trigger points that may be present. In addition to strengthening and stretching exercises, your therapist may want to apply moist heat over your muscle pain.

On occasion your therapist may progress the heat to ultrasound, which is a deeper application of heat. On occasion a massage may help to loosen your muscles. Your therapist may want to do deep, vigorous massage to break up any scar that has developed around your muscle tissue. This form of massage is called myofascial release therapy. Whatever method is chosen, the choice of treatment is usually based on the location of your myofascial trigger point and the sensitivity of the pain over the muscle. The choice of treatment is also based on the expertise of your clinician.

A technique called spray and stretch is sometimes used to decrease myofascial pain. The spray-and-stretch technique involves stretching painful muscle while using a cold spray. This cold spray is a vapocoolant and decreases the pain conduction in muscles from the pain fiber nerve endings. Furthermore, this vapocoolant helps muscles to relax. This form of therapy can provide you with immediate relief of your pain. This type of therapy is used for mildly painful myofascial pain.

The stretch and spray technique is used until your muscle length is back to normal. Because the vapocoolant can cause your muscles to contract, your therapist or chiropractor may immediately apply moist hot packs. These hot packs will rewarm your skin and help you to relax your muscles. After your muscles have been relaxed and rewarmed, the spray and stretch can be repeated. Your therapist or chiropractor will do several cycles of stretch as well as relaxation.

If you still complain of pain and have active trigger points, you may be a candidate to have ischemic compression massage. This type of massage consists of applying a local force to tissues surrounding your trigger point and then releasing it. This maneuver will cause some inflammation around your trigger point. This inflammation will cause your blood vessels to increase in caliber and will increase blood flow to your injured muscle. By increasing your blood flow, you will have an increase in oxygen, glucose, and other nutrients necessary for normal muscle function. This type of therapy is usually used in conjunction with injections of numbing medicine into your painful areas.

Trigger point injections administered by your doctor into your muscles can relax your muscles as well. The volume of anesthetic fluid that goes into your muscle tissue is anywhere from one to three milliliters. This volume of fluid can disrupt the scar that has formed around and within your muscles. Some doctors do not inject any local anesthetic or steroid into your muscle. They use what is called a dry-needle technique. They think that insertion of the needle into your muscle can break up some of the scar about the muscle itself. Dry needling can both be recommended in the treatment of neck pain patients with trigger points in the upper trapezius muscle.[5]

Injection therapy into your trigger points can provide you with significant relief. Other doctors mix a local anesthetic with a steroid. The numbing medicine relaxes your muscle and decreases the pain so that your physical therapist can stretch the muscle back to its original length. The steroid works to take the inflammation out of your muscle cells. There does not appear to be a difference in local anesthetic efficacy as the common local anesthetics seem to be equally effective for trigger point infiltration.[6]

Following injection therapy, your therapist will do spray and stretch. Following the spray and stretch, hot packs will be used to heat the cold muscle from the spray technique. After this is done, your physical therapist will have you move your muscle through its complete range of motion. It is always important that you have a stretching maneuver following your trigger point. Some practitioners use saline or saltwater to inject your muscle. The purpose of the saltwater is to break up the scar around your muscle. Occasionally your doctor will inject you with a long-acting numbing medicine called bupivacaine or Marcaine. Although rare in the healthy volunteers, many patients with lumbosacral radiculopathy have gluteal trigger points, located at the painful side which responds to injection therapy.[7] Myofascial release therapy is emerging as a strategy with a solid evidence base and tremendous pain relief potential.[8]

Acupuncture is another method that can be extremely valuable in the treatment of your myofascial pain syndrome. Acupuncture does not use numbing medicines or steroids. Remember that you can be allergic to some numbing medicines as well as steroids. The acupuncture needle tip can break up some of the scar around your muscle tissues. Furthermore, placement of the acupuncture needle can stimulate your body's productions of endorphins and other natural chemicals that you have stored within your body to decrease your pain.

Acupuncture therapy has been shown to be an extremely viable treatment of a myofascial pain syndrome. Acupuncture therefore, is a treatment option for patients who do not respond to the usual therapies (non-steroidal anti-inflammatory drugs) for musculoskeletal conditions.[9]

Treatment for myofascial pain syndrome typically includes medications, trigger point injections or physical therapy. Antidepressants such as fluoxetine (Prozac), sertraline (Zoloft), and duloxetine (Cymbalta) can be helpful with the chronic pain of myofascial pain syndrome. Anti-seizure medications such as gabapentin (Neurontin) and pregabalin (Lyrica) can also be helpful with the chronic pain of the syndrome. Capsaicin cream, a topical pain reliever derived from chili peppers, may also be helpful with the chronic pain of myofascial pain syndrome. The use of muscle relaxants in patients with myofascial pain muscles seems to be justifiable even though significant research has not been done. Tizanidine may be efficacious.[10]

If you continue to have significant pain associated with your myofascial pain syndrome, another method that can decrease your pain is a botulism toxin injection into your painful muscle. This botulism toxin (Botox) is a gram-negative bacterium. In small doses it can relax or even paralyze small muscle fibers. The relief of the Botox can last up to three months. The problem with the Botox injection is that some individuals develop what appears to be fever and generalized joint pain associated with the bacteria that gets into their bloodstream. Botox injections are used in pain management besides myofascial pain and are used in migraine headaches, myofascial pain syndrome, pelvic pain, and interstitial cystitis.[11]

Sometimes inflammation of your muscle cells can cause you to have pain. Overexertion will lead to a certain degree of inflammation about your muscle cells. For this reason, nonsteroidal anti-inflammatory drugs can decrease your pain. You will probably only need these medications for several days to a week. Over-the-counter ibuprofen is an effective treatment for your muscle pain. Remember that nonsteroidal anti-inflammatory drugs can potentially cause you ulcers. Another drug that you may be prescribed by your doctor is a muscle relaxant. Muscle relaxants can significant decrease your pain. However, these drugs can cause drowsiness, and some of them can cause you to become weak.

With respect to gender specificity, it appears that men suffer more from acute myofascial pain, whereas women suffer more from latent myofascial pain syndromes. Latent myofascial trigger points are more prevalent in women who are not active with respect to aerobic exercise. On the other hand, active trigger points are more prevalent in men who are doing vigorous exercises or who are doing heavy manual labor.

References

1.   Chen CK, Nizar AJ. Myofascial pain syndrome in chronic back pain patients. Korean J Pain. 2011;24(2):100-104.

2.   Kim DH, Yoon DM, Yoon KB. The effects of myofascial trigger point injections on nocturnal calf cramps. J Am Board Fam Med. 2015;28(1):21-27.

3.   Xie P, Qin B, Yang F, et al. Lidocaine Injection in the Intramuscular Innervation Zone Can Effectively Treat Chronic Neck Pain Caused by MTrPs in the Trapezius Muscle. Pain Physician. 2015;18(5):E815-826.

4.   Firmani M, Miralles R, Casassus R. Effect of lidocaine patches on upper trapezius EMG activity and pain intensity in patients with myofascial trigger points: A randomized clinical study. Acta Odontol Scand. 2015;73(3):210-218.

5.   Cagnie B, Castelein B, Pollie F, Steelant L, Verhoeyen H, Cools A. Evidence for the Use of Ischemic Compression and Dry Needling in the Management of Trigger Points of the Upper Trapezius in Patients with Neck Pain: A Systematic Review. Am J Phys Med Rehabil. 2015;94(7):573-583.

6.   Zaralidou AT, Amaniti EN, Maidatsi PG, Gorgias NK, Vasilakos DF. Comparison between newer local anesthetics for myofascial pain syndrome management. Methods Find Exp Clin Pharmacol. 2007;29(5):353-357.

7.   Adelmanesh F, Jalali A, Jazayeri Shooshtari SM, Raissi GR, Ketabchi SM, Shir Y. Is There an Association Between Lumbosacral Radiculopathy and Painful Gluteal Trigger Points?: A Cross-sectional Study. Am J Phys Med Rehabil. 2015;94(10):784-791.

8.   Ajimsha MS, Al-Mudahka NR, Al-Madzhar JA. Effectiveness of myofascial release: systematic review of randomized controlled trials. J Bodyw Mov Ther. 2015;19(1):102-112.

9.   Kam E, Eslick G, Campbell I. An audit of the effectiveness of acupuncture on musculoskeletal pain in primary health care. Acupunct Med. 2002;20(1):35-38.

10.   Manfredini D, Landi N, Tognini F, Orlando B, Bosco M. Muscle relaxants in the treatment of myofascial face pain. A literature review. Minerva Stomatol. 2004;53(6):305-313.

11.   Nodera H. [Use of botulinum toxin for pain therapy]. Brain Nerve. 2008;60(5):503-508.

24. Pain in the Face

Neuralgias or pathology of the nerves of the face has been recognized for centuries. These types of pain, especially trigeminal neuralgia, can be some of the most severe pain that you could ever experience. The pain associated with trigeminal neuralgia has been well defined. Sometimes your facial pain can be idiopathic, which means that there is not a defined cause for your pain. There can be an area of maximum pain in your upper or lower lip. When this area is stimulated by washing your face, talking, or opening and closing your mouth, your pain can be severe. It may last a few seconds to several minutes. If you go untreated, the pain can progress to become severe. You may drool from your mouth. As your pain gets worse, you will be unwilling to open or close your mouth or touch the area that triggers your pain.

A common type of pain syndrome is pain related to temporal mandibular joint disorders. This usually involves the joint between your lower jaw, which is called the mandible, and your temporal bone, which is called your maxilla. When these two bones meet, they form a joint. If you have a temporal mandibular joint (TMJ) disorder, you will probably be referred to an individual who has expertise in this area. This health-care provider will examine the movements of your jaw, your muscles about your jaw, your ligaments, and the way your teeth align. If your pain appears to be related to your TMJ, your specialist will determine whether your problem is within your joint or outside of the joint. This is an important diagnosis because the treatment differs.

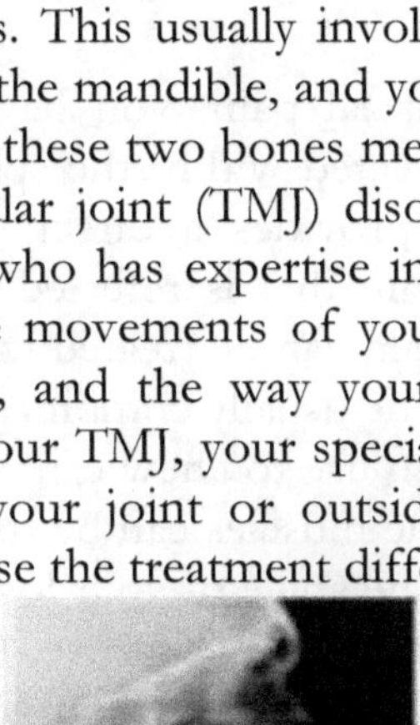

Figure 1. Lateral X ray of face showing facial bones.

Problems outside of your temporal joint are usually related to the muscles that are used to chew. A thorough examination is necessary because your teeth can cause pain to be referred to your face. A third molar, for example, can refer pain to your ear. If you have a history of arthritis, you can have joint problems within your TMJ. You can have dislocations of the small discs within your TMJ. This can result in inflammation as well as dysfunction of your joint and cause persistent and chronic inflammation, which in turn will cause you to have chronic pain. If you do suffer from TMJ, you usually have many problems, including the following: Misalignment of your teeth, emotional stress, poor body mechanics or a history of generalized myofascial pain.

To understand TMJ pain, you should have some knowledge of the anatomy of this joint and how it works. This joint is a true joint. It is composed of cartilage. This type of cartilage in your TMJ can regenerate. Your TMJ is involved in mouth movement. Within your TMJ, you have a disc. Your joint is stabilized by muscles around your joint. The muscles that are involved in chewing that exist around the TMJ are also responsible for TMJ functioning.

Your jaw movement is both up and down as well as some lateral movement. These movements are involved in chewing. You can develop myofascial pain in any of the muscles involved in chewing. You can develop pain of extra-articular origin. This means that your pain is outside of your TMJ joint. If one of your chewing muscles dysfunctions, you can have pain about your joint.

If you have myofascial pain, you have trigger areas which are zones of hypersensitivity located within the spasmodic muscle. If you or your health-care provider provides a direct, constant pressure on the trigger area, it can cause pain that is referred to other areas about your jaw. If this happens, your pain can be treated with a trigger point injection consisting of a local anesthetic usually combined with a steroid.

The muscles that you use to chew can refer pain to your teeth and gums. Pain from some of the muscles can be referred to your upper teeth. If you have muscle pain at the angle of your lower jawbone, your pain can travel upwards to the outer ring of your eye. Other muscles involved in chewing can refer pain to the sides of your head. Sometimes heat and muscle relaxants can relieve some of your pain. Your TMJ muscle pain can originate from psychological causes. Stress, which can cause you to grind your teeth, leading to dental irritation, can cause your muscles to become overactive. This can cause your muscles about your jaw to become spasmodic and can fatigue easily.

If you have TMJ, you will complain of pain about your TMJ as well as muscle spasms and clicking of your TMJ as well as limited motion on attempting to open your mouth. If you are under significant emotional stress, you may clench your teeth especially at night. This can increase the pressure within your TMJ, which can cause you to have abnormal TMJ movement.

You must remember that psychological symptoms such as depression and anxiety occur more among females than males. Also remember that depression and anxiety are associated with increased pain symptoms. Psychological or emotional distress causes more pain symptom reports and also increases the severity of pain. Because females can have greater emotional distress than males, they are predisposed to increased pain associated with TMJ. You also need to be aware that female TMJ patients have a greater need for treatment of their symptoms than males. Depression has been associated with greater pain severity among females, whereas depression causes more activity impairment in males. However, levels of anxiety are associated with increased pain severity. Anxiety can cause greater pain disability in males.

The overall prevalence of TMJ pain was higher for women than for men. For non-Hispanic white women up to age 50, the prevalence was approximately 7% to 8%, but it decreased after age 55. Non-Hispanic black women had much lower prevalence at younger ages which increased thereafter up to 55 to 64 years of age. A similar racial pattern seemed to emerge for non-Hispanic black men, with the lowest prevalence at ages 25 to 34 years, while non-Hispanic white men had a higher prevalence.[1]

The are no differences in the prevalence of degenerative changes in the TMJs in Caucasians and Afro-Americans. The strong correlation found between such changes and occlusal support in women but not in men might be explained by hormonal differences.[2] Males showed less racial/ethnic and age variation.[3]

Only 0.77% overall in a study reported TMJ without any comorbid headache/migraine, neck, or low back pains. Females reported more comorbid pain than males.[4] Hispanic and Blacks reported more than Whites. In addition, 53% of those with TMJ pain had severe headache/migraines, 54% had neck pain, 64% low back pain, and 62% joint pain. Differences in gender and race by age patterns were detected. For females, headache/migraine pain with TMJ pain peaked around age 40 and decreased thereafter regardless of race/ethnicity. Facial pain and jaw symptoms were reported more frequently by Caucasians compared to African-Americans, but they were also reported to have an earlier onset.[5] There were no significant differences in diagnoses between African American and Caucasian women.[6]

In a study in an Israeli Arab group compared with an Israeli Jewish group a comparison of women only in both groups revealed no statistically significant differences with respect to the incidence of TMJ.[7] Studies published as early as 1973 reported greater sensitivity to painful stimuli in individuals with TMJ when compared to the general healthy population. These findings supported the idea that changes in your central nervous system pain regulation could contribute to the onset of your TMJ pain.

This report is important because a greater sensitivity to pain among females, who because of sex differences are associated with an increased risk of developing TMJ. Females have been reported to develop greater jaw pain than males after experimental jaw clenching. The overall rate increased with age and was greater in African Americans and lower in Asians relative to those of white race/ethnicity.[8] The probability of TMD symptoms was strongly associated with concurrent episodes of headache and body pain and with past episodes of TMD symptoms. Episodes of TMD symptoms, headache, and body pain were associated with increases of approximately 10% in probability of analgesic use and health care attendance.

Your ability to control your pain using your body's own opioid system may be gender specific. Beta endorphins in males can inhibit some types of pain that are not seen in females. This data tells us that there are differences in pain regulatory systems in females than in males. For example, if you are female and if you have decreased beta endorphins, you are more prone to develop pain.

You must realize that fibromyalgia is more common in individuals with TMJ than in the general population. Almost 20 percent of TMJ patients meet the criteria for fibromyalgia. However, 75 percent of fibromyalgia patients may have TMJ. Irritable bowel syndrome occurs more commonly if you have TMJ. No differences in age were found between ethnic groups, nor were there any differences in characteristic pain intensity or oral functions.9 There is evidence however, that significant differences exist between men and women in regard to acute TMJ symptoms.[10] The biopsychosocial differences between men and women suggest that some treatments may be more beneficial for women than for men.

Depression is more common in TMJ than in the healthy population. In 1996, and again in 1998, it was reported that TMJ may be a result of stress-related disorders that are characterized by your pain. Be aware that if you have chronic pain, you have a 60 percent chance of having a relative who suffers from chronic pain as well. If one of your parents or an older brother or sister has a history of TMJ, you may be at risk as well for developing this disorder.

If you have an abnormal mouth bite, you can develop pain in your TMJ joint. When your teeth are properly aligned, especially during chewing, your muscles will be of a normal tone. If you have an abnormal bite, your muscles around your jaw can develop areas of spasm. Sometimes your muscles that are involved in chewing fail to relax. This muscle behavior causes you to have myofascial trigger points in your muscles involved with chewing. Not only will you have pain in your muscles and your TMJ, you also will eventually have TMJ dysfunction. Your dental specialist can make a special orthotic device for you that can be placed intermittently which will allow your jaw muscles to relax. This modality will ultimately decrease your myofascial trigger points.

Studies have been done to evaluate the muscles involved in TMJ pain. Most of the muscles that you use to chew can cause you to have pain about your TMJ. Furthermore, if you have TMJ, you can have ringing in your ears and hearing loss as well as pain around your ear. Heat and massage as well as analgesic medications can reduce your TMJ pain. You may want to try a soft diet for a while as well as use nonsteroidal anti-inflammatory medications. Alternating heat packs with ice packs can be of benefit as well. You should also do self-relaxation techniques.

Your nervous habits can result in TMJ pain as well. Do your chew your fingernails or chew on a pencil eraser or have any other habit that keeps your jaw in a forward position for a prolonged period of time? These maneuvers can cause you to have abnormalities that exist in your muscles and can ultimately cause you to have myofascial pain.

If you have an occupation in which you talk on a telephone for a significant amount of time, use a headset. There have been reports of TMJ pain related to individuals holding their telephone on their shoulder for hours at a time. These maneuvers compress some of your muscles, leading to myofascial pain and trigger points. It has been shown that women are more prone to TMJ than men.

The discs in your joints can displace or wear out and cause you TMJ pain. This is called intra-articular TMJ pain. If your disc is displaced forward, you may develop clicking, popping noises when you open and close your mouth. You can also have pain as well as limitation of your jaw movement. Over time you will develop wear-and-tear changes, leading to osteoarthritis of your joint. The capsule around your TMJ can become inflamed as well as deranged.

You should keep a diary as to when your jaw clicks when you open your mouth. The clicking can occur early or late depending on your jaw-opening position. If your disc is dislocated forward, a chronic problem about your joint can occur. You can injure the ligaments about your joint as well as cause further degenerative changes about your TMJ.

These changes can be observed on x-ray. When you get to this point, you will have pain and limited opening of your mouth on the affected side. You will have difficulty eating some foods such as an apple. The disc in your TMJ will not return to its normal position and over time degenerative arthritis called osteoarthritis can occur. This arthritis occurs after prolonged displacement of your TMJ disc. Your pain is most severe with wide opening of your mouth.

A family history of disc displacement may have an effect on the inheritance of TMJ. There is a higher incidence of TMJ among family members of TMJ patients who have a displaced disc in the joint as compared to TMJ patients who do not have a disc displacement.

In the central nervous system there are areas that exist in the spinal cord and the brain that inhibit painful impulses from reaching the pain center in your brain. It is possible that TMJ may be associated with impairment in your inhibitory system. This allows pain impulses from your jaw to reach your brain without being filtered or decreased in intensity.

If you have a decrease in your inhibition in your spinal cord, you will have exaggerated responses to both painful stimuli and psychological stimuli. For some reason, increased pain sensitivity throughout the body is more prevalent in patients with TMJ. The enhanced pain sensitivity noted among patients with TMJ was done in a clinical laboratory setting.

TMJ patients in general have a lower pain threshold than normal subjects for an unknown reason. TMJ patients in general can have more physical and psychological symptoms of stress. TMJ individuals report greater stress than healthy individuals. This finding is important because stress can cause you to clench your teeth.

The clenching of teeth can affect your muscles for chewing as well as your TMJ joint. Tests have been done to determine tension in your chewing muscles. This test, called an EMG, has been done in study subjects. In individuals with TMJ there is a noted increase in the muscle tone in some or all of the muscles involved with chewing. Psoriasis seems to play a role in temporomandibular joint disorders, causing an increase in orofacial pain and an altered chewing function.[11]

TMJ disorders occur in 12 percent of individuals in the United States. The actual cause of TMJ remains unknown. You should note that if you have TMJ, you may have symptoms similar to other chronic pain syndromes. You may have symptoms but not have objective, physiologic findings. Maladaptive behaviors can be seen in TMJ syndromes. If you clench your teeth as a result of stress, you can develop TMJ. If you have TMJ, you may have excessive use of a health-care system. This is because if you have psychological problems, you may focus entirely on your pain. TMJ can be debilitating.

It is a general consensus that you must have pain in order to be diagnosed with TMJ. If you do not have pain associated with your jaw movement, you probably do not have TMJ. Pain is the most important factor for which TMJ patients seek treatment. TMJ can also be seen in children. In children, however, there are no sex differences with regard to frequency of TMJ occurrence.

Both fatigue as well as psychological distress can increase your pain. As time progresses, your pain will become constant. X-rays can identify changes in your TMJ space. Traumatic injuries can also cause you to experience TMJ pain. If you have rheumatoid arthritis, you can develop TMJ pain. Rheumatoid arthritis is usually on both sides of your body, whereas osteoarthritis is usually confined to one side. If you have rheumatoid arthritis, this disease can progress to your TMJs on both sides of your head. In addition to x-rays, you may need a magnetic resonance image (MRI). A CT can also be used to examine your TMJ. At present MRI is the most effective tool for diagnosing TMJ problems. Your TMJ specialist can also inject dye into your joint. This injection of dye, called an arthrography, can help diagnose the disc displacement.

If you have a displacement of your TMJ disc, your mouth will deviate to one side as you open your mouth. If you have popping or clicking, this indicates that you have disc pathology. An important tool for your doctor or dentist to diagnose the source of your pain is with an injection of numbing medicine. If an injection into your TMJ provides you with significant relief, your pain is intra-articular or coming from within the TMJ itself.

However, if injection into your muscle provides you with pain relief, this tells your health-care provider that the pain is coming from outside your joint. Furthermore, by injecting around the nerve that goes to your TMJ, this maneuver can provide information as to whether your TMJ is the source of your chronic pain. These injections are safe.

Surgery is sometimes indicated for the management of a TMJ problem. When less-invasive procedures fail to alleviate TMJ pain, oral surgery procedures can be done. These include using a scope to reposition your discs. Your oral surgeon can also remove your discs. Implantations can be done into your TMJ. Using a scope is less invasive than opening your TMJ joint. You need to remember that the most conservative therapies are usually the best therapies.

Women have more physical and psychological symptoms with TMJ than males. However, in the study, males had greater psychological-related symptoms. TMJ prevalence peaks between the ages of 25 and 44. After age 44, the chance of you developing TMJ decreases with increasing age. For some reason, female patients who develop TMJ were more likely than males to have chronic pain. Studies have shown that sex is a definite risk for the development of TMJ. TMJ is most noted in women during their reproductive years. The reason for this finding is not known. The problem with doing gender-specific studies on TMJ patients is that only a small number of males actually seek treatment for chronic pain.

Higher levels of stress, depression, and anxiety have been reported in the TMJ population in general when compared to healthy individuals who do not suffer from TMJ. You must be aware that psychopathology is strongly associated with generalized muscle pain throughout the body. The psychological disorders reported in TMJ patients are higher in females than males. In other words, females have more depression and anxiety than males. If you have a history of sexual abuse or trauma, you have a higher risk of developing TMJ.

It has reported that close to 50 percent of TMJ patients have histories of sexual or physical abuse. An abuse history makes you more prone for depression and anxiety. An abuse history in general is associated with increased physical as well as psychological symptoms if you suffer from chronic pain. An abuse history is related to your increased pain complaints as well as your psychological disturbances. Sexual abuse has been noted to be associated with an increased risk of generalized muscle pain in females but not in males. Be aware that females are more often the victims of sexual and physical abuse. As a result, the effect of abuse on pain response is more likely to be noted by females than by males.

Hormones play an important part in your development of TMJ. Your ovarian hormones, if you are a female, can be related to TMJ. A study has examined women with TMJ. The prevalence of TMJ occurs in females during their reproductive years. Note that if you are a female that your ovarian hormones are at their greatest peak during your reproductive years. If you take oral contraceptives or have had estrogen hormone-replacement therapy, you are at an increased risk for developing TMJ. If you use oral contraceptives, your TMJ pain can be worse during your menstrual cycle.

If you suffer from premenstrual symptoms, you are more likely to report TMJ than women who do not have any premenstrual symptoms. No one to date knows exactly how sex hormones produce TMJ effects. It is believed that your sex hormones alter pain processing in the nerves in muscles, TMJ joints, gums, and so on. It is interesting to note that estrogen receptors have been defined in the TMJ of animals. No one knows how these receptors affect TMJ. Psychosocial issues are important in the development of TMJ.

Important sex differences exist in the efficacy or treatment for TMJ. The treatment need is higher in women than men. Women in general have more chronic pain severity than men. Female patients are treated more often by oral surgery than males. It is important to note that females have a greater success rate with treatment modalities of TMJ than males. The question that remains to be answered is whether various treatments are gender specific for males and females.

Women are twice as likely as men to experience TMJ. It is believed that hormonal factors as well as psychological pathology and social factors contribute to sex differences in the onset of TMJ. Research continues into the effect of ovarian hormones on the cause and treatment of TMJ. Further research into TMJ in general will increase our understanding of this disorder and may lead to improved treatment of this disorder.

Trigeminal neuralgia is also called tic douloureux. Tic douloureux is defined as a sudden stabbing pain felt in your face. It usually occurs on one side of your face. One of the nerves that supplies sensation to your face is the trigeminal nerve. This is the nerve that comes off of your brain stem. This trigeminal nerve is the cause of your trigeminal neuralgia. If the exit of the trigeminal nerve from your brain stem is depressed by a blood vessel or other tissue, this can be the cause of your pain. Compression of your trigeminal nerve with blood vessels occurs in approximately 80 percent of trigeminal neuralgia.

Sometimes an aneurysm or changes in your bone architecture about the skull can compress your nerve. Multiple sclerosis can contribute to trigeminal neuralgia as well. It is rare for trigeminal neuralgia to occur on both sides of your face but it can happen. Light touch over your face will usually trigger your pain.

As previously mentioned, the incidence of trigeminal neuralgia is twice that in women as seen in men. Usually the first occurrence will happen when you are 40, and it will usually reach a peak by age 50. For some reason the right side of the face is affected more often than the left side.

There are three branches of the trigeminal nerve. One goes to the area around the forehead and eyes. The second goes to the upper jaw. The third goes to the lower jaw. Sometimes pain will occur in the second and third branches of the trigeminal nerve. However, you must realize that the first branch can also be involved, but it is extremely rare to have this branch involved.

When you have trigeminal neuralgia, your pain will be transient. It can last from seconds to minutes. It can occur daily or sometimes once a week or once a month. Your pain will be like an electric shock. It can be of a stabbing nature as well. Between the episodes of your pain, your sensations over your face should be normal. Your trigeminal neuralgia can last for months. However, these painful episodes can subside, or they can return years later.

Your trigeminal neuralgia usually responds to anticonvulsant medications. Tegretol and Neurontin are two drugs commonly used for the treatment of trigeminal neuralgia. Baclofen and Klonopin can help you as well. Injection of numbing medicine with a steroid into areas about your face that trigger your pain can relieve episodes of trigeminal neuralgia. Opioids are usually not needed for the management of pain, but in extreme cases may become necessary. If these modalities do not relieve your pain, your pain is probably due to trigeminal nerve compression, most often by one of your arteries. Your surgeon may refer you to a neurosurgeon for surgical treatment.

Pain in your mouth and face can come from your teeth, jaws, your temporal mandibular joints, your muscles involved in chewing, and from your salivary glands. Your nose and sinuses can also be a source of pain. Another source of pain is trigeminal neuralgia, which is a pathological state involving your trigeminal nerve. A diagnosis of pain coming from your teeth or jaws can be diagnosed accurately.

If you have had recent dental work, hypersensitive teeth from an abscessed nerve root or from a cracked tooth may be localized. This type of pain is aggravated by warm coffee, cold tea, or candy. If your tooth is only cracked, it can cause pain when you bite into something, especially a piece of hard candy. If you have tooth decay that involves the pulp, it can aggravate your pain, but cold can relieve your pain. When the pulp tissue dies, your pain will subside. When you have these symptoms, seek attention from your dentist.

You can also develop pain that comes from your salivary glands. Your parotid gland as well as other salivary glands can be a site of infection. Furthermore, a small stone can block your parotid duct. Your gland toward the bottom of your face and upper neck can swell. Your pain will increase at the sight or smell of food. Sometimes your swelling and pain can decrease after you eat but can recur following another meal. If your stone remains in the duct, it may have to be removed surgically.

You can experience pain that is called atypical facial and oral pain. This type of pain may be related to psychiatric problems. An example of atypical facial pain is phantom tooth pain in which a tooth has been pulled but the individual still reports complaints of pain in the area of the extracted tooth. If you have phantom tooth pain, your dentist may provide you with fillings or different treatments, none of which will provide you with significant relief in most instances.

Your dentist may even extract neighboring teeth. If you have diabetes or have some vitamin deficiencies, you can develop a syndrome that causes you to have a burning mouth as well as a burning tongue. Sometimes psychogenic factors can give you a pain syndrome of this type. Your doctor and dentist will do a thorough physical examination, including x-rays. In many stances, a psychiatric consultation is indicated. Usually tricylic antidepressants such as Elavil will decrease your pain if you have these symptoms. Almost all patients who have an extremity amputated will experience a phantom limb. Phantom phenomena occur after tooth extraction as well.[12]

If you worry a lot, anxiety can cause chronic facial pain. This type of pain can also be associated with a major life change. If you or someone in your family has become ill or if there has been a death in the family or acute stress, you may develop facial pain. You may also have an increased heart rate as well as headaches and breathing difficulties. With an anxiety reaction, you may notice excessive perspiration. Relaxation techniques can help you manage this type of pain. Relaxation techniques such as meditation, yoga, and biofeedback can help you relieve your pain. Some tranquilizers can also help you with this problem as well. If you have more severe psychiatric conditions, you may also have pain.

Schizophrenia and hypochondriasis or other emotional problems can also cause you to suffer facial pain. As with many of the other pain syndromes in this book, there is no one definable treatment for facial pain, especially atypical facial pain. Your health-care provided will obtain a complete history and do a thorough physical examination with the possibility of other tests before initiating definitive treatment. With this information in mind, you can be an extreme help to your health-care provider by keeping an accurate diary of your pain symptoms.

A stroke can also cause you to have pain in your facial area. Be aware that coronary artery disease can also cause you to have facial pain. If you suffer from this type of pain, nitroglycerin can sometimes relieve it. Remember that the pain from a heart attack can go into your jaw. If you have jaw pain without chest pain or pain in your shoulder or arm, your doctor might fail to consider heart attack as the cause.

If you have had a whiplash injury, one of the nerves off of your cervical spine can send nerve branches to the skin over the angle of your lower jawbone. This type of pain can cause you to have significant sharp pain. On occasional local anesthetics and steroids can be used to decrease this pain. You can have facial pain that has been called atypical facial pain or facial pain of a psychological origin. This type of pain is usually associated with psychiatric symptoms. It can be seen in malingers as well as drug abusers.

The diagnosis of oral pain can be difficult. Pain in your mouth and face is common. It is fortunate that in most cases the cause of your pain can be easily determined. However, the anatomy of the area about your face and throat is complex. This is the reason why a diagnosis can be difficult for your doctor. When you have pain in your mouth as well as in your face, the pain comes from nerves that branch off of your brain. These nerves are called cranial nerves. One common cranial nerve frequently involved as a cause of your facial nerve is a major nerve called the trigeminal nerve, which has three branches: ophthalmic, maxillary, and mandibular. Other nerves also can cause you to experience facial pain. Your facial nerves, glossopharyngeal nerve, your vagus nerve, and some cervical nerves go to various parts of your mouth areas and facial areas and can cause you to experience pain.

TMJ and other facial pains can be relatively mild or they can be totally disabling. In the majority of instances, facial pain can be adequately controlled. Sometimes an injection of a numbing medicine with steroid into this painful area can decrease the pain.

If you have had a previous traumatic event or have had some tissue removed surgically, pathological changes may occur in the area of your trigeminal nerve. Sometimes your trigeminal nerve can compress blood vessels in your face. This can be the cause of a sensation of throbbing pain. If you are younger than 40 years of age, you may develop trigeminal neuralgia, which may be related to an underlying disease such as multiple sclerosis (MS) or a tumor.

Another type of facial pain is glossopharyngeal neuralgia. This type of pain has trigger areas around your tonsils or the back of your throat or even at the base of your tongue. The injection of local anesthetics and steroids will not usually provide you with long-term pain relief. These types of neuralgias usually require the use of anticonvulsant medications. Carbamazepine has been used for years for the treatment of trigeminal neuralgia, but now a newer anticonvulsant medication, pregabilin (Lyrica) can be helpful in alleviating your pain.

If over-the-counter pain medications aren't enough to relieve TMJ pain, your doctor or dentist may prescribe stronger pain relievers. Tricyclic antidepressants such as amitriptyline may be used for pain relief. Muscle relaxants are drugs sometimes used to help relieve pain caused by TMJ disorders. If nighttime teeth clenching is aggravating your pain, your doctor might prescribe a sedative such as clonazepam (Klonopin). Glossopharyngeal neuralgia (GN) is a milder disease than trigeminal neuralgia, as indicated by the number of episodes, treatment, and characterization of pain.[13] The right side is affected more often with TN than with GN. Bilaterally was noted less often in trigeminal neuralgia than in GN cases.[13]

Sometimes a radiofrequency heat lesion can be used to destroy the area where your nerves come from your brain to your face. Your neurosurgeon can do surgery within your brain to get your blood vessels away from parts of your trigeminal nerve. In these previous pain conditions, there were no abnormal central nervous system signs. However, you can have facial pain associated with abnormal central nervous system signs. This can be as a result of trauma, infection of bone in your face, or tumors.

Treatment options include: Steroid injections can help reduce inflammation in your facial joints and muscles. Your doctor can inject numbing medications in your painful areas to reduce your pain. In extreme cases, your doctor can perform radiofrequency heat lesion to destroy the area where your nerves come from your brain to your face in order to relieve your pain. Tricyclic antidepressant medications prescribed by your doctor can help relieve your symptoms of pain, as well as serve as an antidepressant. Different doses will be given depending on which it is being used for.

When other methods don't help, your doctor might suggest procedures such as an arthrocentesis which involves the insertion of needles into the joint so that fluid can be irrigated through the joint. Injections into the joint may be helpful. Arthrocentesis is a simple, minimally invasive procedure with a relatively low risk of complications and significant clinical benefits in patients with TMJ disorders.[14]

Injecting botulinum toxin (Botox) into the jaw muscles used for chewing may relieve pain associated with TMJ disorders. Surgery to repair or replace the joint may be of some benefit.

Because of sex differences with respect to the effect of estrogen as well as progesterone on the absorption, metabolism and elimination of medications, drug dosing may fluctuate in the female patient depending on whether or not the female is pre or post-menopausal. They physiological changes that occur during the menstrual cycle can affect the responses of a drug in the female body. You must discuss the effects of your drug with your doctor because the effect of your drug may decrease during menses.

References

1. Isong U, Gansky SA, Plesh O. Temporomandibular joint and muscle disorder-type pain in U.S. adults: the National Health Interview Survey. J Orofac Pain. 2008;22(4):317-322.

2. Magnusson C, Nilsson M, Magnusson T. Degenerative changes of the temporomandibular joint. Relationship to ethnicity, sex and occlusal supporting zones based on a skull material. Acta Odontol Scand. 2012;70(3):207-212.

3. Plesh O, Adams SH, Gansky SA. Racial/Ethnic and gender prevalences in reported common pains in a national sample. J Orofac Pain. 2011;25(1):25-31.

4. Plesh O, Adams SH, Gansky SA. Temporomandibular joint and muscle disorder-type pain and comorbid pains in a national US sample. J Orofac Pain. 2011;25(3):190-198.

5. Plesh O, Crawford PB, Gansky SA. Chronic pain in a biracial population of young women. Pain. 2002;99(3):515-523.

6. Plesh O, Sinisi SE, Crawford PB, Gansky SA. Diagnoses based on the Research Diagnostic Criteria for Temporomandibular Disorders in a biracial population of young women. J Orofac Pain. 2005;19(1):65-75.

7. Reiter S, Eli I, Gavish A, Winocur E. Ethnic differences in temporomandibular disorders between Jewish and Arab populations in Israel according to RDC/TMD evaluation. J Orofac Pain. 2006;20(1):36-42.

8. Slade GD, Sanders AE, Bair E, et al. Preclinical episodes of orofacial pain symptoms and their association with health care

behaviors in the OPPERA prospective cohort study. Pain. 2013;154(5):750-760.

9.   van der Meulen MJ, Lobbezoo F, Aartman IH, Naeije M. Ethnic background as a factor in temporomandibular disorder complaints. J Orofac Pain. 2009;23(1):38-46.

10.   Phillips JM, Gatchel RJ, Wesley AL, Ellis E, 3rd. Clinical implications of sex in acute temporomandibular disorders. J Am Dent Assoc. 2001;132(1):49-57.

11.   Crincoli V, Di Comite M, Di Bisceglie MB, Fatone L, Favia G. Temporomandibular Disorders in Psoriasis Patients with and without Psoriatic Arthritis: An Observational Study. Int J Med Sci. 2015;12(4):341-348.

12.   Schmid HJ. [Phantom limb after amputation--overview and new knowledge]. Praxis (Bern 1994). 2000;89(3):87-94.

13.   Katusic S, Williams DB, Beard CM, Bergstralh EJ, Kurland LT. Epidemiology and clinical features of idiopathic trigeminal neuralgia and glossopharyngeal neuralgia: similarities and differences, Rochester, Minnesota, 1945-1984. Neuroepidemiology. 1991;10(5-6):276-281.

14.   De Riu G, Stimolo M, Meloni SM, et al. Arthrocentesis and temporomandibular joint disorders: clinical and radiological results of a prospective study. Int J Dent. 2013;2013:790648.

25. Angina

Chest pain in both men and women can be serious. According to the American Heart Association, approximately 6.3 million men and 6.6 million women have histories of heart attacks. In the year 2000, more than 500,000 people died from heart disease. Even though minor medical conditions can cause you to have chest pain, if you are having a heart attack, it can be potentially fatal. For this reason, do not take any chest pain lightly. To be safe, seek medical attention whenever you experience significant chest pain.

If your heart muscles do not obtain enough oxygen, some of your heart muscle can become injured and even some of the muscle can die. This can lead to some dysfunction in the remainder of the muscle that is trying to pump blood out of your heart to the rest of your body. The injured muscle can't pump blood efficiently if at all. You can develop angina or a myocardial infarction.

Angina is pain in the center of your chest. Usually angina is relieved by rest. Anginal chest pain in men may spread to the jaws and arms. Numbness and pain radiating from the chest into the left arm is especially characteristic of anginal pain in men. In women with a decrease in oxygen to the heart muscle for some reason, symptoms of angina pain include pressure in the center of the chest accompanied by pain in the neck or arms. Angina or heart pain occurs when the demand for blood by the heart exceeds the supply of the arteries.

A myocardial infarction (heart attack) or death of a segment of your heart muscle occurs following interruption of the blood supply to the heart muscle. A heart attack can cause sudden severe chest pain. There is a danger that your heart could go into an irregular heartbeat called an arrhythmia. If you have a severe arrhythmia, your heart can stop, which is referred to as a cardiac arrest.

If you have interruption of the blood flow going to your heart, you can have irreversible injury to your heart muscle. This injury usually begins within 20 minutes from the time of the loss of blood flow to your heart muscle. Therefore, if you think that you are having a heart attack, contact your local emergency room or your doctor. If your pain is severe, go directly to your emergency room by ambulance.

The extent of your heart muscle injury is related to the amount of obstruction that you have in your heart vessels. It is also related to the length of time that your heart muscle is without blood flow. You will probably have other vessels in your heart that supply your heart muscle. This is called collateral circulation. This collateral circulation can get some blood flow to your muscle that is without blood flow. When your heart muscle is without oxygen and when your heart muscle dies, the electrical conduction of impulses through the muscle is decreased or stopped. This is the mechanism by which your heart develops abnormal heart beats.

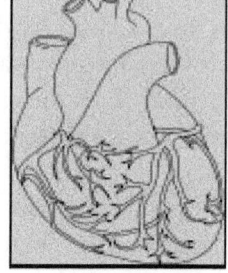

Figure 1. **The heart is a muscle that pumps blood throughout your body.**

It is a diagnostic problem for your doctor to determine whether you are suffering from chest pain from your heart or from another structure. You need to be aware that not all chest pain is heart related pain. Pain in your chest can also come from pneumonia, cancer, or pleurisy (an inflammation of the lining of the lung). Diseases of the esophagus can also cause you to have chest pain, as can shingles.

Angina pectoris is chest pain that results from decreased oxygen from your heart muscle. Angina pectoris is usually pain under your breastbone. You may perceive discomfort instead of pain or pressure. The pain, if it is present or the pressure can radiate to your neck or arm which is usually the left arm. Shortness of breath may also be reported. Angina pectoris is usually elicited by physical exertion.

Occasionally psychological stress can cause you to have angina pectoris. The stress can cause your heart rate to increase, which increases your oxygen demand. If you are worried about an impending speech that you have to give, this could cause you to have anxiety with an increase in your heart with the possibility of developing angina.

Climbing stairs can also cause you to have angina pectoris if you have some obstruction of your arteries that supply blood to your heart muscle. You may develop angina when you awake in the morning. Exposure to cold air can cause angina. You could even develop angina after meals. Angina comes on quickly and can last for up to 15 minutes. It usually resolves with rest or with nitroglycerin.

Under high time pressure, but not under low time pressure, implicit physicians' biases regarding Blacks and Hispanics led to a less patient serious diagnosis. In addition, implicit biases regarding blacks led to a lower likelihood of a referral to specialist when physicians were under high time pressure.[1] The results suggest that when physicians face stress, their implicit biases may shape medical decisions in ways that disadvantage minority patients. Significant differences have been shown between races in an emergency department setting but not between genders with respect to chest pain for the time to the first EKG and percent of patients receiving cardiac catheterization and echocardiography.[2] Blacks waited longer than whites for an EKG and were less likely to receive cardiac catheterizations but more likely to receive echocardiography.

To understand the mechanics of chest pain associated with angina attacks, you need some basic knowledge of coronary heart disease. Coronary heart disease is the major cause of death in not only the United States but also in most industrialized countries. Coronary artery disease can cause you or one of your family members to have a sudden stoppage of his or her heart. Coronary artery disease can be a cause of angina.

Over time coronary artery disease can also cause you to have a heart attack (myocardial infarction). There has been a decrease in the number of deaths from coronary artery disease over the past three decades. This is probably related to the treatment of high blood pressure as well as the medications as well as surgical treatments. Lifestyle changes such as diet, exercise, and stopping smoking tobacco can decrease the incidence of coronary artery disease.

Coronary heart disease is usually related to atherosclerosis, which can occur in your heart arteries as well as other arteries throughout your body. Atherosclerosis is a build-up of fat and other materials in the walls of arteries that causes them to become narrowed. This entity is caused by many factors. If you are over 60, a man, and have a family history of coronary artery disease, you are prone to develop this disease. If you are hypertensive and have an elevated cholesterol and smoke, you are at a higher risk for developing atherosclerosis. If you are obese and have a sedentary lifestyle, your risk for atherosclerosis is increased.

At first, you will develop a buildup of a type of "bad" cholesterol called low-density lipoproteins (LDL) in the walls of your blood vessels about your heart. These low-density lipoproteins eventually can calcify. This calcification will narrow the lumen, or diameter of your blood vessels, causing a decrease in the amount of blood that can pass through them.

This is similar to calcium building up in your plumbing in your residence. If you repetitively deposit calcium in your pipes, eventually your pipes will close off. The same analogy is true for the blood vessels in your heart. When you have a deposit of calcium in your blood vessels, your heart will still pump blood through these vessels. It takes a decrease in the diameter of your blood vessels by approximately 70 percent to decrease your blood flow.

Many diverse factors lead to the progression of atherosclerosis. Increasing age and a family history of coronary artery disease may predispose you to develop this entity. The male sex is an important risk factor for developing coronary artery disease and for having a heart attack, but coronary heart disease is also the leading cause of death in women over 50 years of age. Women will generally have their symptoms approximately 10 years later than men. The risk of coronary artery disease increases with the use of birth control pills and with the onset of menopause. However, the risk of coronary artery disease could be increased with hormone therapy following the onset of menopause.

If you have an elevated blood pressure, you are also at risk for developing coronary artery disease. In fact, hypertension is a major risk factor for developing this disease. If you have a family history of hypertension or if you are beginning to increase your blood pressure, you may to need to change your lifestyle. You will need to stop smoking. If you are obese, you will need to decrease your weight.

Sodium restriction is important for the control of your hypertension, which can ultimately decrease coronary artery disease. Aerobic exercise is also necessary to decrease your risk for developing coronary heart disease. Exercise is extremely important if you have risk factors for developing coronary artery disease. Smoking is another factor that can cause you to be at a high risk for developing coronary artery disease.

You are probably aware that your cholesterol level must not be allowed to become elevated because it can increase your risk of developing coronary artery disease. If you have high levels of low-density lipoprotein cholesterol, you have an elevated chance of developing coronary heart disease. If your cholesterol is elevated, your doctor will help you reduce your cholesterol with both diet and with pharmacologic management.

You must monitor your diet for fat intake. You must significantly decrease your intake of saturated fats. If you eat out a lot at fast-food restaurants, calculate the amount of fat present in the foods that you are consuming. The total fat grams will be listed on the package of the food that you are consuming. Fast-food restaurants also list the fat content of their food in the restaurant and on their websites. Strive to decrease your fat intake. Your doctor can tailor a proper diet for you. However, you must follow this diet. You are probably beginning to realize that you can do things to decrease your chance of developing angina and decrease your chance of having a heart attack.

Plaques (deposits of fat and calcium in your blood vessels) are usually the most common causes of obstruction to blood flow in your arteries about your heart, but other factors can also cause obstruction of blood flow in your heart. Vegetations, small growths that can develop on the valves in your heart from infections, can extend up to your coronary arteries and cause them to become blocked. Diseases such as rheumatoid arthritis can affect the caliber of your coronary arteries.

You must be aware that if you have had or need radiation therapy for cancer treatment, that radiation therapy can cause you to have coronary artery disease. Cocaine use has become more and more prevalent in the United States. However, cocaine use can make the arteries in your heart to go into spasm. Cocaine can accelerate the deposition of fat and calcium in your blood vessels, which can cause you to have angina as well as a heart attack.

Sometimes a decrease in the blood flow in your arteries about your heart can lead to decreased blood flow to the heart muscle tissue, and a decrease in oxygen to your heart will cause a possible injury to your heart muscle. Your heart muscle is dependent upon a balance of oxygen supply as well as demand. At rest, your heart should receive adequate oxygen or you may complain of chest pain. However, if you run a mile or run up steps, the oxygen demand to your heart muscle is increased.

The blood vessels that deliver the blood carrying oxygen to your heart must provide your heart muscle with an adequate blood flow. If your blood vessels are narrowed, your heart cannot get enough blood carrying oxygen to your heart muscle. As a result, some of your heart muscle could become injured and die. This is what happens to your heart muscle when you suffer a heart attack (or myocardial infarction, MI). If you are doing any exercise or aerobic activity and if you develop chest pain, stop the activity that you are doing immediately.

You will usually develop chest pain when your heart oxygen demand exceeds the supply of oxygen that your blood vessels are supplying to your heart. Usually if your heart begins beating faster, the increase in oxygen demand is met by an increased blood flow in your arteries about your heart. The small arteries around your heart muscle will increase their diameter to provide your heart with more oxygenated blood. If your vessels cannot dilate, your heart will not receive enough oxygen and you will experience pain in your chest. Fat and calcium within your heart vessels will restrict the amount of blood that goes to your heart.

Men may have chest pain with radiation of pain to their left arms. A recent study of women finds that fatigue and sleeplessness are accurate predictors of an impending heart attack. Exhaustion, sleep deprivation, and nausea were frequently seen in women who were having impending heart attacks. Fatigue and sleeplessness are warning signs for heart attacks in women. It is thought that this research will alter the way doctors diagnose and treat women who are likely to suffer heart attacks. The appearance of fatigue and sleeplessness in addition to nausea and vomiting in addition to women's heart attack risk factors should alert the doctor that a woman needs to be thoroughly examined for the possibility of a heart attack. Furthermore, women should not ignore these warnings.

It is not uncommon for women workaholics to have heart attacks. If you are a woman and under a lot of stress and you have severe exhaustion but can't sleep and develop nausea as well as sweating, you should go to a hospital emergency room. You must note that in this study that was recently released, 43 percent of the women who had heart attacks and were surveyed did not have any chest pain during their heart attacks.

However, more than 70 percent of the women who had heart attacks reported feeling unusual fatigue. These new findings differ from the previous findings that chest pain was the most important symptom for identifying heart attacks in both men and women. Other, previously discounted symptoms such as fatigue, sleeplessness, nausea, anxiety, and shortness of breath are important signs of heart disease as well.

In this study, 48 percent of women reported sleeplessness, whereas 42 percent reported shortness of breath. Thirty-five percent of women in the study complained of anxiety. These symptoms interfered with the daily activities of the women in the study. The study was sponsored by the National Institute of Nursing Research. It involved 515 women. The women in the study were mostly Caucasian. These women had been diagnosed with a heart attack within the previous six months prior to entering the study. The results of this study indicate that women should be thoroughly checked for coronary artery disease.

Women, however, should look beyond the results of this study and look at other risk factors such as whether they smoke, are overweight, or have high cholesterol levels. Furthermore, diabetes and a family history of heart disease can make them prone to heart attacks as well. The results of this study are important because numerous studies have shown that men on the other hand experience chest pains before a heart attack. There are physiologic differences between men and women that may account for these differences in symptoms associated with a heart attack.

Hormones are different for men and women, and women have smaller arteries that supply their heart muscles. These physiologic differences may account for the differences in heart attack symptoms. You need to realize that heart disease is the number one killer of women as well as men in the United States. When woman have a heart attack, they are more likely to die than men. They are also more likely to have a repeat heart attack within a year as opposed to men.

The results of this study that we described are important because usually we think of angina as chest pain. Different types of angina have been described that can occur in both men and women.

Stable angina is angina that is chronic and is usually caused by physical activity or emotional stress. Stable angina is usually heart-related pain relieved by rest or nitroglycerin. Unstable angina, on the other hand, can increase with rest. Other types of unstable angina can occur at low activity levels. Unstable angina may not be responsive to nitroglycerin. Sometimes you can develop spasms of your arteries that supply your heart muscle. This type of spasm is called Pinzmetal's angina and can be relieved frequently with nitroglycerin.

Stable angina is a term used to describe pain that is predictably caused by narrowing of coronary arteries and a given stress to your heart. For example, walking two flights of stairs or chasing a bus for half a block. The pain is predictable in terms of its severity, how long it lasts, and what brings about relief (such as a single tablet of nitroglycerin placed under the tongue). On the other hand, unstable angina describes a new pattern of pain not previously experienced, for example, pain previously felt after a flight of stairs is now suddenly experienced at rest. Unstable angina is a medical emergency that should be immediately evaluated by a doctor.

As you can see, an adequate and accurate history of your pain is extremely important for your doctor. If you are suffering from angina or suffering a myocardial infarction, an adequate history can help your doctor make an accurate diagnosis so that you can receive the appropriate treatment. I recommend that you write down all of your symptoms. Write down what you were doing when your pain occurred. If you are having only anxiety and fatigue, write down what you were doing before the onset of your symptoms. Remember that other symptoms of other medical problems can be confused with angina pectoris.

Pain that remains in one area and is not referred to other areas and is stabbing and fleeting is usually not angina pectoris, but it is very important to remember that all chest pain can be a sign of heart attack or angina and should be urgently evaluated by a doctor, especially that which has never before been experienced or is associated with nausea and vomiting, sweating, fatigue, or shortness of breath. Your doctor will do a physical examination on you. Your heart rate and blood pressure can be normal, although heart pain will often cause an increase in heart rate and blood pressure.

You can have an irregular heartbeat. Sometimes your doctor will hear a new heart murmur that was not present before your angina attack. In many instances during an angina attack your EKG, a tracing of the electrical activity of your heart, will show signs of cardiac injury. However, it is also possible that your EKG can be completely normal, and this finding does not rule out heart attack or angina.

If you are having chest pain and your EKG appears normal, your doctor may do an echocardiogram or administer radioactive dye and do a heart perfusion study. Your doctor may take a sample of your blood to have it analyzed for any elevations of your heart enzymes. If you have heart muscle damage, the injured tissue will release chemicals. If these so-called heart isoenzymes are increased, this may be a sign that you are having a heart attack. If you have a history of risk factors for coronary artery disease and if your symptoms are stable, your doctor may do a pharmacologic stress test.

A dobutamine echocardiogram study may be done. You will be given a drug that will increase your heart rate. You will be monitored with a continuous EKG to see if there are any changes on your EKG that suggest decreased perfusion to your heart muscles. Occasionally your cardiologist may want to do a coronary angiogram, which is a test that uses a dye to assess the extent of your coronary artery disease.

A chest pain syndrome that may be more prevalent in women is an entity called syndrome X. If you have this syndrome, you may have an exaggerated response of the small arteries that go to your heart muscles.

This exaggerated response is constriction of the diameter of your arteries. When this happens, you have decreased blood flow going to your heart. Usually women that suffer from this illness have a generalized increase in their body pain overall. This disease is undergoing further research at present.

As mentioned previously, women can have myocardial infarctions without having any chest pain. This can also be true in men. In other words, painless myocardial infarctions can occur in both sexes. These painless myocardial infarctions are usually discovered on routine EKGs.

As stated, women need to be educated as to the symptoms based on evidence obtained from studies including men and women. You must know that women have significantly greater back and jaw pain when it does occur as well as nausea and vomiting than men when they present with symptoms of acute coronary syndromes. If you have these symptoms, you may be having a heart attack and you must seek medical attention immediately. Men have more chest pain as well as sweating when they are having a heart attack. Essentially men and women can experience the same symptoms, but the proportions of the symptoms are more prevalent in women than men.

The prevalence of the cardiac syndrome X is higher in women when compared to men. Estrogen deficiency has been shown to play a major role in the origin of cardiac syndrome X. Estrogen has properties on blood vessels that can increase the diameter of the blood vessels. The results of this study demonstrate that the blood vessels in your heart can be modified by sex hormones. A further study reveals that an estrogen deficiency contributes to the development of angina and that in women this angina can be treated with estrogen supplements.

Men are more likely to be hospitalized for unstable angina than women. Angiography was underused in a publicly insured population. Improved access to coronary angiography among minority populations with multiple coronary risk factors is needed.[3]

Research has demonstrated a smaller proportion of women who suffer from angina have coronary artery disease than men who have angina. At one time it was thought that these findings contributed to the perception that chest pain was less serious in women. However, we now know that chest pain is serious in both men and women. Research continues to demonstrate that heart disease, which has not always been considered a serious problem for women, is now a serious problem for women. With more women smoking today, the incidence of heart disease has risen. Approximately 240,000 women in the United States die from heart disease each year. Heart disease is the second-leading killer of women under age 55.

Cancer is the primary reason why women die. However, by age 55 heart disease causes more deaths in women than cancer. Did you know that one out of two American women will die of heart disease or stroke? Just like men, women should not smoke. Men and women should be aware of their blood pressures, cholesterol levels, and their blood sugar levels.

Studies have shown that if women control their weight and work with their doctor to control their blood pressure and modify their lifestyle, they can minimize the risk of heart disease and minimize the risk of having a heart attack. Be aware that if you are overweight, you run the risk of having an elevated blood pressure. The elevated blood pressure can cause you to have a heart attack. The problem in this country is that obesity is increasing and is near epidemic.

Almost 50 percent of adults in the United States are overweight. Furthermore, about 30 percent of the youth in the United States are overweight. These findings suggest that more individuals will develop high blood pressure and eventually more individuals will develop coronary artery disease and one can expect that there will be more deaths related to myocardial infarction.

Women have not been included in research studies done on the heart until recently. The reason for this was that most premature heart attacks occurred in men before age 55. Women who develop heart disease at older ages were not included in the studies. Furthermore, researchers eliminated women in their earlier studies because it was thought that women's hormones could alter the results of the studies on the incidence of heart attacks and deaths. The good news is that there have been inclusions of women in studies of coronary artery disease following the institution of the Women's Health Initiative about 10 years ago.

Studies are being done to evaluate hormone-replacement therapy for the prevention of heart disease. It is known that estrogen does affect the caliber of the arteries that go to your heart and also affects the muscles in the walls of your arteries. Estrogen may also have an effect on your blood's ability to clot. If your blood clots too readily, you can have stoppage of the blood flow in your coronary arteries. The estrogen hormone may have an affect on your body's ability to form clots. Estrogen therapy can be associated with a stroke and the risks of this therapy must be discussed with your physician.

Aspirin can affect your body's ability to clot and, if you are having angina or if you suspect that you are having a heart attack, aspirin can be lifesaving. Current studies are being done examining the effects of nutrients for the prevention of heart disease. The prevalence of myocardial infarction and unstable angina, revascularization rate and extent of coronary artery disease differ significantly among chest pain patients of different ethnic groups. These findings have important clinical implications and support consideration of ethnicity in risk stratification and determination of the patient management strategy in patients with symptoms suggestive of myocardial infarction.

Remember that angina is not a heart attack. Angina is your body's warning to you that something is wrong and only means that some of your heart muscle is not getting enough blood temporarily. Angina does not mean that your heart muscle is suffering permanent damage. A heart attack, on the other hand, occurs when the blood flow to your heart muscle is suddenly and permanently cut off. This will cause damage that is usually permanent to your heart muscle. If you have angina, it means that you have an underlying coronary heart disease.

When you have an angina attack, you are at an increased risk of having a heart attack. South Asian ethnicity might result in a higher atherosclerotic vascular risk compared with white ethnicity.[4] Calcified atherosclerotic plaque is less prevalent and less severe in African-Americans relative to European Americans.[5]

Your angina is treated by controlling your risk factors. This includes decreasing your blood pressure if you are hypertensive. It also means that you should stop smoking cigarettes. If your cholesterol is elevated, you must follow your doctor's instructions to reduce the cholesterol and take any cholesterol-lowering drugs that your doctor may prescribe. If you are overweight, strive to exercise and reduce the fat in your diet.

If you take these steps, you will reduce the possibility that you will have a heart attack. Do not overdo physical activity. Use alcohol only in moderation, if at all. If angina occurs after eating a large meal, avoid large meals and avoid foods that leave you feeling stuffed. Angina can be controlled by medications. The prevalence of myocardial infarction and unstable angina, revascularization rate and extent of coronary artery disease differ significantly among chest pain patients of different ethnic groups.[6] These findings have important clinical implications and support consideration of ethnicity in risk stratification and determination of the patient management strategy in patients with symptoms suggestive of myocardial infarction. The "classic" signs and symptoms of acute MI may not be classic for all racial and ethnic groups.[7]

Even though physical activity is helpful to you in most instances, in people with pre-existing heart disease physical exercise can precipitate a heart attack and should only be conducted under the direction of your doctor. Remember if you have unstable angina or chest pain at rest, you will probably need hospitalization for intensive medical therapy. Aspirin and heparin can be given to decrease the clotting factors of your bloodstream.

If you have angina, these drugs can decrease the progression of angina to a heart attack. If you suspect that you are having a heart attack, seek immediate medical attention. Most deaths associated with an acute heart attack occur during the first hours following the onset of the heart attack. Ethnic groups differ in their pain-reducing behaviors. For whites, pain intensity and interference were the strongest predictors of pain-reducing behaviors. For African Americans, total pain sites, as well as interference and frustration, were significantly associated with pain-reducing behaviors, while among Hispanics, worry and frustration were the strongest predictors for total pain-reducing behaviors.[8]

Call your emergency medical service if you suspect that you are having a heart attack. Most emergency medical technicians can recognize the symptoms of a heart attack. You will require oxygen. Nitroglycerine and morphine will be administered to you. If your heart rate is abnormal, these professionals can treat your abnormal heart rate as well. Your EKG can be sent by telemetry by your emergency medical technician to a local emergency room so that the emergency room doctor can make a diagnosis of your heart rhythm and recommend any treatments that may be immediately necessary.

It is important that blood is restored to your heart muscle. Sometimes your blood flow to your heart muscles can be increased by administering therapy to you that will break up blood clots in your heart blood vessels. Streptokinase is one drug that can be used in this situation. You will be confined to bed for 24 to 36 hours. You will be placed in a cardiac care unit. Your activities will be gradually increased.

There are enzymes that are released into your bloodstream when you have heart muscle damage. These enzymes will be monitored by your treating doctor. There might be some differences in how triage nurses approach the management of patients with chest pain on the basis of gender and ethnicity.[9]

Nitroglycerin is a commonly prescribed drug for the treatment of angina. Nitroglycerin will relieve your angina pain by making your blood vessels going to your heart wider. The increased blood flow will permit more oxygen to go to your heart. This increased oxygen will keep up with the demand of your heart. You should take nitroglycerin when you have the onset of discomfort. Other medicines such as beta blockers can be used to slow your heart rate and decrease the contraction of your heart muscle. This will conserve oxygen.

Propanolol (Inderal) is an example of a beta blocker. Calcium channel blockers (Verapimil) affect the calcium in your muscle cells. Calcium channel blockers such as Verapamil can decrease the incidence of you having angina as well as a heart attack. Ethnic differences in pain-reducing behaviors were explored. For whites, pain intensity and interference were the strongest predictors of pain-reducing behaviors. For African Americans, total pain sites, as well as interference and frustration, were significantly associated with pain-reducing behaviors, while among Hispanics, worry and frustration were the strongest predictors for total pain-reducing behaviors.[8]

If medication fails to control your angina, coronary artery bypass surgery is sometimes necessary. A blood vessel is grafted onto your blocked artery. This allows your blood flow to bypass the blockage so that blood can go to your heart muscle to provide your heart muscle with needed oxygen. Your surgeon can use an artery inside your chest or take a vein from your leg.

Another treatment that can be used to increase your artery size is called balloon angioplasty. This involves insertion of a catheter that has a tiny, tiny balloon on the end of it into an artery either in your arm or your leg. The balloon is inflated briefly to widen your vessel in places where your arteries are narrow. Work with your doctor to develop an exercise plan. A physical therapist can work with you and observe you while you are doing some exercise. You may start with a 5-minute walk and increase your exercise 5 minutes per week until you reach a 30-minute walk. Among blacks, dyslipidemia, diabetes, and smoking were independently associated with premature CAD.[10]

Among Hispanics, dyslipidemia, male sex, and family history of CAD were independently associated with premature CAD. Smoking was the only risk factor in whites, and no independent risk factor was identified in Asian Indians.

The diagnosis and treatment of angina is extremely important because there are more than 500,000 deaths in the United States related to coronary artery disease every year. Over 1 million new and repeat cases of heart attack occur each year. Approximately 44 percent of these patients die. Almost 13 million individuals who have angina or a heart attack are still living. The number of men and women living are almost equal.

Since 1990, the death rate from coronary artery disease has actually decreased. More than 6 million people in the United States suffer from angina. Another study was done that revealed that 400,000 new cases of stable angina occur each year. The incidence of angina is greater in women than men. Furthermore, the incidence of angina in women over age 20 was highest in African American women followed by Mexican American followed by Caucasian women.

The same is true for racial differences in men. For patients with undifferentiated chest pain, overall race, sex, and age differences were explained by higher rates of aspirin administered to older men with chest pain. No race, sex, or age differences for acute myocardial infarction or unstable angina were noted.[11] Higher rates of adverse events among women with obstructive coronary artery disease, regardless of ethnicity, as well as high rates of angina readmission however have been reported.[12]

If you have persistent angina that is refractory to treatments, your pain-medicine doctor could place a catheter in your epidural space. This device is called a dorsal column stimulator. It provides electrical current to the back of your spinal cord. This current could decrease your chest pain. It is used frequently in Europe for angina that is refractory to other treatments. Atherosclerotic plaque as measured by using coronary CT angiography, differ between African American and white patients, with relatively more noncalcified disease in African Americans and more calcified disease in white individuals.[13]

Another type of procedure that can increase your blood flow is called a stent. A stent is a surgical procedure, but it is a minor procedure compared to open heart surgery. Stents are implanted through your veins with a catheter. The stent expands when it is placed. The stent will provide better blood flow at the location of your artery where the blood flow is decreased. Your chest wall is not opened to have this procedure done.

Stents that are being used currently are coated with heparin to prevent clotting within the stent. The purpose of the stent is to permanently hold your blood vessel open. This procedure like placement of the balloon into your coronary arteries is a relatively safe procedure and can be extremely effective.

Smoking increases your risk of coronary artery disease. If you are obese, you should make dietary changes to decrease your cholesterol and weight. Nitroglycerin and other vasodilator medications will make the blood vessels going to your heart larger, therefore increasing the amount of oxygen that your heart receives.

If your heart rate is too fast, your doctor may prescribe beta blockers, such as propranolol, to slow your heart rate and decrease the contraction of your heart muscle to help conserve oxygen. Your doctor may prescribe you a calcium channel blocker, such as Verapamil, to decrease your incidence of having angina or heart attack.   Exercise regimens prescribed by your doctor may be necessary to strengthen your heart muscles. Surgical interventions such as coronary artery bypass surgery, balloon angioplasty and stent placement may be needed to improve blood flow to your heart if medications are not successfully treating your condition.

References

1.   Stepanikova I. Racial-ethnic biases, time pressure, and medical decisions. Journal of health and social behavior. 2012;53(3):329-343.

2.   Bell PD, Hudson S. Equity in the diagnosis of chest pain: race and gender. Am J Health Behav. 2001;25(1):60-71.

3.   Barnhart J, Bernstein SJ. Is coronary angiography underused in an inner-city population? Ethn Dis. 2006;16(3):659-665.

4.   Brister SJ, Hamdulay Z, Verma S, Maganti M, Buchanan MR. Ethnic diversity: South Asian ethnicity is associated with increased coronary artery bypass grafting mortality. J Thorac Cardiovasc Surg. 2007;133(1):150-154.

5.   Divers J, Wagenknecht LE, Bowden DW, et al. Ethnic differences in the relationship between pericardial adipose tissue and coronary artery calcified plaque: African-American-diabetes heart study. J Clin Endocrinol Metab. 2010;95(12):5382-5389.

6.   de Hoog VC, Lim SH, Bank IE, et al. Ethnic differences in clinical outcome of patients presenting to the emergency department with chest pain. European heart journal. Acute cardiovascular care. 2015.

7.   Lee H, Bahler R, Park OJ, Kim CJ, Lee HY, Kim YJ. Typical and atypical symptoms of myocardial infarction among African-Americans, whites, and Koreans. Crit Care Nurs Clin North Am. 2001;13(4):531-539.

8.   Hastie BA, Riley JL, Fillingim RB. Ethnic differences and responses to pain in healthy young adults. Pain Med. 2005;6(1):61-71.

9.   Shapiro SE, Howard PK. Does gender and ethnicity impact initial assessment and management of chest pain? Adv Emerg Nurs J. 2011;33(1):4-7.

10.   Izadnegahdar M, Mackay M, Lee MK, et al. Sex and Ethnic Differences in Outcomes of Acute Coronary Syndrome and Stable Angina Patients With Obstructive Coronary Artery Disease. Circ Cardiovasc Qual Outcomes. 2016;9(1):S26-35.

11.   Takakuwa KM, Shofer FS, Hollander JE. Aspirin administration in ED patients who presented with undifferentiated chest pain: age, race, and sex effects. Am J Emerg Med. 2010;28(3):318-324.

12.   Becker ER, Rahimi A. Disparities in race/ethnicity and gender in in-hospital mortality rates for coronary artery bypass surgery patients. Journal of the National Medical Association. 2006;98(11):1729-1739.

13.   Nance JW, Jr., Bamberg F, Schoepf UJ, et al. Coronary atherosclerosis in African American and white patients with acute chest pain: characterization with coronary CT angiography. Radiology. 2011;260(2):373-380.

26. Complex Regional Pain Syndrome

Complex regional pain syndrome (CRPS) is the newest name for the confusing conditions of reflex sympathetic dystrophy and causalgia.[1] Reflex sympathetic dystrophy (RSD) can be a devastating entity for you, especially if it is not diagnosed and treated within a timely fashion. Reflex sympathetic dystrophy usually affects one of your extremities (arms or legs) but also can affect your face. Reflex sympathetic dystrophy is now called complex regional pain syndrome. The complex regional pain syndrome is a painful disorder that can occur in an extremity after any type of injury, or even spontaneously.[2]

Females are affected at least three times more often than males. The highest incidence occurs in females in the age category of 61-70 years. The upper extremity was affected more frequently than the lower extremity and a fracture was the most common precipitating event. A medical history of a migraine and osteoporosis were associated with CRPS.[3]

Reflex sympathetic dystrophy is serious, painful, and potentially disabling. Pain associated with this entity is throbbing, burning, or aching. You can have pain just to touch. You can have swelling of your extremity as well as either warmth or coldness depending on the phase of your RSD and sweating. Your hair may grow faster on the extremity with RSD at first, only to slow down as the disease progresses. Your extremity will sweat. It can turn color. The nails in your affected limb can grow faster on the extremity that suffers from reflex sympathetic dystrophy.

Reflex sympathetic dystrophy usually occurs following an injury. However, a heart attack or stroke can cause you to have reflex sympathetic dystrophy. It can be seen in the knee as well as in the shoulder. In a study of reflex sympathetic dystrophy, 40 percent of the cases followed an injury to a muscle or a nerve. Simple bruises or sprains can trigger reflex sympathetic dystrophy. Fractures accounted for 25 percent of reflex sympathetic dystrophy cases.

Twenty percent of the RSD patients were postoperative on an arm or leg, whereas 12 percent occurred after a heart attack. Three percent occurred after a stroke. Approximately 37 percent of patients in the study had emotional disturbances at the time of the onset of the reflex sympathetic dystrophy. It is not clear why complex regional pain syndrome (CRPS) develops in some patients but not in others, despite similar initiating events.[4] Stressful life events are more common in the CRPS patients.5 However, three out of four cases undergo resolution.[6] Open wounds, sprain and strain, superficial injury, contusion, and nerve and spinal cord injury are main injury mechanisms. Injury in the extremities confers a higher risk of CRPS.[7]

It was once thought that reflex sympathetic dystrophy was an emotional problem. However, studies have shown that many people do not suffer from emotional problems at the time of onset of reflex sympathetic dystrophy. Would you become anxious or depressed if you had constant severe pain that decreased your daily activity and disrupted your sleep? To prevent you from having permanent disability, treatment needs to be started immediately. Treatment usually consists of oral medications as well as injection therapy by an anesthesiologist using local anesthetics.

Steroids may also be used effectively to treat RSD. If your symptoms persist, sometimes you will need surgery to remove the offending nerves causing your pain. Remember that early diagnosis and treatment can significantly improve your outcome. Further research in the exact cause of this disease and the appropriate treatment continues. Increased systemic gene-related peptide levels in patients with acute CRPS suggest neurogenic inflammation as a pathophysiologic mechanism contributing to vasodilation, edema, and increased sweating.[8]

If you have had reflex sympathetic dystrophy, it may have been called another condition. It is now called a complex regional pain syndrome. At one time it was called post-traumatic sympathetic dystrophy, algodystrophy, Sudeck's atrophy, transient osteoporosis, and post-traumatic vasomotor syndrome. The shoulder/hand syndrome was also used to describe reflex sympathetic dystrophy following a heart attack or a stroke.

If you sustained actual nerve damage, your reflex sympathetic dystrophy is called causalgia. Sympathetically maintained pain (SMP) is a symptom of neuropathic pain conditions defined as the pain component that is relieved by specific sympatholytic procedures. If sympatholytic procedures have no influence on the pain, the symptom is called "sympathetically independent pain" (SIP).

A previous definition of causalgia was referred to the syndrome associated with known nerve injury, whereas reflex sympathetic dystrophy included those patients whose pain and associated symptoms were followed by a variety of causes. Injury associated with causalgia was more severe, whereas that associated with RSD was relatively minor. Now reflex sympathetic dystrophy is referred to as complex regional pain syndrome I, whereas causalgia is referred as complex regional pain syndrome II. Causes of both of these syndromes include fractures as well as dislocations.

Reflex sympathetic dystrophy and causalgia were originally described by Dr. Mitchell, a neurologist during the Civil War. He noted that some soldiers who had injuries to their hands or feet developed a syndrome that consisted of burning pain, pain to touch over the skin of the injured extremity, shiny skin, and skin that had different colors consisting of either redness or a blue cyanotic color.

Blue or cyanotic discoloration usually occurs when skin or other tissues do not get enough blood and oxygen. Mitchell also noted that the pain in the extremity was out of proportion to the injury. For example, if you sustained a sprain to your ankle, you would expect to have some pain. However, if you develop reflex sympathetic dystrophy, the pain is excruciating and unbearable. Mitchell noted the onset of reflex sympathetic dystrophy following gunshot wounds. The exact cause of reflex sympathetic dystrophy remains under investigation.

It was originally hypothesized that if your sympathetic nervous system became hyperactive, this hyperactivity was at least one of the causes of reflex sympathetic dystrophy. Your sympathetic nervous system is one component of your autonomic nervous system. The other component of your autonomic nervous system is called the parasympathetic nervous system. Your autonomic nervous system regulates your circulation and your breathing as well as your stomach and bladder functions. You have no control over your autonomic nervous system. This distinguishes it from your peripheral nervous system which is usually under your control.

Because it is thought by some medical clinicians that your sympathetic nervous system can have some role in the onset of reflex sympathetic dystrophy, you must have a basic understanding of this system in order to understand reflex sympathetic dystrophy. Your sympathetic nervous system fibers emerge from your mid back part of your spinal cord. On the other hand your parasympathetic fibers come from your brain stem as well as your lower sacral areas. Your sympathetic nervous system sends sympathetic nerve fibers to the blood vessels in your head and neck as well as to your skin and muscles in your arms and legs. These fibers also go to your heart, your lungs, and your esophagus.

Furthermore, fibers can go to your stomach, pancreas, liver, gallbladder, and your intestines. Your kidneys, ureter, uterus, bladder, and prostate can all be affected. In your extremities, sympathetic fibers go to your blood vessels as well as your sweat glands and hair follicles. Remember that your hands and feet can sweat profusely if you have reflex sympathetic dystrophy and the hair on your arms and legs can grow faster or fall out. Your sympathetic nerve fibers can restrict circulation in certain areas of your body.

Your sympathetic nervous system can also change the chemical environment of your muscle tissue as well as your other nervous system tissue and sensitive the small pain fibers in these different tissues. You must also realize that your sympathetic nervous system is linked to emotional states. Therefore, your sympathetic nervous system plays an important role in the psychological aspects of pain. Sometimes if your doctor blocks your sympathetic nerve pathways, you can have some relief of your reflex sympathetic dystrophy.

When you have an injury to your extremity, for example, you will have pain impulses that go to your spinal cord as well as your brain. The impulses that are going to your spinal cord and brain are initiated by pain fibers in your tissue. These pain fibers are both enhanced and inhibited at all levels of your brain and spinal cord. Your tissues produce pain-producing as well as pain-enhancing chemicals. This causes your nerves to transmit pain impulses onto your spinal cord and ultimately to your brain. However, in your spinal cord you have chemicals that can stop or attenuate the pain impulses.

You also have what are called descending pathways, which are essentially nerves with chemicals that decrease the transmission of pain signals before they reach your brain. To modulate your pain, there must be checks and balances within your nervous system. Remember that pain is a warning to your brain that something is wrong at a particular place in your body.

However, your body has normal mechanisms to lessen your pain. When you suffer from reflex sympathetic dystrophy, your pain-producing chemicals and nerves are much stronger than the aspects of your nervous system that are able to decrease the pain. Over time the part of your nervous system that decreases your pain becomes unable to function properly. At this time, your pain becomes overwhelming and disabling.

Chemical substances in your tissues activate your pain fibers. These chemicals cause your blood vessels to increase their diameter. When this happens, you will have warmth in your painful area as well as redness and increased temperature. As your blood vessels enlarge, you may also have swelling in your tissue. Chemicals such as acetylcholine, potassium, and serotonin can stimulate pain in your tissues.

However, when these chemicals are in your brain or spinal cord they do not cause pain. Histamine in your tissues can also be a chemical that can cause you to have pain. However, histamine is being used in creams to decrease your pain in your skin and muscles. Further studies have shown that the release of histamine into your spinal cord can decrease your pain as well. The mechanisms by which histamine either cause pain or help relieve pain remain to be studied and elucidated.

Prostaglandins are also released if you have injury to your tissue. As mentioned previously, prostaglandins themselves do not produce pain; when they are around pain nerves, however, they sensitize these nerves to pain. Prostaglandins can intensify any inflammation that you may have and increase the action of bradykinin on your nerve endings. Substance P in your tissues can be a cause of significant pain. It is important for you to realize that there are many pain producing chemicals especially in reflex sympathetic dystrophy.

The reason for this polypharmacy is that many chemicals combine to cause your pain associated with your reflex sympathetic dystrophy. If you have increased sweating associated with reflex sympathetic dystrophy, this implies that your sympathetic nervous system has become overactive. However, if your reflex sympathetic dystrophy persists over time, you will notice that the sweating in your hands or feet can significantly decrease. It is believed that with chronic reflex sympathetic dystrophy that the sympathetic reflexes do not remain active.

In 1916, it was noted that the pain could be relieved by surgically removing some of the sympathetic fibers that innervate the affected extremity. This surgeon also noted that patients who had his procedure had some pain relief and had decreased sweating and improvement in their skin color. This surgeon then thought that the sympathetic nervous system was involved in the etiology of reflex sympathetic dystrophy. Over time the treatment of reflex sympathetic dystrophy included repetitive sympathetic blocks or removal of the sympathetic nerves, either surgically or by chemicals such as phenol.

Sympathetic blocks involve placing a local anesthetic about the bundles of nerves which exist outside of your central nervous system. These nerve bundles which are called ganglia are in your neck as well as your lower back. The ganglion in your neck influences your arm pain while your ganglia in your lower back influence RSD pain in your leg.

Early description of reflex sympathetic dystrophy included injuries without obvious nerve damage. Causalgia, on the other hand, was the description given to symptoms of reflex sympathetic dystrophy where a nerve had been actually injured, such as in a gunshot wound that was described by Dr. Mitchell during the Civil War. Sprains and strains can also be a cause of these syndromes as well as bursitis and tendonitis. Arthritis can also cause either reflex sympathetic dystrophy or causalgia. If you are a female and have had a mastectomy, you may develop reflex sympathetic dystrophy. If one of the veins in your legs has been occluded, you may also develop reflex sympathetic dystrophy. After placement of a cast on your arms and legs, you may develop reflex sympathetic dystrophy and/or causalgia. Some individual have developed these syndromes following the onset of shingles. Head injuries and strokes can also cause you to have reflex sympathetic dystrophy or causalgia.

A rare but devastating form of reflex sympathetic dystrophy can occur after a tooth extraction. Heart attacks can be associated with reflex sympathetic dystrophy of your upper arms. Painful reflex sympathetic dystrophy like symptoms can occur around your perineum (the area between the anus and urinary outlet) following surgery around this area.

Remember that sympathetic nerve fibers go to all parts of your body and, therefore, all parts of your body can be affected. The problem with reflex sympathetic dystrophy is that in many instances it is either over diagnosed or underdiagnosed. A consensus conference, therefore, was held by doctors and scientists from all over the world.

These individuals have compiled the diagnostic criteria for complex regional pain syndrome. The results of their meeting stated that complex regional pain syndrome describes a variety of painful conditions. The painful conditions must exceed the duration of the expected clinical course of the inciting event. For example, if you sustain an ankle sprain, your pain should be gone in several weeks. If your pain becomes severe and remains for several months, this suggests that you may have a complex regional pain syndrome. The problem with the two types of complex regional pain syndrome is that they can progress over time.

For you to be diagnosed with RSD, you should have the following happen: An initiating traumatic event to your tissue. The onset of spontaneous pain to touch as well as pain to a noxious stimulus that lasts longer than expected may indicate RSD. Your pain must be global. For example, if you have injured your hand, you may have an injury to one of the nerves in your hand. For example, your ulnar nerve will give you pain or numbness in your last two fingers of your hand. This is the definition of a neuritis, which means inflammation of a nerve. This is not RSD.

RSD means that the whole hand (global) is painful and not just in the distribution of one nerve. Evidence of swelling of your extremity becomes evident with either an increase or a decrease in your skin blood flow as well as alterations in the color of your skin and sweating. The diagnosis of RSD must be excluded by the existence of other conditions that could account for the degree of your pain and dysfunction. For example, arthritis and inflammation can give you pain that is similar to that of reflex sympathetic dystrophy.

For you to be diagnosed with causalgia, also known as complex regional pain syndrome II, you will have the above mentioned symptoms but you should also have a documented nerve injury. Furthermore, for the diagnosis of both of these entities, you should have documented temperature changes noted on the skin over the area of your reflex sympathetic dystrophy. Remember that the diagnosis of CRPS cannot be made if you do not have pain. This is because CRPS is a pain syndrome by definition. Most of the time your pain will be of a burning nature.

Your pain will develop after a traumatic event or after immobilization such as casting. Your pain will be on one side. Only rarely can reflex sympathetic dystrophy spread to another extremity. The onset of your symptoms usually occurs within a month from your surgery or trauma. You do not have reflex sympathetic dystrophy if you have anatomical, physiological, or psychological conditions that would cause your pain and dysfunction in your affected extremity. Remember that infection or arthritis are diseases that can mimic the symptoms of RSD. These entities can cause you to have significant pain. If you have behavioral problems, your behavioral problems can be a cause of pain.

If you become extremely anxious, you can have sweating associated that one normally sees in reflex sympathetic dystrophy. If you have complex regional pain syndrome, light touch or deep pressure should cause you pain. Cold applications to your skin can worsen your pain. Movement of your joints can also cause pain. You skin should be shiny. Your nails should grow faster on the side of the reflex sympathetic dystrophy. At first your hair will grow faster on the side of your reflex sympathetic dystrophy but eventually your hair pattern will decrease and you may even lose hair in this area
. Tremors or spasms should be noted on the side of your reflex sympathetic dystrophy. If you have complex regional pain syndrome, you should also have complaints of stiffness at the joints where your fingers

meet your hand or where your toes meet your foot. Remember that the complex regional pain syndrome is usually over diagnosed. Unfortunately, some doctors will call shoddy surgery RSD. This condition is rare. However, when it does occur, it must be treated immediately. If you have any of these symptoms mentioned in this chapter, notify your doctor.

Following surgery, reflex sympathetic dystrophy is a difficult entity to diagnose and treat. Studies on reflex sympathetic dystrophy, for example, following hand surgery can vary from less than 1 percent to 15 percent of all patients. As previously stated, reflex sympathetic dystrophy is often accompanied by dysfunction of your sympathetic nervous system, which results in changes in the blood flow to your skin of your affected limb. It was noted in 1946 that reflex sympathetic dystrophy needs to be diagnosed early because the treatment is more effective if you have an early diagnosis.

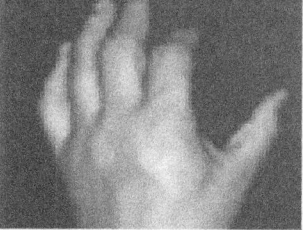

Figure 1. RSD frequently causes swelling.

In other words, early treatment positively affects your outcome. Blockade of your sympathetic nervous system is most effective for the treatment of your complex regional pain syndrome if it is performed within the first four to six weeks from the onset of your symptoms. These blocks become less effective the longer you wait to treat your complex regional pain syndrome.

After surgery, the clinical diagnosis of RSD is often delayed because RSD can resemble normal postoperative states. If you have had hand surgery, for example, you can expect to have pain, swelling, and loss of function as well as the other symptoms associated with reflex sympathetic dystrophy. However, these symptoms should be gone by six weeks. At one time, it was thought that a three-phase bone scan was useful for the diagnosis of complex regional pain syndrome.

Studies were done as early as 1981. Individuals also used the three-phase bone scan for monitoring the progress of RSD. This imagery is related to the distribution of a radioactive isotope throughout the body, and a nuclear medicine doctor will note the distribution of this radioactive isotope in the affected extremity. The distribution of the radioactive isotope is dependent upon blood flow as well as the activity of the bone. The problem with this test is that it has not been shown to be as good as previously assumed. Furthermore, if your three-phase bone scan is negative, this does not mean that you do not have reflex sympathetic dystrophy.

The three-phase bone scan is positive in only 53 percent of the individuals with RSD. The three-phase bone scan is of little value in monitoring the course of the treatment of your complex regional pain syndrome. A three-phase bone scan may be effective for staging the early or late forms of RSD. Magnetic resonance imaging (MRI) can aid in the diagnosis of RSD by identifying swelling in the center of your bone. This bone marrow edema is characteristic of complex regional pain syndrome. This study is more reliable than a three-phase bone scanning or plain x-ray exams.

Skin temperature differences in the arms and legs are extremely useful for the diagnosis of complex regional pain syndrome. Contact and infrared thermography have both been recommended for the diagnosis of reflex sympathetic dystrophy, but the problem with thermography is that it can be influenced not only by skin blood flow but also by the temperature of the room environment as well as by your muscle and your deep tissue metabolism. A new method called laser Doppler imaging is effective for the diagnosis of complex regional pain syndrome. The study is important because the results of this study are influenced by your superficial blood flow. Your superficial blood flow is under the control of your autonomic nervous system. Other studies are being developed, which include plethsmography and capillaroscopy. Another device to evaluate reflex sympathetic dystrophy is called the quantitative pseudomotor axon test. This test is time-consuming and is currently available only in several academic centers. However, the results of this test are accurate.

There are different phases of reflex sympathetic dystrophy. A test that measures all three of these phases is necessary. The only one to date that will detect all three phases is the laser Doppler device. After you have sustained an injury to your extremity, the blood vessels to your extremity become bigger. This allows more blood flow to go to your extremity. Your hand or foot will, therefore, feel warm and may appear to be red. This phase usually occurs within the first month of your injury. A three-phase bone scan at this time will demonstrate increased isotope activity in your extremity, which indicates phase I reflex sympathetic dystrophy.

As your RSD progresses, the blood vessels to your extremity will decrease in size. They go from the enlarged diameter to a normal appearing diameter. This is phase II. A three-phase bone scan will, therefore, appear normal at this time. A laser Doppler study, on the other hand, will reveal an abnormality of your sympathetic nervous system. You will have some swelling as well at this time and global pain about your extremity and sweating of your extremity as your sympathetic nervous system becomes overactive. This phase can progress on to phase III.

During this phase, your blood vessels become extremely small and you have decreased blood flow to your hand, foot, or your affected extremity. This will cause your skin to become cold. By this time, you will notice that your skin has become shiny and that the sweating in your hand or foot may have increased. A three-phase bone scan at this time can detect a significant decrease in your blood flow to your extremity. Your treating doctor should try and prevent you from progressing through these phases.

As stated previously, an early diagnosis and treatment will prevent this progression to the worst phase. After you have reached phase three of reflex sympathetic dystrophy, the disease is irreversible. The success rate for phase I is extremely high, which does decrease as you progress to phase II. This is the reason why you should keep an accurate and thorough pain diary. Your symptoms of your pain will provide some suggestion to your doctor as to what phase of reflex sympathetic dystrophy that you are in. In all the phases, you will need an occupational therapy evaluation to attempt to desensitize the pain in your skin and to preserve normal range of motion in your hand, foot, arm, leg, and so on.

With RSD, pain is noted in 84 percent of individuals longer than 12 months. Ninety-one percent have temperature differences in their extremities after 12 months. Recurrence with exercise was noted in 97 percent of patients. Fifty-five percent continued to have swelling after 12 months. Muscle spasms were noted in 42 percent of individuals. Sweating was noted in 40 percent of patients. Nail growth continued in 52 percent of individuals, whereas hair patterns were present in only 35 percent of patients.

Be aware that on rare occasions RSD can spread into more than one extremity. This observation suggests that an individual may have a predisposition to develop RSD. If you have chronic RSD, you can have skin infections associated with persistent swelling of your skin as well as blood vessels that can spontaneously rupture. You may have a change in skin pigmentation and your fingernails or toenails on the affected extremity can become clubbed. The frequency of reflex sympathetic dystrophy shows a peak of the incidence of this entity around 50 years of age. However, you must be aware that both children and elderly individuals can develop RSD.

The distribution of RSD between men and women is almost equal for individuals younger than 50 years of age. However, for those over 50 years of age there is a predominance of reflex sympathetic dystrophy noted in women. Even though some investigators have questioned the existence of the sympathetic nervous system's influence on the pain associated with reflex sympathetic dystrophy, there is clinical evidence that this influence does actually exist. This led investigators to describe two types of pain. One is sympathetically maintained pain and is pain associated with chemicals released by the sympathetic nervous system.

The other type of pain is sympathetically independent pain, which is not associated with the chemicals liberated by the sympathetic nervous system into the bloodstream. Other types of pains can be responsive to sympathetic blockade. This type of blockade with a local anesthetic can even decrease pain associated with peripheral nerves. Sympathetically maintained pain usually has a decrease in your pain component following a sympathetic block. Sympathetically maintained pain can be seen in other entities besides reflex sympathetic dystrophy. It may be seen in neuropathies, phantom limb pain, and shingles as well as neuralgias. The onset of reflex sympathetic dystrophy can occur at any time following a traumatic event. There is a case report of reflex sympathetic dystrophy beginning one year after a fracture occurred. It was thought at one time that RSD could occur without any trauma. This is no longer thought to be true.

Exact causes of reflex sympathetic dystrophy continue to be studied. It is thought that there is a sympathetic nervous system component that causes you to have pain when you develop reflex sympathetic dystrophy. Your nerve ending develop an abnormal sensitivity to the chemicals that are liberated by your sympathetic nerve fibers.

If you have had a nerve injury, your nerve will attempt to regrow and will sprout small sensory pain fibers. Sometimes as your nerves attempt to grow together, the area where they come together can be extremely painful. Where the nerve endings come together can cause an extremely painful area called a neuroma. This neuroma is sensitive to the chemicals released by your sympathetic nervous system.

Most medical investigators report that over time the sympathetic nervous system becomes less involved in the maintenance of reflex sympathetic dystrophy syndrome. As mentioned earlier in this chapter, you can have reflex sympathetic dystrophy that does not involve a nerve injury. In 1996, it was reported that the peripheral nervous system as well as the central nervous system is involved in the progression of RSD.

With this type of pain, your pain receptors may be stimulated by a sympathetic nervous system biochemical such as norepinephrine or through the release of prostaglandins. Prostaglandins will sensitize your nerve endings to other substances that are in your tissues. The prevalent theory is that pain associated with reflex sympathetic dystrophy is mediated by prostaglandins.

Because many individuals have no decrease in their pain when they have sympathetic blocks in both reflex sympathetic dystrophy and causalgia, many investigators question the existence of any sympathetic involvement in these pain syndromes. In 1995, it was proposed that inflammation with the release of prostaglandins function was the cause of pain in both RSD and causalgia. Furthermore, evidence indicates an inflammatory basis for the loss of bone mass that occurs in reflex sympathetic dystrophy.

The COX-2 enzyme may be responsible for the pain associated with reflex sympathetic dystrophy. This is the reason why many doctors today treat reflex sympathetic dystrophy with the new COX-2-inhibiting drugs such as Celebrex. Furthermore, there may be an interaction between COX-2 enzyme and stimulation of the sympathetic nervous system. Even though your injury usually occurs in your arms or legs, there can be distorted information processing within your spinal cord. In other words, changes in your spinal cord can occur secondary to your nerve injury in your arms or legs. Small inhibitory nerves in your spinal cord, called internuncial neurons, may be ineffective if you develop reflex sympathetic dystrophy.

The evidence for vitamin C to prevent CRPS in patients with distal radius fractures fails to demonstrate a significant benefit.9In addition to your central nervous system (composed of your brain and spinal cord) as well as your peripheral nervous system, which is composed of nerves outside of your brain and spinal cord, you also have a sympathetic nervous system. Studies have shown that females are more vulnerable to sympathetically mediated pain than males.

The chemicals that are involved that cause you to have reflex sympathetic dystrophy may be potentially affected by your sex hormones.

It is believed that your hormone status at the time of your trauma is important for the development of the pain associated with reflex sympathetic dystrophy. The present data do not support the hypothesis the RSD patients, relative to other pain patients, are uniquely disturbed in psychosocial functioning.[10]

The effects of reflex sympathetic dystrophy on the central processing in your central nervous system may be the basis for the spread of reflex sympathetic dystrophy to your other extremities. Many recommendations for the treatment of reflex sympathetic dystrophy and causalgia exist. Because there are so many different treatments proposed, you should be aware that no single treatment is superior to the others. Remember that no treatment for complex regional pain syndrome is consistently successful.

It is known that early recognition and active treatment of the complex regional pain syndrome improves your outcome. For example, injections of local anesthetics about your sympathetic nervous system can alleviate your symptoms of reflex sympathetic dystrophy long term. These types of injections must be done early in the onset of your symptoms of reflex sympathetic dystrophy. The injections can be done in your stellate ganglion, which provides sympathetic fibers to your arms, or the injections can be done in the lumbar sympathetic ganglion, which supplies sympathetic fibers to your legs. Combined treatment of conventional physiotherapy and aerobic exercises may be an excellent synthesis for this syndrome in these patients.[11]

Because disuse of your extremities can contribute to the onset of reflex sympathetic dystrophy, your doctor will institute occupational therapy for you. This type of therapy emphasizes range of motion. As stated previously, the new COX-2-inhibiting drugs can be helpful in decreasing your pain associated with complex regional pain syndrome. Sympathetic sweat responses and skin vasomotor reflexes were evaluated in CRPS-1 patients.[12] Reduced responses of these fibers may reflect underlying damage to the sympathetic postganglionic fibers.

A clonidine patch can be used to decrease your pain. This patch is usually used to treat high blood pressure. However, the patch does decrease the sympathetic nervous system chemicals that can be released if you have reflex sympathetic dystrophy. The patch is usually worn for one week before it is changed. The evidence for vitamin C to prevent CRPS in patients with distal radius fractures fails to demonstrate a significant benefit.[9]

Steroids administered by mouth have been shown to be effective for the treatment of reflex sympathetic dystrophy. Steroids will decrease inflammation caused by prostaglandins. If your pain is severe, your doctor will probably prescribe a narcotic drug for you. Depending on the severity of your pain, your doctor will prescribe a mild narcotic such as Darvocet or a stronger narcotic such as Methadone. Anticonvulsive medications can be helpful in decreasing your pain. Gabapentin (Neurontin) or pregabalin (Lyrica) is frequently used now for the treatment of pain associated with your complex regional pain syndrome.

Narcotic medications administered into your spinal fluid can help decrease your pain. Sometimes a morphine pump, which sends a narcotic into your spinal fluid, needs to be implanted to control your RSD pain. Clonidine, which is frequently administered by a patch over your skin, can also be administered into your epidural space for the control of your pain as well. Antidepressant medication such as amitriptyline has also been shown to be effective in the management of pain associated with reflex sympathetic dystrophy and causalgia.

Amitriptyline increases certain chemicals in your central nervous system that are helpful in decreasing the amount of pain that reaches your brain. Implantation of a wire attached to a battery into your epidural space can also provide you with significant pain relief. This apparatus is called a dorsal column stimulator. Spinal cord stimulation is the most effective treatment for CRPS, which is proven resistant to medical management.[13] Psychological intervention is also helpful because of the severity of the pain associated with reflex sympathetic dystrophy, you can develop fear, anxiety, and depression. Psychological intervention including the use of biofeedback and sometimes hypnosis can successfully be used to treat your pain.

C-fiber afferent substance P signaling chronically supports spinal neuroglial activation after limb fracture and that glial activation contributes to the maintenance of central pain fiber sensitization in CRPS.[14] Treatments inhibiting glial activation and spinal inflammation may be therapeutic for CRPS.

Early in your symptoms of RSD, your doctor can inject local anesthetic near your ganglion to relieve pain in your sympathetic nervous system. Local long-acting anesthetic injections may be needed in your areas of discomfort to help relieve your pain. Steroids can help reduce inflammation caused by prostaglandins. Your doctor may prescribe clonidine to help control your pain. Antidepressant medications prescribed by your doctor can increase certain chemicals in your central nervous system that are helpful in reducing the amount of pain impulses that reach your brain.

Because of sex differences with respect to the effect of estrogen as well as progesterone on the absorption, metabolism and elimination of medications, drug dosing may fluctuate in the female patient depending on whether or not the female is pre or post-menopausal. The physiological changes that occur during the menstrual cycle can affect the responses of a drug in the female body. You must discuss the effects of your drug with your doctor because the effect of your drug may decrease during menses. Some RSD patients may benefit from psychological therapy, such as biofeedback, to help treat the fear, anxiety, and depression they may feel because of their pain condition.

Intravenous lidocaine is used to block the sodium channels in neuronal membranes, thus stopping initiation and conduction of impulses associated with neuropathic and inflammatory pain in RSD.[15] If you have RSD, it may be advisable to avoid caffeine. Gabapentin produced dose-related inhibition of mechanical hyperalgesia over a 3-week period, and this effect was blocked by concomitant caffeine administration 1 week after injuries in animals.[16]

It has been suggested that a possible genetic diathesis exists in RSD patients with poor treatment outcomes. Genes conferring susceptibility to RSD may be present in individuals who develop RSD.[17] Physical therapy is widely recommended as a first-line treatment. The efficacy of local anesthetic sympathetic blockade as treatment for CRPS I is questionable.[18] Some Mexican females may have a genetic predisposition to severe sympathetically maintained neuropathic pain syndromes.[19]

References

1.   Bushnell TG, Cobo-Castro T. Complex regional pain syndrome: becoming more or less complex? Man Ther. 1999;4(4):221-228.

2.   de Mos M, de Bruijn AG, Huygen FJ, Dieleman JP, Stricker BH, Sturkenboom MC. The incidence of complex regional pain syndrome: a population-based study. Pain. 2007;129(1-2):12-20.

3.   de Mos M, Huygen FJ, Dieleman JP, Koopman JS, Stricker BH, Sturkenboom MC. Medical history and the onset of complex regional pain syndrome (CRPS). Pain. 2008;139(2):458-466.

4.   Demir SE, Ozaras N, Karamehmetoglu SS, Karacan I, Aytekin E. Risk factors for complex regional pain syndrome in patients

with traumatic extremity injury. Ulus Travma Acil Cerrahi Derg. 2010;16(2):144-148.

5.   Geertzen JH, de Bruijn-Kofman AT, de Bruijn HP, van de Wiel HB, Dijkstra PU. Stressful life events and psychological dysfunction in Complex Regional Pain Syndrome type I. Clin J Pain. 1998;14(2):143-147.

6.   Sandroni P, Benrud-Larson LM, McClelland RL, Low PA. Complex regional pain syndrome type I: incidence and prevalence in Olmsted county, a population-based study. Pain. 2003;103(1-2):199-207.

7.   Wang YC, Li HY, Lin FS, et al. Injury Location and Mechanism for Complex Regional Pain Syndrome: A Nationwide Population-Based Case-Control Study in Taiwan. Pain Pract. 2015;15(6):548-553.

8.   Birklein F, Schmelz M, Schifter S, Weber M. The important role of neuropeptides in complex regional pain syndrome. Neurology. 2001;57(12):2179-2184.

9.   Evaniew N, McCarthy C, Kleinlugtenbelt YV, Ghert M, Bhandari M. Vitamin C to Prevent Complex Regional Pain Syndrome in Patients With Distal Radius Fractures: A Meta-Analysis of Randomized Controlled Trials. J Orthop Trauma. 2015;29(8):e235-241.

10.   DeGood DE, Cundiff GW, Adams LE, Shutty MS, Jr. A psychosocial and behavioral comparison of reflex sympathetic dystrophy, low back pain, and headache patients. Pain. 1993;54(3):317-322.

11.   Topcuoglu A, Gokkaya NK, Ucan H, Karakus D. The effect of upper-extremity aerobic exercise on complex regional pain syndrome type I: a randomized controlled study on subacute stroke. Top Stroke Rehabil. 2015;22(4):253-261.

12.   Poudel A, Asahina M, Fujinuma Y, et al. Skin sympathetic function in complex regional pain syndrome type 1. Clin Auton Res. 2015;25(6):367-371.

13.   Gopal H, Fitzgerald J, McCrory C. Spinal cord stimulation for FBSS and CRPS: A review of 80 cases with on-table trial of stimulation. J Back Musculoskelet Rehabil. 2015.

14.   Li WW, Guo TZ, Shi X, et al. Substance P spinal signaling induces glial activation and nociceptive sensitization after fracture. Neuroscience. 2015;310:73-90.

15.   Rickard JP, Kish T. Systemic Intravenous Lidocaine for the Treatment of Complex Regional Pain Syndrome: A Case Report and Literature Review. Am J Ther. 2015.

16.   Martins DF, Prado MR, Daruge-Neto E, et al. Caffeine prevents antihyperalgesic effect of gabapentin in an animal model of CRPS-I: evidence for the involvement of spinal adenosine A1 receptor. J Peripher Nerv Syst. 2015;20(4):403-409.

17.   Mailis A, Wade J. Profile of Caucasian women with possible genetic predisposition to reflex sympathetic dystrophy: a pilot study. Clin J Pain. 1994;10(3):210-217.

18.   Bussa M, Guttilla D, Lucia M, Mascaro A, Rinaldi S. Complex regional pain syndrome type I: a comprehensive review. Acta Anaesthesiol Scand. 2015;59(6):685-697.

19.   Vargas-Alarcon G, Alvarez-Leon E, Fragoso JM, et al. A SCN9A gene-encoded dorsal root ganglia sodium channel polymorphism associated with severe fibromyalgia. BMC Musculoskelet Disord. 2012;13:23.

27. Raynaud's Phenomenon

Maurice Raynaud was a French doctor who died in 1881. He described a syndrome wherein the skin of the fingers or toes of some of his patients became white in color or blue in color, and these patients complained of moderate to severe pain after exposure to cold temperatures or as a result of emotional stress. Raynaud described his patients as complaining of burning pain, numbness, swelling in their extremities, as well as excessive sweating. This condition is now called Raynaud's phenomenon (RP). Raynaud's phenomenon is characterized by episodic constriction of the small arteries. The phenomenon is an exaggerated response to cold or other triggers, and eventually results in reduced blood flow to certain areas of the body. The disorder most commonly affects the fingers and toes, the ears, and the tip of the nose. The tongue may also be affected.[1] RP may affect from 5% to 10% of the U.S. population. RP is more common in women than in men. Raynaud's phenomenon most often affects young women between the ages of 15 and 40. The incidence of RP is higher in colder climates and varies among ethnic groups.

Diseases that contribute to Raynaud's disease or phenomena include obstructive arterial disorders, vascular disorders, and scleroderma. Drug intoxications as well as some cancers and neurological entities can cause Raynaud's disease. Furthermore, thermal or occupational trauma, especially vibration trauma, can also cause Raynaud's disease. Raynaud's disease is a vascular pain. It is also a complex form of pain. Raynaud's disease can last a few minutes to hours. The average length of attack is 5 minutes to 60 minutes. Raynaud's is usually a symptom of another disease, such as lupus, scleroderma, rheumatoid arthritis, or atherosclerosis.

It may also be caused by taking certain medicines, using vibrating power tools for several years, smoking, or having frostbite. The primary form is the most common. It most often starts between age 15 and 25. It is most common in: women and people living in cold places. The secondary form tends to start after age 35 to 40. It is most common in people with connective tissue diseases, such as scleroderma, Sjögren's syndrome, and lupus. Primary Raynaud's phenomenon is often so mild a person never seeks treatment.[2] Community-based data suggest that identification of RP among African Americans should raise consideration of possible comorbidity, particularly cardiovascular disease.

Secondary Raynaud's phenomenon is more serious and complex. It is caused when diseases reduce blood flow to fingers and toes. In women, the onset of RP is more commonly at an early age and is associated with a family history of RP suggesting genetic factors may play a role, as may hormonal and emotional factors. RP secondary to autoimmune disease is also more common in women than in men.

In contrast, the prevalence of RP in men increases with increasing age and smoking and is more likely to be secondary to occupational exposures such as vibration or atherosclerotic peripheral vascular disease than in women. revealed a significant difference in the prevalence of RP between 2 ethnic groups living in the same geographic region. The risk factors associated with RP show considerable sex differences, RP being mostly constitutional in women and occupational in men.[3]

You can have obstruction of both your arteries and veins of your limbs. When this happens you have what is called Burger's disease. This disease is caused by swelling of the small arteries and veins in your extremities. The painful symptoms that you note are a result again of decreased oxygen flow to your tissues. When your blood supply is decreased, which happens in Burger's disease, your oxygen to your tissue is significantly decreased.

You will develop pain in the calves of your legs. If the oxygen deficit is extremely low, your nerves to your legs will suffer injury. This nerve injury will cause you pain as well as lack of oxygen to your extremity muscles. If your pain is severe, you may not experience relief with rest. If your tissues are deprived of oxygen for a long time, you can develop ulcerations in your skin and also develop gangrene.

Another problem with your blood vessels that can cause you to have pain is Takayasu's syndrome. This syndrome is due to inflammation or swelling of your small arteries of the upper part of your body, including your eyes. It occurs more in young girls as well as young women. More than 60 percent of individuals complain of weakness and fever as well as joint pain and pain in the upper extremities. When this pain occurs, you will soon develop the pain about the arteries that are inflamed. This disease can progress to even cause you to have angina pectoris. If this angina pectoris progresses, you may have a heart attack as well.

Temporal arteritis is another inflammation of the large arteries, especially around your temples. Inflammation of one or both of these arteries can cause you to have a significant headache. It can also involve other branches of your carotid artery. Temporal arteritis occurs usually if you are over 55 years of age. Temporal arteritis is more common in women than in men. Occasionally if you have temporal arteritis you will have headaches that are occasionally unbearable. Your headache will begin over your involved arteries. As stated, the pain mostly begins about your temples. However, this disease can also affect your occipital arteries. These are the arteries that are toward the back of your head and approximate an area where the back of your skull meets your neck.

You may have tenderness to touch over the swollen and inflamed arteries. The areas around your inflamed arteries are extremely sensitive to firm touch. You may even have decreased blood flow to your jaw muscles. Therefore, when you chew you may have significant pain in your jaw muscles. Temporal arteritis can affect arteries in multiple locations throughout your body. You may develop a flulike syndrome with generalized muscle pain as well as fever and weakness. The muscle pain can progress and involve your neck, shoulders, and pelvis as well as your legs. The arteries are usually affected on both sides of your body. You can also have decreased blood flow to your organs. This will cause a decrease of blood flow to your organs, resulting in significant pain. Your small arteries throughout your body are called arterioles.

Sometimes the diameter of your arterioles can significantly decrease. This change in your vessel diameter is called vessel constriction. Your fingers and toes may change color. With a decrease of oxygen to your tissues, you will experience a burning pain. With a prolonged decrease in blood flow to your tissues, you may develop abnormal shocking sensations in your extremities including your fingers and toes.

Raynaud's disease is a disorder of your fingers, toes, nose, ears, and sometimes your tongue. When you have symptoms, you will suddenly experience a decrease in your blood flow to these areas. You will have color changes of your skin, especially on your fingers and toes, with exposure to cold or emotional stress. As stated previously, cold on your face can also cause changes in your fingers and toes. Many people use the term Raynaud's disease to include Raynaud's phenomena. This disease is classified as one of two types: primary and secondary. Secondary Raynaud's disease is also called Raynaud's phenomena.

Primary Raynaud's disease has no underlying medical problem and is mild and causes fewer complications than secondary Raynaud's disease. Approximately 50 percent of people diagnosed with Raynaud's disease are primary Raynaud's disease and 50 percent are Raynaud's phenomena. Women are five times more likely than men to develop primary Raynaud's disease. Most patients develop Raynaud's disease before age 40. Be aware that 30 percent of individuals with primary Raynaud's disease progress to secondary Raynaud's disease. Approximately 15 percent of individuals with primary Raynaud's disease do improve. The secondary Raynaud's disease or Raynaud's phenomena is essentially the same as primary Raynaud's disease but secondary Raynaud's disease occurs in individuals who have predisposing factors.

We have mentioned the associated diseases that you can have if you have secondary Raynaud's disease. Primary Raynaud's disease can be later classified as a secondary Raynaud's disease after a predisposing underlying disease has been diagnosed. This observation is seen in 30 percent of patients. A secondary type of Raynaud's disease is more complicated and severe. This type of Raynaud's disease is more likely to worsen. We have mentioned diseases that can predispose you to secondary Raynaud's disease, including scleroderma, SLE, rheumatoid arthritis, and polio. For some reason, herniated discs and spinal cord tumors as well as cerebrovascular accidents and polio can progress to Raynaud's disease.

The syndromes that we have mentioned are related to lack of oxygen to tissue. If you have decreased oxygen to your tissue, you will develop pain. The pain may be intermittent or it can be constant. Your pain will be constant if the oxygen flow to your muscles and nerves in your extremities is severely compromised. If you have decreased blood flow to your muscles, you will have areas in your muscles that are painful. These painful areas will mimic myofascial trigger points. If you have decreased blood flow to your tissues as well as inflammation with the release of prostaglandins, your pain can become severe. Prostaglandins sensitize your pain transmitting fibers.

In the 1800's Raynaud described a condition in which fingers and toes became cold and painful following exposure to cold temperatures or as a result of emotional stress. Consequently, Raynaud's phenomenon refers to symptoms of decreased blood flow in the fingers and toes. Eighty percent of individuals who have Raynaud's disease are female.

Usually Raynaud's disease occurs before age 35. The prevalence in the general population in the United States approaches 5 percent for this disease. If you have Raynaud's disease, usually you have normal arteries. The painful symptoms that you experience with this disease are again related to a decrease in oxygen to your tissues. Usually these symptoms are reversible. Sometimes if you have underlying systemic diseases, you can develop Raynaud's disease.

In your fingers, toes, nose, and ears, you have small blood vessels or arteries that transmit blood and oxygen to your tissues. If you have Raynaud's disease, these vessels become extremely small. This is called vasoconstriction. When your Raynaud's disease crisis is over, your blood vessels will appear normal.

If your hands become cold, you may develop Raynaud's disease. If you live in a cold environment and have to shovel snow off of your walkway, your hands will become cold. If your hands or your feet become cold, this will cause the internal diameter of your blood vessels to decrease. When this happens, your blood vessels can vasoconstrict, causing you to have significant pain. As your extremities become colder, the blood flow to your fingers, toes, ears, and nose can completely stop. As your toes and fingers become warm again, your blood vessels reopen. It is recommended that you dress warmly to avoid extreme cold exposure.

Cold on your face also can trigger Raynaud's phenomena in your hands. This observation suggests that there is an abnormality in your area of your brain that controls temperature regulation. This will develop pain in your veins. You can have inflammation in one of your veins. Sometimes this inflammation can decrease the blood flow in your vein. Your vein can be red and tender as well as firm to touch.

You may develop pain at rest. If you have a stoppage of blood in your veins, it can form a clot. You may develop pain in your calf muscle noted when you bend your foot up toward the ceiling. You may develop pain in your muscles and tendons in the leg that has the occlusion of blood flow in the vein. If the blood flow in your vein has returned, you can still have pain that remains in your legs. You can also develop pain in your muscles that mimics myofascial trigger points.

Any time that you have an effect on the blood flow to any of your tissues caused by the syndromes that mentioned, you can develop reflex sympathetic dystrophy. The reason for this development of this potentially disabling disease is unknown. If reflex sympathetic dystrophy occurs, your skin will become shiny and you will develop sweating in your hands or on the soles of your feet. Your bone density will decrease. This is due to the lack of blood flow to your bones.

When your bone blood flow decreases, minerals and calcium do not reach the bone. Your bone will become weak as a result. This can make you prone to fractures of your bone. Your muscles may shrink in size and you may even develop tremors. Sometimes sympathetic blocks with local anesthetics performed by your anesthesiologist can relieve these painful symptoms.

Raynaud's disease can also be associated with connective tissue disease. This disease can be related to connective tissue diseases such as scleroderma, systemic lupus erythematosus, rheumatoid arthritis, dermatomyositis, and polyarteritis. These are all connective tissue disorders. Connective tissue is the supporting tissue or framework of your body. It is formed of different substances that contain different kinds of cells.

Vibration trauma associated with chainsaws and jackhammers can predispose you to developing Raynaud's disease. Repetitive motion movements that can cause carpal tunnel syndrome can also predispose you to develop Raynaud's disease. Electrical shocks and persistent exposure to extreme cold can also lead to the development of Raynaud's disease. The prevalence of Raynaud's phenomena in the general population can be up to 15 percent of the population.

If you work with vibratory tools such as jackhammers, you are prone to Raynaud's disease. The problem is that this aspect of Raynaud's disease will be permanent even if you stop working with a vibratory tool. This is an industrial disease and is eligible for workmen's compensation benefits in most states. In some instances, Raynaud's disease is so mild that it is no more than a nuisance, whereas sometimes you can have severe enough pain to require you to take narcotic medications.

The exact cause of Raynaud's disease remains speculative. It can be caused by hyperactivity of your sympathetic nervous system. Furthermore, it could be caused by your body's increased sensitivity to chemicals that are circulating in your bloodstream. There are receptors on your blood vessel walls. Some of these receptors are called alpha receptors. With the stimulation of these receptors, the internal caliber of your blood vessels can significantly close. If you have an increased number of these receptors on your blood vessels, you could develop Raynaud's disease.

You need to be aware that there are three phases of Raynaud's disease. When you are first exposed to cold, your small arteries contract and your fingers, toes, ears, or the tip of your nose and tongue become pale and white. This observation occurs because you are deprived of blood. Remember if you have an increased blood flow to your tissues, the tissue will appear red. After your oxygen is deprived, your blood vessels will expand. It is the veins that expand most.

The veins carry blood that has minimal or no oxygen. This will give your blood a bluish tint. The area of the low-oxygen-carrying blood will appear blue. The area also feels cold to touch. When your arteries begin to dilate, the blood flow is increased. Oxygen is increased and your tissue color will appear normal. Putting your extremities in a warm environment will cause your blood vessels to expand. As the blood vessels expand, you may experience a throbbing pain.

As previously stated, females are more likely to develop Raynaud's disease than males. Studies are now being done attempting to correlate Raynaud's disease with caffeine consumption as well as some dietary habits. The predisposition to develop Raynaud's disease may be genetic. Risk factors for developing Raynaud's disease do differ between males and females. Smoking is associated with Raynaud's disease only in males. Alcohol abuse can be associated with Raynaud's disease only in women. These observations tell you that there must be different mechanisms that influence the onset of Raynaud's disease.

Menopause and changes in your sex hormones can alter your blood flow to minimal levels in your digits as well as your ears and nose. If you have adult onset diabetes mellitus, your blood vessels may not dilate normally. Some individuals with diabetes are, therefore, prone to develop Raynaud's disease.

Be aware that extreme cold will cause the muscles in the walls of your small arteries to contract. If you have a decrease in blood flow to your tissues, you have decreased oxygen as we have reiterated which will cause you pain. However, if you do suffer from Raynaud's disease, the amount of constriction of your arteries is extreme as compared to others who do not have Raynaud's disease. If you have Raynaud's disease, you will have a more severe constriction of your blood flow. Remember that anxiety and emotional distress can increase the activity of your sympathetic nervous system, which causes your blood vessels to constrict as well.

If you live in a cold area, wear a hat that covers your ears or wear earmuffs. If you are sensitive to cold, use drinking glasses that are insulated. You must also wear gloves before putting your hands into a freezer. The thermal regulatory control of your skin blood flow is vital to the maintenance of your normal body temperature. The sympathetic nervous system controls your skin blood flow. If you are exposed to cold, your sympathetic nervous system will cause your vessels to constrict. You can have other predisposing factors to cause you to have Raynaud's disease. Living in a cool, damp climate can predispose you to Raynaud's disease. Hypertension can also have an effect as well as excessive sweating.

If you have a history of migraine headaches, you have an increased incidence of developing Raynaud's disease. Operating any machinery that vibrates can make you subject to Raynaud's disease; and if your fingers are subject to continuous physical stress such as typing or if you are a professional pianist, you can develop Raynaud's disease as well.

Rare symptoms of Raynaud's disease can occur as well. There has been a case reported of a 38 year old female who had Raynaud's disease in her right upper extremity but also developed Raynaud's disease in her right nipple. She would develop pallor about the nipple and her pain on occasion would become unbearable.

If your Raynaud's disease is severe and chronic, you will develop deep ulcers in your skin. If your Raynaud's disease persists, you may develop gangrene, which can cause you to have an amputation of your affected digits. If you sustain a cut to your hands or your feet, notify your doctor if the cuts do not heal in a reasonable time. The treatment for Raynaud's disease can include calcium channel blockers, drugs that increase the caliber of your blood vessels. Your doctor will decide what treatment will best suit you. You should take vitamin C as well as E. Garlic has been shown in some noncontrolled studies to be effective.

Your connective tissue can be classified as dense or loose. Adipose tissue is an example of lose connective tissue. Connective tissue can be elastic. Cartilage and bone are connective tissues. Your blood can be regarded as a connective tissue. For some reason that is not totally known, connective tissue diseases can be associated with Raynaud's disease. For example, Raynaud's phenomenon is seen in 90 percent of patients with scleroderma, 30 percent of patients with rheumatoid arthritis, and 30 percent of patients with Sjogren's syndrome. Scleroderma is essentially a disorder of a smooth muscle. This is a connective tissue disease that can be associated with esophageal reflux because of the effect of smooth muscle in your esophagus.

Scleroderma also affects your skin. By definition, it is called "hard skin." It is uncommon. Scleroderma is classified according to the degree of your skin thickening. Scleroderma is most common in adults. However, it can be seen in children. The hallmarks of scleroderma are light skin and Raynaud's phenomena.

Scleroderma is a generalized disorder of the small arteries as well as the connective tissue. Not only can your gastrointestinal tract be affected but also your lungs, your heart, and your kidneys. Most all patients who have scleroderma have Raynaud's disease. Patients with scleroderma can have pallor of the digits following cold exposure or emotional stress. Your fingers and toes can turn blue followed by redness in addition to burning pain and tingling. Raynaud's phenomena associated with scleroderma can affect your toes, fingers, ears, nose, and even your tongue. You can get gangrene in your fingers and toes and end up with an amputation. Swelling can be seen over your hands and feet. Over time, thinning of your skin can occur. The thinning of your skin is easily noted over joints. Usually scleroderma begins before age 40 and is more common in females. Approximately 80 percent of scleroderma patients are females.

Scleroderma can affect the kidneys and cause you to have kidney failure. Scleroderma can also affect your heart and cause some arrhythmias about your heart. You may need an echocardiograph if you have chest pain. This test can reveal some thickening around the outer wall of your heart. You will have muscle pain as well as joint pain if you have scleroderma. You will have stiffness in the morning. Systemic lupus erythematosus is a disease of unknown cause. It can also be associated with Raynaud's disease. Systemic lupus erythematosus (SLE) is caused by your body's production of antibodies that injure the tissues of some of your organs in your body. The symptoms can come and go. You may have a rash develop on your face. However, SLE can be life threatening if it involves your internal organs. SLE can cause you to have failure of your kidneys or hemorrhage as well as a pulmonary disease.

If you suffer from vasculitis (inflammation of your blood vessels) you can develop Raynaud's symptoms. Usually SLE occurs between ages 16 and 55. SLE occurs more frequently in women. It is more prevalent in African American as well as Asian women. The triggering of your antibodies to attack your tissue is unknown. In some individuals, ultraviolet light can trigger the disease. This disease is usually inherited. This disease is caused by your antibodies. If your antibodies are deposited in your kidneys, you can have irreversible kidney damage.

Antibodies can attack your red blood cells as well as your platelets. If your platelets become low, you can develop bleeding problems. If you have SLE, you will develop fatigue as well as muscle pain and arthritis. These symptoms can disappear only to come back at a later time. The rash that you develop over your face looks like a butterfly shape. Individuals with SLE are prone to develop Raynaud's disease. There is no known cure for SLE. Your generalized pain in your joints will be treated with analgesics. Approximately 30 percent of individuals with SLE will develop Raynaud's disease associated with SLE.

Arthritis is another disease that associated with Raynaud's disease. Rheumatoid arthritis is a chronic inflammatory disease that affects various organs. However, rheumatoid arthritis mostly affects the joints between your bones. You will notice changes in your hands, feet, elbows, neck, and so on. No one knows why rheumatoid arthritis occurs. It can be due to a accumulation of some of your white cells caused by a substance in your bloodstream. Rheumatoid arthritis will cause invasion of your cartilage, and your cartilage will be degraded and also your bone will be affected by rheumatoid arthritis. Rheumatoid arthritis is destructive.

Inflammation and pain can occur around your tendons as well. Rheumatoid arthritis affects 5 percent of Native Americans. Otherwise, the rheumatoid arthritis affects between 1 to 2 percent of the population. Because Raynaud's disease is associated with rheumatoid arthritis, occasionally you may need sympathetic blocks with local anesthetic. Rheumatoid arthritis can affect your skin, eyes, lungs, and heart as well as your nervous system. Rheumatoid arthritis can also affect the arteries that supply blood to your heart muscle.

Dermatomyositis is an inflammatory disease that can affect your muscle. You will have muscle pain and tenderness. This disease is accompanied by a rash. The rash occurs on your upper eyelids. You may have some swelling around your eyes as well. You can have redness about the knuckles of your fingers. This disease can affect almost any organ system in your body. You can have involvement of the muscles of your fingers and toes. The muscles in your legs can become weak. This disease, like SLE, can be caused by an abnormality in your immune system. Raynaud's phenomena can become prominent if you have dermatomyositis. Your muscles will become weak. The diagnosis of this disease can be done by taking samples of your muscle.

Polyarteritis nodosa can also be associated with Raynaud's disease. This disease is caused by inflammation or swelling of the walls of your blood vessel. This disease can affect blood vessels of any size as well as in any location. It usually occurs between ages 40 and 50. Men are affected more than women. Your kidneys can be affected. If the disease progresses, you can develop kidney failure. This disease can affect your arteries going to your heart and can cause you to have a heart attack. It may cause abdominal pain and bleeding. This disease can affect your nervous system as well. It can cause you to have weakness as well as loss of sensation. As stated previously, it can be associated with rheumatoid arthritis.

Raynaud's disease can also be associated with carpal tunnel syndrome. The carpal tunnel syndrome causes one of the nerves at your wrist (median nerve) to be trapped and compressed. You can develop burning pain and tingling in your hand. Usually this affects the first three fingers of your hand. The symptoms usually occur at night. Sometimes if you shake your hand, the pain will go away. Not only can Raynaud's phenomena be associated with carpal tunnel syndrome, but other disorders can be associated with the carpal tunnel syndrome as well, including rheumatoid arthritis, gouty arthritis, and trauma.

If you have a thoracic outlet syndrome, you may develop Raynaud's disease as well. Like the carpal tunnel syndrome, the thoracic outlet syndrome compresses nerves. The nerves from your spinal cord that go to your arms must pass through an outlet between your neck and shoulders. This outlet can be compressed by one of your ribs or by bone, muscles, or other tissues. You can have abnormal sensations in your fingers called parathesias. You may develop weakness of your hand muscles. Sometimes surgery can help this syndrome. If you have this syndrome, you may also be prone for Raynaud's phenomena as well. Be aware that pressure caused by crutches can compress nerves and vessels that go throughout your arms to your hands and fingers. Chronic use of crutches can contribute to the onset of Raynaud's phenomena.

In spite of all these diseases associated with Raynaud's disease, there is no reliable method of provoking Raynaud's phenomena. In other words, there may be some time during a day, month, or year that you develop the symptoms associated with Raynaud's phenomena.

The diagnosis of Raynaud's disease involves several components. The first component is that color changes must occur during the attacks provoked by cold or emotional stress. Another criterion is that these episodes must occur for at least two years. If you have no disease that decreases your blood flow to your tissues, the third criteria is that the attacks must occur in both the hands and the feet. Another criteria is that there should be no other cause for these episodes.

A diagnosis of Raynaud's disease can be confirmed by a cold stimulation test. The temperature of your fingers and toes is taken. Your hand and/or your foot is then placed in a container of ice water for 20 seconds. After your extremity is removed from the water, your temperature is immediately recorded. Your temperature is taken every five minutes until it returns to a normal baseline level. Normal individuals recover their temperature within 15 minutes. If you have Raynaud's disease, it will take you longer than 20 minutes to reach your baseline temperature.

Vibration delivered to the hand and arm by industrial pneumatic tools is a common cause of vascular and neurovascular problems, including cold-induced vascular spasm (vibration white finger) and peripheral neuropathies with paresthesias, dysesthesias, and sensory abnormalities.[4] A decade ago, the US Public Health Service estimated that 1.2 million American workers were at risk. Differentiation of primary and secondary Raynaud's phenomenon from the thoracic outlet syndrome and from the carpal tunnel syndrome pose potential diagnostic difficulties.

These community-based data suggest that identification of RP among African Americans should raise consideration of possible comorbidity, particularly cardiovascular disease.[2] The rate of Raynaud's phenomenon in a Japanese population was higher than male and female Caucasians.[5] Studies with standardized laboratory measurements of skin blood flow suggest an influence of female sex hormones on vasospasm. However another study shows that most females do not experience an important subjective influence of sex hormonal status on vasospastic attacks.[6]

The laser Doppler scanning is now helpful for the diagnosis of Raynaud's disease. Blood flow can be measured about your fingers and toes. Laser Doppler scanning is usually correlated with your finger blood pressure. Skin blood pressure results can determine diagnosis of Raynaud's disease more accurately than the laser Doppler study. The laser Doppler study can be useful as well.

There are no good laboratory tests that will give you a diagnosis of Raynaud's disease. Currently there is no known way to prevent the development of Raynaud's disease. As a result, there is no known cure for this disease. A newer drug is being studied for the treatment of Raynaud's syndrome. This drug is isosorbide mononitrate. The isosorbide mononitrate was shown to be effective in the treatment of the symptoms associated with Raynaud's disease in 19 women.

Further research needs to be carried out to evaluate the effects of this drug compared to a placebo control. As you now see, Raynaud's disease can fluctuate from being a mild nuisance to a severe disabling disease that can result in loss of fingers or toes. Research continues in diagnosis and treatment of this disease. If you suspect that you are developing Raynaud's disease, seek medical attention from a doctor knowledgeable in the diagnosis and treatment of this disease.

Since ancient times, Chinese medical texts have described problems of hands and feet as a result of severe cold. Chinese doctors have prescribed herbal remedies. Sometimes bitter orange and honey-baked licorice can be of benefit according a traditional Chinese medicine specialist. If you want to utilize Chinese herbal medicine for the treatment of your Raynaud's disease, consult a specialist in this field. Fish oil supplements may possibly decrease some of the symptoms associated with mild Raynaud's disease. It is believed that this effect is due to the anti-inflammatory property of the fish oils.

Avoid triggers that cause you to develop Raynaud's disease. Keep your extremities warm. You Use layered clothing. Use rubber gloves or mittens under your regular gloves. Regular gloves allow heat to escape in extremely cold weather. If you are inside, wear socks as well as comfortable shoes. You should not smoke or use any tobacco products. Also avoid the use of any vibrating tools. You must learn to manage your stress. Regular exercise can increase blood flow to your tissues and reduce stress. Relaxation techniques and biofeedback may be of extreme benefit to you if you suffer from Raynaud's disease.

There is a distinct predominance of females whose mean age of onset is significantly lower than that of males.   Blacks have significantly more sclerodactyly, leukopenia, anemia, and hyperglobulinemia than whites. This study Indicates that when patients with Raynaud's phenomenon are separated into major groups as described, demographic, clinical, and laboratory features characterize each group.[7]

Vitamin E, magnesium, and fish oils can be of some benefit. Herbal medicines are currently being studied to determine their effects on the treatment of Raynaud's disease. Cayenne pepper and ginger may possibly enhance circulation to your painful areas. Again, further research is indicated for the effective herbal medicines on the prevention of Raynaud's disease. Pain can be associated with Raynaud's phenomena.

Nicotine can decrease the internal diameter of the vessels in your body. A class of drugs used to treat hypertension called beta blockers can also be associated with Raynaud's phenomenon. The exact reason for this observation remains unclear at present. Beta blockers can decrease your heart rate as well as your strength of contraction of your heart muscles. Side effects of beta blockers can result in cold extremities. This may be the reason that you can develop Raynaud's phenomena.

A class of drugs called ergots is used for the treatment of migraine headaches. This class of drugs can also be used for vascular headaches as well as cluster headaches. An example of this drug is Wigraine. This drug can cause constriction of your blood vessels. A decrease in the blood flow and oxygen to your tissues can precipitate Raynaud's phenomena. Any drug that stimulates the sympathetic nervous system, such as dopamine, can cause your blood vessels in your body to constrict. An example of a sympathetic stimulating drug is dopamine.

Dopamine can be used to increase the strength of your heartbeat if you have had heart failure. However, drugs that stimulate your sympathetic nervous system also constrict your blood vessels. Raynaud's phenomena have been associated with use of drugs that stimulate your sympathetic nervous system.

When you have a sympathetic injection with a local anesthetic in your sympathetic nerves, the blockade of your sympathetic fibers to your arteries will cause your arteries to become bigger in diameter. This will increase the blood flow to your painful tissues, which in turn increases the oxygen to your nerves and muscles as well. This is the mechanism why sympathetic blocks can decrease your pain. If you have a decrease in blood flow to the tissues we have described, chemicals in your body that cause pain are released. Histamine, kinins, 5-Hydroxytriptamine, and substance P are released. Substances will transmit pain to your spinal cord, which will eventually reach the pain-processing center in your brain.

Smoking is associated with Raynaud's disease. Smoking also constricts your blood vessels, depriving you of oxygen and causing pain.[8] Avoid vibrating tools such as jackhammers and jigsaws. Repetitive motion movements can predispose you to carpal tunnel syndrome and Raynaud's disease. Avoid any triggers that cause your pain, such as extreme cold. Stay warm by dressing in layers. Be sure to wear gloves if you are outside. It is important to keep your skin temperature warm and regulated.

If your skin becomes cold, your sympathetic nervous system will cause your blood vessels to constrict can cause you pain. Perform relaxation and biofeedback techniques to reduce your stress level. Regular exercise can increase blood flow to your tissues and reduce stress. NSAIDs such as ibuprofen may reduce any swelling and pain that you have. Take any medications as prescribed by your doctor. Injections of local anesthetic into your sympathetic nerves may relieve some of your pain.

References

1.   Zeni S, Ingegnoli F. [Raynaud's phenomenon]. Reumatismo. 2004;56(2):77-81.

2.   Gelber AC, Wigley FM, Stallings RY, et al. Symptoms of Raynaud's phenomenon in an inner-city African-American community:

prevalence and self-reported cardiovascular comorbidity. J Clin Epidemiol. 1999;52(5):441-446.

3.   Valter I, Maricq HR. Prevalence of Raynaud's phenomenon in 2 ethnic groups in the general population of Estonia. J Rheumatol. 1998;25(4):697-702.

4.   Cherniack MG. Raynaud's phenomenon of occupational origin. Arch Intern Med. 1990;150(3):519-522.

5.   Harada N, Ueda A, Takegata S. Prevalence of Raynaud's phenomenon in Japanese males and females. J Clin Epidemiol. 1991;44(7):649-655.

6.   Bartelink ML, Wollersheim H, van de Lisdonk E, Thien T. Raynaud's phenomenon: subjective influence of female sex hormones. Int Angiol. 1992;11(4):309-315.

7.   Velayos EE, Robinson H, Porciuncula FU, Masi AT. Clinical correlation analysis of 137 patients with Raynaud's phenomenon. Am J Med Sci. 1971;262(6):347-356.

8.   Dreyfuss D, Calif E, Stahl S. [the Adverse Effects of Smoking on the Hands]. Harefuah. 2015;154(5):327-329, 338.

28. Shingles

Shingles is an infectious disease caused by a virus that causes herpes zoster and affects some of the nerves that go into your spinal cord. One or more nerves can be affected. Usually the shingles pain stays on one side of your body. Sometimes shingles will affect your lower extremities. The virus is called varicella zoster. Chicken pox is caused by the same virus that will cause you to have shingles. This virus will remain in the area that connects your spinal nerve and your spinal cord. This area is called your dorsal root ganglia. This virus typically reactivates when people are older than 50. This reactivation usually occurs after your immune system has been weakened, usually by another viral infection such as the flu or common cold. It is possible that genetic variation may explain some portion of varicella-zoster virus reactivation.[1] If you have cancer, you may be prone to develop shingles as well.

Sometimes there is no known reason why you develop shingles. If you have had contact with an individual who has had chicken pox, there is a chance that you could develop shingles. However, this scenario is rare. You need to be aware that shingles does not increase during seasonal chicken pox outbreaks. When the virus is reactivated in your dorsal root ganglia, it goes along your nerves to your nerve endings. The virus at this time will cause your skin to develop lesions. Herpes zoster is more common in women, the elderly and immunosuppressed individuals.[2]

You need to be aware that any part of your central nervous system can be affected by this virus. In rare cases, this virus can even affect your brain; this is called encephalitis. The virus has been reported in some cases to affect the sympathetic ganglia as well, which can cause severe burning pain. This will cause you to have symptoms that mimic reflex sympathetic dystrophy symptoms. The prevalence of herpes zoster is significantly different among races with Whites having a higher incidence than Blacks.[3,4]

If you have Hodgkin's disease, you risk developing shingles. If you have a history of cancer of your breasts, lungs, or gastrointestinal tract, you run an increased risk of developing shingles. Early reports indicated that men and women were affected at the same rate. However, more recent studies have reported that men are affected more frequently than women. If you are debilitated, you also run the risk of developing shingles. Immunosuppressed patients are at increased risk for herpes zoster, but incidence in solid organ transplant patients is very high.5 The Black race has a decreased the risk of zoster in late life significantly.[6,7]

Following chicken pox, antibodies are made in your body to fight the chicken pox virus. This is the reason why you usually do not get chicken pox again. If your immune system is compromised for any reason, however, your body's ability to combat the virus is greatly reduced. This is the reason why you may develop shingles. If your immune system appears to be attacked, your body will immediately fight the shingles virus.

After you have had the onset of shingles, you may develop post-herpetic neuralgia. This is a chronic pain syndrome that occurs following the onset of shingles. When you have the onset of shingles, you will have blisters as well as burning sensations in your skin where the infected nerves run. When you develop post-herpetic neuralgia, which can persist for years, however, your skin lesions usually heal. If you are between the ages of 40 and 60, the chances of you developing post-herpetic neuralgia are 20 percent.

If you are over 60 years of age, your chance of developing post-herpetic neuralgia will increase to 50 percent. Post-herpetic neuralgia is a difficult entity to treat. Post-herpetic neuralgia can cause you to have agonizing pain as well as suffering. Some individuals have even committed suicide to escape this terrible pain. Sometimes you can develop burning pain associated with the herpes zoster virus. However, it may be some time before your skin lesions appear.

Before you develop a skin rash, the diagnosis of herpes zoster is difficult to make. After your skin lesions erupt, the diagnosis is easier to make. If you have pain in your mid back, you may be incorrectly diagnosed with a coronary artery disease or pneumonia. If your doctor wants to confirm your diagnosis, the virus should be isolated from your pustules no later than seven days after they erupted.

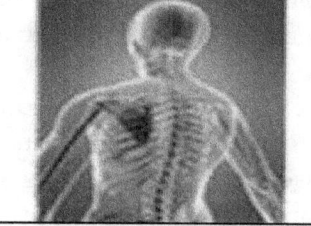

Figure 1. Shingles pain occurs in any nerve of your spinal cord.

If you are suffering from post-herpetic neuralgia, you may have difficulty with sleep because of your torturous pain. Your activities will be decreased. As a result of continuous pain, loss of sleep, and the inability to socialize, you may easily become depressed. Your post-herpetic neuralgia may be confused with other medical diseases. However, you must keep a documented history of your shingles onset. You must tell your doctor if you have had lesions on your skin. By the time you see your doctor, you may still have the skin lesions or you may have scarring of your skin. The problem with the post-herpetic neuralgia is that it can affect your central nervous system, which includes your spinal cord and brain.

Be aware that if you have severe burning pain that develops on one side of your body, you may or may not have a skin eruption but you can have shingles. Sometimes the lack of a skin eruption confuses doctors as to whether you actually have the onset of shingles, because skin lesions are so common. If you do develop skin eruptions, the lesion will begin as redness. The redness over your skin will turn to blisters. The blisters can form pus. Eventually these lesions on your skin break down. A crust then forms. If your skin, in addition to your nerves, is affected by the virus, you may develop scars as well as loss of skin pigment about the infected site.

Be aware that the virus can travel to your eyes. If you or anyone in your family has developed shingles and begins to complain of eye pain, this is a medical emergency. You must contact an ophthalmologist immediately. If left untreated, you may be blinded by the virus. The incidence of shingles is approximately 4 to 5 cases per 1,000 people.

The chance of you developing shingles increases with your age. Usually when you have a viral infection, you will build up antibodies in your body that will help to fight the virus. The problem with shingles is that you do not appear to have developed antibodies to this virus that caused the initial episode of shingles. In other words, you run the risk of developing shingles after your initial case of shingles has resolved. Be aware that psychological stress can also trigger the onset of shingles. If you have a history of a prolonged use of steroids, you may also be prone to develop shingles. For reasons yet unknown, the Caucasian race appears to have a higher incidence of shingles than other races.

Your chest will be most affected by shingles. Nerves that come off of your spine at your mid back are called thoracic nerves. These thoracic nerves may be affected by the virus, causing an outbreak of shingles in your chest. Your chest is most commonly affected (50 percent of individuals who develop shingles experience chest effects). A nerve coming off of your brain that distributes branches to your face called the trigeminal nerve is the next most common nerve affected. Next the nerves off of your neck (called the cranial nerves) are affected, followed by the nerves coming off of your spinal cord that go to your legs (called the lumbar nerves). As you can see, shingles can affect nerves all over your body.

Different types of laboratory tests are available to diagnose acute herpes zoster. As noted previously, virus recovery from your tissue and blood can provide a rapid diagnostic tool for early diagnosis. Occasionally, the virus can be recovered from the back of your throat. Different types of diagnostic tests that use various stains are available. After these scrapings are stained, they may show diagnostic material in your cells. Many doctors advocate taking a small amount of your tissue (called a punch biopsy) so that they can do an examination under a specialized, high-powered microscope called an electron microscope. This is an extremely reliable test and it can provide a diagnosis of whether you have the herpes zoster virus before you develop blisters on your skin.

Be aware that not every patient who develops shingles has severe, incapacitating pain. You may only complain of itching. On the other hand, you may complain of the most horrible pain that you could ever imagine. Your pain can be either constant or it can be intermittent. It is the constant, severe, horrible pain that predisposes individuals to suicide to escape this torment. The problem with this disease is that you could have excruciating pain to touch. This poses a problem if you are trying to sleep.

You would have difficulty lying on a mattress without having severe pain. It is interesting to note if those younger than 50 years of age rarely develop prolonged pain after the acute onset of shingles. You also need to know that if you are over 50 years of age and develop shingles that your pain is usually worse (and that your post-herpetic neuralgia pain is also worse than for individuals who are younger than 50 years of age).

After you have been diagnosed with shingles, your doctor will probably treat you with antiviral agents. Acyclovir, famciclovir, and valacyclovir can be used for the treatment of your viral infection. Antiviral medications are used to decrease the intensity and duration of your shingles and are used to prevent the chronic pain associated with post-herpetic neuralgia. Be aware that you can still have the onset of post-herpetic neuralgia even after treatment with these antiviral agents.

Pain associated with post-herpetic neuralgia can be described as aching, burning, or stabbing. The worst pain is pain that is triggered by light touch such as clothing, bathing, or lying on a mattress. Sometimes cold weather or cold water can worsen your pain. Post-herpetic neuralgia is a dreaded complication of shingles.

If you develop shingles and if your pain lasts longer than six weeks after your skin lesions have disappeared, you have developed post-herpetic neuralgia. Be aware that a certain proportion of individuals who develop post-herpetic neuralgia will improve over time with no treatment.

If you have post-herpetic neuralgia, the chances are that you will have improved by 12 months. Approximately 30 percent of individuals who develop post-herpetic neuralgia still complain of pain after one year. Two percent of individuals who suffer from post-herpetic neuralgia will have pain longer than five years.

Anxiety and depression are psychological factors that can affect your shingles as well as your post-herpetic neuralgia. As mentioned previously, stress can play an important role in the development of both shingles and post-herpetic neuralgia. Psychological stress in some instances can decrease your immune system, making you prone to develop shingles. Many individuals who have abnormal behavioral patterns will become preoccupied with their pain. Usually these individuals are critical of health-care providers who have tried to help them relieve their pain. These individuals may also have narcotic tolerance.

It appears that post-herpetic neuralgia affects the smaller nerves that cause you to have severe, burning pain. For some reason, on occasion your sympathetic nervous system can become overactive. This over activity of your sympathetic nervous system can cause blood vessels that are going to your tissue to decrease their diameter (constrict). This will cause your tissue to have a decrease in its blood flow. The decrease in blood flow decreases oxygen as well as nutrients to your tissue.

This lack of tissue oxygen can cause you to have pain. The decreased oxygen can cause release of pain-producing chemicals at the nerve endings in your tissues. The lack of oxygen to your nerves can affect the larger nerves that transmit the stabbing pain.

A significant problem associated with post-herpetic neuralgia is that these large nerves can be damaged and actually disappear. When these nerves are gone, there are no impulses to fight the burning impulses transmitted by the small nerves called C fibers.

Sometimes as your nerves are being damaged by the virus that causes post-herpetic neuralgia, these nerves can become hyperirritable, causing you to suffer significant pain. You must understand that this virus can injure and destroy the nerves that it affects. When your nerves become injured, they can develop areas of sensitivity at the site of nerve destruction. These sites can become hyperirritable and as a result can cause you to have significant, horrible pain.

These injured nerves, as they attempt to heal, can develop sprouts. It is these sprouts that can become extremely sensitive. These sprouts of hypersensitivity can occur at any location on your nerve. Studies have shown that these nerves can conduct spontaneous pain impulses. This increase in nerve electrical activity can recruit other pain transmitting nerves around your lesion. In other words, there can be a magnification of the amount of pain (because the pain is combined) that you will suffer.

A potential problem exists for you in that some family members or even some doctors do not believe that you are suffering severely. Doctors who do not frequently treat post-herpetic neuralgia can be reluctant to give strong analgesic medications. These doctors think that over time you may become addicted to narcotic medications. Be aware that severe pain can have significant adverse effects on your body. It can increase your blood pressure, your pulse, and even decrease your immune system. Your blood vessels can decrease in their caliber. All of these changes can ultimately affect your heart as well as your kidneys and your psychological make-up. Therefore, you and your doctor must decide whether you are to be prescribed a narcotic pain medication.

Remember that both pain medication and chronic suffering can have adverse effects on your body. Most pain-medicine doctors believe that your pain should be managed appropriately. If you follow your pain-medicine doctor's instructions, your chances of becoming addicted are extremely small. When you have the acute herpes zoster attack, your pain is usually localized to the affected nerves. You may have fever as well as weakness and fatigue. At this time, your pain could be shooting, dull, or even burning. Your skin eruptions usually occur approximately four days later. As stated previously, the herpes zoster virus can go not only to your sensory nerves but also the nerves that go to your muscles. As a result, the muscles that are in your chest can be paralyzed.

Also muscles in your arms or legs can be paralyzed if the virus is in these nerves. You may not have paralysis, but you will experience weakness. Usually your weak muscle symptoms are reversible. If you have the initial stage of the viral infection, you are suffering viral replication. This means that the virus in your system is replicating rapidly. Your immune system is usually depressed. As the disease progresses, your immune system should be able to fight the virus. As you go into a third phase, your body will continue to fight the virus with your antibodies. However, it is at this time that you could have permanent nerve changes.

Shingles recurs in 8 percent of individuals. Usually the shingles will occur at the same site affected previously. After you have developed crusts, these lesions will fall off in five to six weeks. After they have fallen off, they will leave an irregular scar. You may not have any feeling about the scar. If you have suffered from post-herpetic neuralgia for six months, the chance of a complete cure is remote. As discussed previously, you can have pain associated with post-herpetic neuralgia, but you can also have dysesthesias. These are uncomfortable, unpleasant sensations but are not true sensations.

As noted earlier in this chapter, herpes zoster can be associated with a loss of your larger fibers that conduct sensation. Older patients in general have a loss of these larger fibers. Therefore, when they develop post-herpetic neuralgia their pain can be more severe than a younger individual who has a greater number of these large pain fibers. Remember, the initial stage of the infection is a viral replication. The virus duplicates itself rapidly. This is the reason why an antiviral medication must be administered as early as possible after the diagnosis has been made to decrease the rate of this replication. Not only is the virus recovered from blisters, it can also be recovered from the bloodstream. Occasionally, the virus can get into the fluid that surrounds your spinal cord and ultimately cause you to have meningitis. Type II diabetes is associated with an increased risk of developing shingles, is particularly high in adults 65 years and older and moderately increased in adults under 65 years of age.[8]

Doctors of different specialties treat shingles. You may be treated by your primary care doctor or a dermatologist. You may have to go to an emergency room because of severe pain and be treated by that doctor. You may also be referred to a pain-medicine specialist. Psychologists are also valuable in the management of your pain. All of these health-care providers can significantly help you manage your pain. You may find that each of these providers uses a different modality for the treatment of your pain. This is not to say that any one of these treatments is entirely wrong nor does it mean that any of these methods provided by different health-care providers are entirely correct.

If you are elderly, you also have a predisposition to depression. Pain management in elderly individuals is unique because you may present with multiple underlying medical problems in addition to your pain problem. This makes the management of your post-herpetic neuralgia challenging. The correct diagnosis must be made before any treatment is initiated. If you are taking multiple drugs, remember that drugs can interact. Therefore, an accurate diagnosis must be made prior to initiating pain management. [9] The efficacy of vaccines recommended for older-aged adults is consistently greater for females than for males.[10]

As you age, your body will respond differently to different drugs. Furthermore, the distribution of the drugs in your body will change. Elderly individuals in nursing homes may have difficulty communicating their pain. This lack of communication can make it extremely difficult for a pain-management doctor or a primary care doctor to manage a painful post-herpetic neuralgia syndrome. Adults with peptic ulcer disease are at increased risk of shingles independently compared with the general population.[11] If you are a family member of an elderly individual, help your relative's doctor by providing that doctor with a detailed history of the onset, duration, and severity of the post-herpetic neuralgia. Elderly cancer patients run a higher risk of developing shingles than those without cancer.[12] The rates of shingles related complications are significantly higher for hematologic than solid cancer patients.

Lotions, different types of patches, nonsteroidal anti-inflammatory drugs, antidepressants, and muscle relaxants may all be needed to control your pain. You may even need injections of numbing medicines into your nerves. Placement of local anesthetics around your sympathetic nerves may be of benefit in reducing your pain, especially if the injection is done soon after the onset of your pain.

Zoster vaccine is recommended for prevention of herpes zoster among adults aged 60 years and older. The zoster vaccine coverage is higher in this insured population than previously reported in the US general population, but it remains low. Significant racial/ethnic disparity was observed and worsened even among individuals with relatively equal access to zoster vaccination.[13] For vaccination to be improved among those least likely to be up-to-date on recommended adult vaccines, efforts also are needed to identify adults who do not have a regular provider or insurance and who report fewer health care visits.[14]

Immunosuppressed patients are at increased risk for herpes zoster , and is noticed in solid organ transplant recipients.[5] Black race elderly patients had decreased risks of zoster in late life.[15] There is a risk of malignancy following an episode of herpes zoster in both men and women and in all age groups 18 years and over.[16] The risk is greatest during the first 180 days following the diagnosis of herpes zoster.

Topical agents are frequently used to treat shingles pain. These agents accelerate the healing of your skin and can decrease the pain associated with the shingles virus. However, topical anesthetics administered at the time that you develop shingles will not affect the development of post-herpetic neuralgia. Compresses or Burrow's solution or calamine lotion placed directly over your painful site can decrease the pain associated with acute herpes zoster.

A patch has been developed for the treatment of shingles. This patch has proven to be extremely useful in the management of shingles and post-herpetic neuralgia pain. A local anesthetic called lidocaine is placed within a patch system. The lidocaine is placed within an adhesive. The adhesive binds to your skin. The lidocaine that is in this patch is dispersed through your skin and travels to your painful, hyperirritable nerve endings. When this drug reaches your nerve endings, it calms your painful nerves. Note that this patch will not cause you to have numbness about your skin. If you are numb, you could injure the tissue. You may lie on the tissue not knowing that you are injuring your tissue. This is the reason why you do not want to be numb for any length of time about your skin.

Another type of transdermal (skin) drug-delivery system is a clonidine transdermal patch. This is placed over the area of your maximal pain. This drug is a drug that controls an individual's blood pressure. If you are suffering from post-herpetic neuralgia, however, your nerve endings may release certain chemicals that increase your pain. Scientists have demonstrated that the use of a clonidine transdermal patch can decrease components of your burning pain. This type of patch is changed on a weekly basis. One advantage of these patches is that they provide you with a constant blood drug level. If you take pills, you have peaks and troughs in your bloodstream after taking the pill and after the pill is excreted from your body. In contrast, the patch provides a constant flow of the drug.

If you are elderly, remember that the clonidine patch is a blood pressure patch. It can decrease your blood pressure. If you get out of a chair or out of bed too quickly, you may become dizzy (a result of orthostatic hypotension). Orthostatic hypotension could cause you to become dizzy and fall. If you have been prescribed this patch, be aware of this side effect.

You may need to take pills by mouth. If you are elderly, you must be aware that changes exist in your body with respect to target organ sensitivity to drugs. This means that the receptors that sit on the cells of some of your organs may not be as responsive to certain drugs as they would be if you were much younger. As you age, the absorption of drugs through your gastrointestinal system decreases as your age increases. On the other hand, some drugs are passively absorbed through your gastrointestinal system. This means that there will be no change in your blood level.

Drugs such as tricyclic antidepressants are passively absorbed through your gut. Tricyclic antidepressants are frequently used for the management of pain associated with post-herpetic neuralgia. As a matter of fact, tricyclic antidepressants are used to treat a variety of chronic pain syndromes. The exact mechanism by which these drugs decrease your pain is unknown. The pain-relieving effect of amitriptyline (Elavil) has been shown in rats to decrease pain caused by certain nerves.

The correct dose of amitriptyline needed by elderly patients suffering from post-herpetic neuralgia is currently unknown. Higher doses definitely produce a greater decrease in your pain. However, the problem with using higher doses is that you may develop a significant decrease in your blood pressure. This is similar to that caused by clonidine. If you become dizzy and fall, you could fracture your hip or one of your other bones. If you become sedated with this drug, another tricyclic antidepressant will be substituted.

Some doctors advocate the use of sedatives for relaxation and to help you sleep in addition to your other medications. If you are elderly, it may be wise for you to refrain from using drugs such as Valium. Valium can have long-acting effects. If you are elderly, Valium is not readily metabolized or excreted. If you take enough of this drug, you may become excessively sedated and even stop breathing. If you have significant sleep deprivation and are becoming agitated as a result of sleep deprivation, a shorter-acting and less-potent drug may be of some benefit to you. A drug called temazepam may have some advantage as a sedative for you. Lyrica (pregabilin) can be helpful in relieving your pain.

You may benefit from the administration of a nonsteroidal anti-inflammatory drug because you may have a portion of your pain caused by your prostaglandins. An example of this drug is ibuprofen. The new COX-2 inhibitors may be somewhat safer for you because their incidence of side effects is less than the older NSAIDs. Because the virus does cause inflammation in your nerves and surrounding tissues, you can benefit from the use of nonsteroidal anti-inflammatory drugs.

It is best to try to avoid narcotics unless they are absolutely indicated. Some narcotics, such as Demerol and Talwin, are associated with psychiatric side effects. It is best to avoid these two drugs in the geriatric population. If narcotics are to be used, mild narcotics should be initiated, as previously stated. Tramadol has been successfully used in a geriatric population. Morphine is commonly used for severe pain.

Baclofen, which does stimulate some receptors in your spinal cord, can decrease the pain associated with post-herpetic neuralgia. It can also relieve any muscle spasms that occur as a result of this painful entity. Amantadine is a drug that can also provide some relief for the management of post-herpetic neuralgia. It is an anti-Parkinson's medication. However, it also has NMDA receptor antagonist activity. These receptors can cause you severe pain when they are activated. If you suffer from post-herpetic neuralgia, you may not feel like eating.

Baclofen, Amantadine, and Elavil can decrease your burning pain associated with post-herpetic neuralgia while anticonvulsant medications can lessen your sharp, shooting pain. Another topical drug that is sometimes used is capsaicin cream. It can be purchased over the counter and can also be purchased by prescription at a higher concentration.

This substance is found in hot peppers. It depletes and prevents the re-accumulation of substance P in your nerves. However, this medication does cause burning. The burning sensation caused by the capsaicin prevents some individuals from using this drug. However, it can provide excellent benefits. It takes several days to deplete the substance P in your nerve endings. Sometimes a transcutaneous electrical nerve stimulator (TENS) can be helpful. The TENS unit, however, is not frequently prescribed because on occasion it could worsen the pain associated with shingles.

If you are experiencing pain in your chest wall, for example, your doctor may place an injection into the nerve that provides sensation to your chest. This nerve is called the intercostal nerve. The type of block that is used to relieve your pain depends on the type of pain that you have. The pain associated with post-herpetic neuralgia can be somatic, sympathetic, or central. The somatic pain follows a certain nerve that is affected. Sympathetic pain can decrease the blood flow to your tissues and causes you to have a burning pain. Central pain is a result of rewiring of your central nervous system. For this type of pain, you need a different type of block.

Sometimes an epidural injection using local anesthetics can provide relief. Further research is being done to evaluate the effects of the administration of epidural ketamine for the treatment of your pain. For your acute lesions, just an injection under the skin with a local anesthetic can provide pain relief. The different type of nerves that can be injected with a local anesthetic include your trigeminal nerve, your brachial plexus, the nerves under your ribs (called intercostal nerves), as well as your sciatic nerve.

It has been shown that sympathetic nerve blocks, if done early, can relieve pain associated with shingles and can also decrease the incidence of developing post-herpetic neuralgia. To be effective, they should be performed within the first two months after the onset of your symptoms. Stellate ganglion blocks are used for pain in your head, neck, and arms. Thoracic epidural blocks are used for pain in your mid back and chest wall, whereas lumbar sympathetic blocks are used for the management of post-herpetic neuralgia pain in your lower extremities. The purpose of nerve blocks is to interrupt your pain impulses and to facilitate therapy and to help you increase your daily-living activities. Nerve blocks should be used if your pain is becoming too severe and cannot be controlled by non-narcotic medications.

An implanted spinal cord stimulator has been demonstrated to be effective for the management of post-herpetic neuralgic pain that is refractory to all other modalities. The goal of the stimulation is to decrease your pain by at least 50 percent. If you do obtain adequate pain relief, the stimulator is implanted permanently surgically. For pain that persists in your arms or legs and is refractory to other treatments, a nerve stimulator can be placed in your extremity to provide you with pain relief. Chemical substances that disrupt nerves have been used since 1930 for the treatment of post-herpetic neuralgia.

If all the previous modalities fail to provide you with relief, a narcotic pump can be placed within your body. The pump consists of a reservoir about the size of a hockey puck. It is connected to a tube that runs into the fluid that surrounds your spinal cord. Essentially this pump gives you a drop of a narcotic drug every minute or so and is another way of controlling your pain. The drug-delivery system is refilled approximately every 45 days. Before placing this pump, your doctor will do a trial of morphine and compare it to a salt solution to see whether you actually obtain pain relief from this device.

There is no single standard surgical procedure that is effective for the treatment of post-herpetic neuralgia. A procedure called a dorsal root entry zone (DREZ) lesion has been shown to be effective for the management of post-herpetic neuralgia in some patients. Sometimes a neurosurgeon can interrupt your pain pathways by doing a procedure in your spinal cord.

Varicella vaccine is safe, effective, and cost-effective in adolescents, and adults. Breakthrough cases of varicella infection are significantly milder than wild-type varicella infection.[17] No severe adverse events have been reported following vaccination, and the incidence of herpes zoster is less in vaccinees than in individuals who have had natural varicella infection.

References

1. Tseng HF, Smith N, Marcy SM, Sy LS, Chao CR, Jacobsen SJ. Risk factors of herpes zoster among children immunized with varicella vaccine: results from a nested case-control study. Pediatr Infect Dis J. 2010;29(3):205-208.

2. Sundstrom K, Weibull CE, Soderberg-Lofdal K, Bergstrom T, Sparen P, Arnheim-Dahlstrom L. Incidence of herpes zoster and associated events including stroke--a population-based cohort study. BMC Infect Dis. 2015;15:488.

3. Joon Lee T, Hayes S, Cummings DM, et al. Herpes zoster knowledge, prevalence, and vaccination rate by race. J Am Board Fam Med. 2013;26(1):45-51.

4. Dworkin RH. Racial differences in herpes zoster and age at onset of varicella. J Infect Dis. 1996;174(1):239-241.

5. Pergam SA, Forsberg CW, Boeckh MJ, et al. Herpes zoster incidence in a multicenter cohort of solid organ transplant recipients. Transpl Infect Dis. 2011;13(1):15-23.

6. Schmader K, George LK, Burchett BM, Pieper CF. Racial and psychosocial risk factors for herpes zoster in the elderly. J Infect Dis. 1998;178 Suppl 1:S67-70.

7. Schmader K, George LK, Burchett BM, Pieper CF, Hamilton JD. Racial differences in the occurrence of herpes zoster. J Infect Dis. 1995;171(3):701-704.

8. Guignard AP, Greenberg M, Lu C, Rosillon D, Vannappagari V. Risk of herpes zoster among diabetics: a matched cohort study in a US insurance claim database before introduction of vaccination, 1997-2006. Infection. 2014;42(4):729-735.

9. Lu PJ, Euler GL, Harpaz R. Herpes zoster vaccination among adults aged 60 years and older, in the U.S., 2008. Am J Prev Med. 2011;40(2):e1-6.

10. Fink AL, Klein SL. Sex and Gender Impact Immune Responses to Vaccines Among the Elderly. Physiology (Bethesda). 2015;30(6):408-416.

11. Chen JY, Cheng TJ, Chang CY, et al. Increased incidence of herpes zoster in adult patients with peptic ulcer disease: a population-based cohort study. Int J Epidemiol. 2013;42(6):1873-1881.

12.   Yenikomshian MA, Guignard AP, Haguinet F, et al. The epidemiology of herpes zoster and its complications in Medicare cancer patients. BMC Infect Dis. 2015;15:106.

13.   Hechter RC, Tartof SY, Jacobsen SJ, Smith N, Tseng HF. Trends and disparity in zoster vaccine uptake in a managed care population. Vaccine. 2013;31(41):4564-4568.

14.   Williams WW, Lu PJ, O'Halloran A, et al. Surveillance of Vaccination Coverage Among Adult Populations - United States, 2014. MMWR Surveill Summ. 2016;65(1):1-36.

15.   Schmader K, George LK, Burchett BM, Hamilton JD, Pieper CF. Race and stress in the incidence of herpes zoster in older adults. J Am Geriatr Soc. 1998;46(8):973-977.

16.   Iglar K, Kopp A, Glazier RH. Herpes zoster as a marker of underlying malignancy. Open Med. 2013;7(2):e68-73.

17.   Chartrand SA. Varicella vaccine. Pediatr Clin North Am. 2000;47(2):373-394.

29. HIV pain

The acquired immune deficiency syndrome (AIDS) is known to be caused by the human immunodeficiency virus (HIV). Pain from other diseases and infections can be worsened by the HIV virus and AIDS. It is important for you to understand how AIDS is developed and what complications can come about in someone with this devastating and debilitating syndrome. Although it has many facets, pain resulting from AIDS and HIV can be controlled. To understand AIDS, you should know what a virus is and how a virus is replicated. A virus is a biological particle that is composed of a genetic material called DNA or RNA and a protein. A virus is not considered to be a living organism. Viruses are organisms that are essentially between living and nonliving things. Viruses can take over the genetic machinery of a cell or cells that they infect. By taking over the whole cell that they infect, they ultimately control the genetic machinery of the cell. The genetic machinery directs the cell's fate.

A virus can replicate itself within a host cell or do nothing once it infects the host cell. When a virus replicates itself in a host cell, thousands or even millions of copies of itself can be released from the cell and then go on to infect other cells. HIV, for example, can enter your body from unsafe sex practices or contaminated blood, enter your cells, and make millions, billions, and even trillions of copies of itself that go on to infect other cells in your body.

A virus, therefore, is a highly effective means of causing you to develop and have an infection. A virus will consist of either RNA or DNA that is encased in a protein outer coat, which is called a capsid. If the virus gets into your body, it can cause a disease unless it is attacked by your antibodies. A virus that causes a disease is called virulent. If the virus gains entrance into your body but does not cause a disease, it is called a temperate virus. It is not clearly understood why a virus will be temperate or virulent.

Viruses are not considered living organisms, as previously stated. The cells in your body reproduce naturally. A virus, on the other hand, can reproduce only by invading one of your cells. The virus then uses your chemicals and other structures within your cell, referred to as genetic material, to make more viruses. A virus cannot reproduce unless the virus is able to invade one of your cells. The virus in your cells acts essentially like a parasite. If the virus is outside of your cell, it is the lifeless particle that has no control of its movement. It is spread randomly through the wind, in water, food, by blood, or by body secretions.

With respect to HIV, blood and body secretions are important mechanisms by which this virus spreads from one person's body into someone else's body. The science of virology is relatively new. A virus was first isolated in 1935. Electrophoresis is now used to examine different properties of a virus. Electrophoresis is a process that separates molecules based on their electrical charges. Different types of viruses exist depending upon the genetic material that it contains. HIV, which is the causative virus of AIDS, is very complex. HIV has two strands of RNA inside of it. These two RNA strands are surrounded by two layers of a protein. A layer of fatty substances surround the inner proteins. Proteins with sugar chains attached to them are located within the fatty layer. The protein sugar complex on the fatty layer forms the outer coat of the virus.

Viruses in general are classified as DNA viruses or RNA viruses, depending on whether RNA or DNA is within the viral structure. In other words, a virus contains either RNA or DNA, but never both. The difference between an RNA virus and a DNA virus is the fashion in which they change the genetic machinery of the cell that they infect. When the virus is inside of your cell, a DNA virus usually produces new RNA, which in turn makes more viral proteins. On the other hand, the DNA from the virus that has infected your cell may join the DNA of your cell and then direct the synthesis (creation) of more new viruses. An RNA virus works in a different fashion. An RNA virus can enter your cell and make new proteins directly. The polio virus is an RNA virus.

You need to know that in a normal, nonviral cell such as a cell in your skin or muscle, DNA is needed to make RNA. The HIV virus is a different type of virus, called a retrovirus. In a retrovirus, RNA makes DNA with the help of an enzyme. This new DNA then makes new RNA. The RNA then makes the proteins that become part of new viruses. Now that you understand what a virus is, you need to understand what a vaccine is. Vaccines can be important for the treatment of HIV and AIDS.

In 1881, Louis Pasteur grew a weakened form of the rabies virus. He knew that if he could inject a weakened form of the virus he could help the body to use its mechanisms to fight the rabies virus and prevent it from replicating. If you are given a weak form of a virus, you will not have the symptoms normally associated with a virus such as fever and chills. Louis Pasteur showed that a single injection of a weak virus could provide you with future immunity from a normal infectious virus.

Following injection of a weak form of a virus into your body, your body will construct antibodies to destroy not only the weakened virus (vaccine) but also the strong infectious form (virulent form) of the virus.

Louis Pasteur's original experiment is the basis of the development of vaccines to combat viral infections. When a virus, such as HIV or any other virulent virus attacks one of your cells, first the virus attaches to your cell. The virus will attach itself to the outer membrane of your cell at an area called a receptor site. When the virus attaches to your receptor site, the virus will release an enzyme that weakens a spot on the wall of your cell membrane. After the virus has weakened the outer wall of your cell, it will then inject the RNA from itself into your cell through the hole in your cell wall.

Sometimes the whole virus can go right through the hole in your cell wall without just injecting its RNA. When the virus is inside of your cell, the HIV complex can make RNA, which in turns makes DNA. The DNA can then take complete control of your cell. The DNA can tell your cell to make new DNA, which is an RNA that is needed to make new viruses.

When the new viruses are made, an enzyme is released that destroys the outer wall of your call. When this wall is destroyed, the new viruses that have been made within your cell are now released into your body. These viruses will go to infect different cells of different tissues within your body at this time. As this process progresses, you can see how you can develop a viral infection.

You develop fever, chills, joint pain, muscle pain, and so forth. Be aware that when the new virus is made from the original virus, your cell that was infected by the virus will then be destroyed. You need to also know that when a new virus infects your cell, it does not cause immediate cellular destruction. Remember that a temperate virus does not cause a disease immediately. Therefore, even though a virus is within your cell or cells, it may take time for it to do any damage to your cell. This example is the reason why HIV can be present in the body for some time before causing symptoms. HIV is classified as a retrovirus, as stated previously. The majority of the other viruses that commonly cause people to become sick are either DNA or RNA viruses. A retrovirus more commonly infects animals.

Most viral infections are contracted from particles in the air or from touching infected individuals. The retrovirus that can cause AIDS can be transmitted by one of three means: exposure to infected blood products, sexual contact with infected people or an infection from a mother to her baby. The infection with this virus appears within two to six weeks following infection.

Early symptoms of infection with HIV are much like flu symptoms and include muscle pain, joint pain, headaches, as well as a sore throat and fever. Antibodies to the HIV virus develop in your body within three to six months of your infection. Later symptoms, which take up to 10 years to develop, as those of AIDS, result from the destructive effects of HIV on your immune system and are characterized by unusual types of pneumonia, cancer, central nervous system infections, and other problems.

Changes in your immune system will eventually occur after you have been infected with the HIV virus. After the HIV virus enters your cell, the virus can set up a chronic infection in which new virus particles are constantly produced. You may develop some antibodies to the virus. When the level of your body's antibodies decreases, you can develop AIDS.

Progression to AIDS, which is a syndrome following infection with the virus, can begin with a low red blood cell count. Other factors can be necessary for you to contract the HIV infection and for the development of progression to AIDS. There are four high-risk groups for developing AIDS, as follows: homosexual and bisexual men, hemophiliacs and transfusion recipients, intravenous drug abusers and children born to infected mothers.

Homosexual and bisexual men account for approximately 37-40 percent of the reported cases of AIDS in the United States. However, this number is increasing. The majority of women with AIDS in the United States are in childbearing years. The number of individuals with AIDS does not take into account the high number of HIV-infected asymptomatic women. Remember that an HIV infection takes time to develop AIDS. The risks for a woman to expose herself to the HIV virus are through unsafe sex practices, intravenous drug use, and transfusions. A significant number of HIV-infected women have given birth to HIV-infected babies.

There is speculation that pregnancy can accelerate the disease progression of HIV. If you are pregnant and have HIV, you may develop symptoms two to three years after the delivery of your baby. This rate of AIDS development is faster than for homosexual men or intravenous drug users; approximately 40 percent of asymptomatic carriers of the virus in these categories will develop AIDS. The AIDS virus will decrease your lymphocytes, which are cells that normally exist in your bloodstream.

Lymphocytes are important mediators of your immune system. These cells help fight the development of various diseases. The average time of onset of your viral infection to development of AIDS varies months to years with a mean time of approximately 10 years.

Health-care providers cannot test an individual for HIV without permission. To check you for an HIV infection, your doctor must obtain an informed consent from you. Informed consent is a legal requirement and means that your doctor must inform you that you will be tested for HIV. You must sign an agreement that gives your doctor the right to do this test. Without your informed consent, your doctor is violating your patient rights. Informed consent is required in most states before you can be tested for HIV. If you received blood products between 1987 and 1995, you are at an increased risk of developing AIDS. If you have active tuberculosis, you run a higher risk of contracting the HIV virus. If you are a health-care worker who performs invasive procedures such as starting intravenous catheters, surgery, and so on, you are at a risk of being exposed to the virus as well.

It is not the invasive procedure itself that poses the risk for HIV, but the risk of a dangerous blood exposure while performing such a procedure. Furthermore, if you are a health-care provider and have had a needle stick, you again run the risk of exposure to the virus. If the needle puncture produces minimal blood exposure, the chance of you becoming infected is rare. If you are in any of these higher-risk categories, you should have your blood tested for the virus.

The name for the initial viral test performed is ELISA (enzyme-linked immunoabsorbent assay). If you have a positive screening test using ELISA, the infection with the HIV complex is confirmed with a repeat ELISA test as well as another test called a Western blot test. A doctor will usually not report a positive ELISA test to you until your Western blot test has been confirmed to be positive. If you are pregnant and have been infected with the HIV virus, the incidence of a premature birth is increased as well as mental retardation of your baby.

You also run the risk of having a low-birth-weight baby. Otherwise, there is no evidence that the HIV virus affects the outcome of your pregnancy if you have no symptoms. Remember that if you have been infected by the HIV virus and do give birth, your baby has a chance of developing AIDS. Because HIV can be transmitted sexually, if you are positive for the virus you should be screened for other sexually transmitted diseases such as gonorrhea and syphilis.

You may need to be tested for the hepatitis virus as well as Chlamydia infection. If you have the HIV virus, you should be immunized with some vaccines for other diseases. You can develop a pneumococcal infection, which can cause pneumonia. It is recommended that you receive a pneumococcal vaccine. Revaccination after five years should be considered. You should also have the hepatitis B virus vaccine. HIV-infected individuals are at a higher risk of becoming carriers of the hepatitis B virus after having an acute hepatitis B virus infection.

You may also need to be tested for the hepatitis C virus. HIV virus infection is characterized by a deterioration of your body's immune system. This deterioration in your immune system will cause you to develop AIDS. Cells in your immune system are disabled and are killed during the infection. You have important immune cells in your body called CD4+T. During the HIV infection, the number of these cells progressively declines. When these cells fall to a critical level, you are vulnerable to infections as well as cancers.

The HIV virus induces AIDS by causing the death of the CD4+T cells in your body. These cells are important for the normal function of your immune system. The AIDS virus also interferes with their normal function. When this happens, your ability to fight other infections is diminished. HIV virus is called a slow virus. This means that the course of infection with the HIV virus has a long interval between the initial infection and the onset of the AIDS symptoms. Some of the conditions that HIV/AIDS can cause: fever and night sweats, loss of appetite, nausea and vomiting, chest pain related to pneumonia, chronic sinus infection with headache, tumor on your spinal cord, meningitis with neck pain and headaches, painful lesions in your mouth, hepatitis with abdominal pain or burning or piercing pain in your arms or legs.

After you are infected by the HIV virus, in two to four weeks you will have flulike symptoms. The HIV virus is unique in that it escapes your body's immune responses. Once infected, you can progress to AIDS in an average of 10 years. Combinations of three or more anti-HIV drugs called highly active antiretroviral therapy can delay the progression of the HIV disease for prolonged periods.

As your body's immune system is overwhelmed, increased quantities of the virus enter your bloodstream from your cells that were infected. With the increased use of agents for erectile dysfunction, there have been increases in sexual activity among older adults. With this increase in sexual activity, the number of HIV and AIDS cases has increased drastically. This virus can cause you to have a neuropathy. A neuropathy is a lesion in your nerves in your body that are outside of your spinal cord and brain.

AIDS can cause you to have a painful neuropathy. Neuropathy associated with AIDS can be intermittent or constant. The pain can vary in severity from mild to severe. The pain can be burning, shooting, aching, or stabbing. It is believed that the HIV virus can cause nerve damage, which is the cause of your neuropathy. You can develop headaches from HIV virus meningitis. Also you can have abdominal pain related to gastrointestinal disease and chest pain related to pneumonia.

The use of receiving an influenza vaccine is if you have AIDS is controversial. There is a chance that this vaccine could promote HIV replication for up to three months following your vaccination. You should also be considered for a vaccination against the Haemophilus influenza pneumonia. If you have the HIV virus, you run the risk of being infected with the varicella zoster virus. If you are exposed to chicken pox or shingles, you may need an antiviral medication. You should have a tuberculosis test in addition to the other recommended tests. This test is called a PPD test, which is a protein extract from cultures tuberculin bacteria. This test will tell if you have been in contact with tuberculosis. It takes 48 to 72 hours for this test to become positive. If you have a positive test, you should receive tuberculosis treatment, which consists of treatment with an antituberculin drug or drugs.

If you have been infected with the HIV virus, you run the risk of other bacterial infections. You can develop a bacterial infection causing purple colored lesions about your skin. You can also develop gastrointestinal infections as well as pulmonary infections. You can develop a salmonella infection as well as bacterial pneumonia. Bacterial pneumonias occurs frequently in HIV-infected patients.

These bacterial pneumonias can be a result of a streptococcus pneumonia or an H. influenzae pneumonia. Some of these infections can be resistant to antibiotics. If you have syphilis and are HIV infected, treatment failures are common. You need to know that syphilis can affect your central nervous system. When this happens, your doctor will do a spinal tap to diagnose whether you are developing neurosyphilis. You are at a risk of developing not only tuberculosis but you are also at risk for developing a fungal infection in addition to all of the other diseases described.

A common fungal infection is candidiasis. This fungus can affect your mouth, esophagus, and your vagina (if you are a woman and have HIV). These fungal infections are common in HIV-infected individuals.

The severity of a fungal infection as well as the other diseases mentioned depends on your degree of suppression of your immune system. Oral and vaginal fungal infections usually respond to topical therapies. You can also develop a fungal infection of your central nervous system. The cryptococcus neoformans fungal infection is the most common cause of central nervous system fungal infections in patients who have developed AIDS.

You can develop headaches as well as fever and have significant changes in your mental status. To make this diagnosis, your doctor will do a spinal tap on you. Your doctor will measure your spinal fluid pressure by placing a needle into your spinal fluid to see whether you are having excessive pressure on your brain. You may need repeated spinal fluid taps followed by removal of some of your spinal fluid to decrease any pressure that could be affecting your brain. Som

e fungal infections are more prevalent in certain areas of the United States. You can also develop a histoplasmosis fungal infection if you live around the Ohio Valley, although this type of infection is not limited to this area. You can develop a fever, weight loss, and an enlargement of your liver and possibly your spleen. This fungus can affect your bone marrow and decrease some of your blood cells.

Another fungal infection that is prevalent in the southwestern United States that can cause you problems is the coccidioides immitis. This fungal frequently affects the lungs. Aspergillosis is another fungus that can infect you. When these different organisms affect your body, you can have generalized pain, including muscle pain, joint pain, and headaches. If you have increased pressure in your spinal fluid that is compressing your brain, you can have severe headaches.

Of course, with pneumonia, you will expect to have chest pain associated with a bacterial or fungal infection. One of the leading causes of death in individuals with AIDS is the pneumocysdis carinii pneumonia. This is the most common infection in AIDS patients and is the leading cause of death in this patient population. Not only does this disease affect your lungs, it can affect other parts of your body as well.

If you have AIDS, you can also develop tumors associated with AIDS. These tumors include Kaposi's sarcoma as well as Hodgkin's and non-Hodgkin's lymphoma. Another type of infection that you can develop is a protozoan infection. Protozoa is an infectious agent. You can develop a parasite infection caused by a protozoon. Protozoa will get into your cells. When inside your cells, protozoa will use what it needs from your cell so that the protozoa can survive. Protozoa is composed of one cell.

They are microscopic in size but are larger than a virus. The protozoa can multiply within your body. A protozoa infection example is toxoplasma gondii, which can cause a serious infection of your central nervous system. You can present to your health-care provider with a severe headache as well as other abnormalities of your nervous system. Cryptosporidium is an infection that can give you chronic diarrhea. Usually this parasite can be observed in your stool. Other protozoeal infections can cause you to have chronic diarrhea as well. Another protozoa that can cause generalized infections in your body is the strongyloides protozoa.

Gender differences between men and women are noted. With respect to AIDS, women's bodies differ from men's bodies. Drug companies are doing studies to see whether there is any evidence that women respond differently to the AIDS drugs. Women progress to AIDS at the same rate as men but it only takes half the viral infection that it took to infect men. It is now known that there are gender differences in HIV.

A study in Kenya revealed that women were often infected by multiple virus variants as opposed to men. In other words, the HIV infecting the men appeared to be of one type of HIV virus, whereas women have several different variants of the virus. It was speculated that the virus was mutating faster in women than in men. Women naturally have more cells in their bodies that recognize and attack the HIV virus.

It is thought that women's stronger immune response than men to the virus could force the virus to mutate or it is possible that women have a greater infection of the virus than men. In other words, women probably get a larger dose of the virus when they are infected than men. If women are infected with more versions of the HIV virus, this could mean that they would react differently to different drugs or to different vaccines. Women who are infected with the smaller number of the HIV virus became sick at the same rate as did men.

It has been reported by the American Civil Liberties Union that there are civil rights violations against individuals who have HIV and AIDS. The ACLU related that individuals are being fired, rental agreements are destroyed, and they receive inadequate care when they relate that they have HIV or AIDS. It is estimated that 900,000 people in the United States have AIDS or HIV. They are denied medical treatment and are discriminated against in their workplace. They have difficulty getting into nursing homes as well.

In New York, an AIDS mortality rate per 10,000 persons age 15 to 64 was studied. AIDS was among the five leading causes of death for men age 25 to 54 and the leading cause of death for men age 30 to 39. For women AIDS was the fourth leading cause of death for women age 25 to 29 and the second leading cause of death for women age 30 to 34. Premature mortality was noted to be 10 percent in men age 15 to 64 and 3.6 percent for women. Condom use has been recommended as a method to prevent HIV transmission.

Public health professionals have been concerned about the devastation caused by HIV and AIDS in the developing world. It is estimated that 10 percent of people in South Africa are infected with HIV. These rates are higher in other African countries. In Africa, for some reason, the HIV virus passes from women to men at a higher rate of efficiency than is observed in the West. In the year 2000, then President Clinton declared the world AIDS epidemic a threat to U.S. national security.

It is estimated that if 1 million people in the United States now have HIV or AIDS, approximately 500,000 of them are either untreated or undiagnosed. Drugs for the treatment of AIDS are constantly being developed. Essentially, AIDS has gone from being an immediate sentence of death to a chronic manageable disease.

Currently Russia has the fastest growing epidemic of AIDS, thought to be because of intravenous drug use. Epidemics are now beginning in China. The rate of AIDS cases and deaths did slowdown, which was attributed to successful antiretroviral therapy. The problem with some of the drug therapy is that some individuals either develop a resistance to the drugs or they experience side effects from the drugs and stop taking them.

With the increased use of agents for erectile dysfunction, there have been increases in sexual activity among older adults. With this increase in sexual activity, the number of HIV and AIDS cases has increased drastically. The problem that has arisen in the United States is that many adults over age 50 are not protecting themselves against AIDS. Some of these individuals do not think that they are at risk for HIV infection. The incidence of AIDS in individuals over 50 continues to increase in the United States. In women over 50, the number of new AIDS cases more than doubled between 1991 and 1996.

In older men, the increase was similar. An effective vaccine against HIV infection continues to be researched. That one "magic bullet" remains to be developed. Some of the vaccines currently being studied provide protection for some individuals but not all. Between 1991 and 1995, there was a 63 percent increase in women diagnosed with AIDS. The increase in HIV infection in men was noted in younger women who date older men. When HIV and AIDS was first made known in the 1980s, it was a disease of gay men as well as a disease of people who had received blood transfusions or individuals who shared needles for injecting drugs. An increasing number of women with AIDS have been reported, and the exposure to the HIV virus was through heterosexual sex.

An study was published in 2005 that included African Americans males and females as well as white males and females with reference to ethnicity and its effects on fatigue in patients with HIV/AIDS. Moderate to severe fatigue intensity was reported by patients with HIV/AIDS. Women, Hispanics, the disabled and those with inadequate income or insurance reported higher fatigue intensity scores than other individuals.1 Prevention of HIV in women is being emphasized. As you can see from this chapter, the HIV infection with a progression to AIDS is a devastating disease. However, as new treatments are being discovered, if you have the HIV infection, your quality of life will be greatly improved. You must, however, remember that the drugs to treat AIDS are extremely powerful drugs but they do not render a cure for the HIV infection.

Your pain can be treated with narcotic drugs as well as antidepressants and anticonvulsant medications such as Neurontin. Mexilitine may also help to control your pain. Exercise therapy is sometimes beneficial for the management of your pain. It is believed that exercise can increase your body's endorphins, which in turns helps to manage your pain. HIV-related pain becomes increasingly severe as the disease progresses.

Drugs used to treat the HIV infection can cause neuropathic pain. It is estimated that 30 percent of the neuropathic pain syndromes suffered by individuals who have the HIV disease are caused by drugs to attack the HIV virus. Neuropathic pain in the HIV-infected patient in most instances can be adequately controlled. In treating AIDS-related pain, your doctor should direct attention to your emotional distress, your depression, and anxiety, which can also be seen if you suffer from AIDS.

Overall the AIDS incidence and mortality have continued to decline, probably because of new therapies, especially antiviral therapies. However, for women the benefits have been shown to be less than for men. It has been reported that there is gender-based discrimination in the treatment of women with HIV infections. It is also reported that there is insufficient attention to the medical community's response to women's HIV risks. Among people diagnosed with HIV infection, females had a disproportionately high premature mortality from HIV/AIDS.

There are ethnic disparities in the clinical manifestations of HIV-related neuropathies including pain and the susceptibility to neurotoxic antiretrovirals and distal sensory polyneuropathy pain.[2] Despite financial eligibility, racial minorities, especially African-Americans, were disadvantaged in their access to healthcare services during their last months of life.[3] Risky sexual behavior" accounts for the majority of new HIV infections regardless of gender, age, geographic location, or ethnicity.[4]

HIV disproportionately affects young men who have sex with men.[5] In general, men tended to partner with others of the same race, HIV was more prevalent among men of color, and race acted independent of whether one would engage in behaviors that would put them at highest risk for transmitting HIV.[6] The heterosexual transmission of HIV has affected middle-aged African American women at alarming rates.[7,8]

Older individuals can have HIV/AIDS as well as younger individuals. All patients had known dates of initiation of highly active antiretroviral therapy. It was observed that women aged 50 years or more were less likely to experience gastrointestinal symptoms but more likely to experience general malaise, neurologic or other symptoms compared with women less than 40 years of age. Only neurologic symptoms had a higher prevalence among older men who had sex with men. Caucasian women generally had the highest prevalence of symptoms, and African American women had the lowest prevalence.[9] By race/ethnicity, in the United States, Blacks/African Americans continue to experience the most severe HIV burden, followed by Hispanics/Latinos.

Ongoing distress, coupled with limited support, leads to a life in which many people living with HIV endure their pain in silence and experienced profound loneliness.[10] To improve the quality of life and health of these individuals, we cannot focus solely on the individual, but must also focus on the local community and society as a whole. Clinical trials of smoked and noncombustible marijuana are needed to determine the role of cannabinoids as a class of agents with potential to improve quality of life and health care outcomes among patients with HIV/AIDS.[11]

Exercise therapy will help release endorphins that can help inhibit your pain. Prescriptions such as anticonvulsants, antidepressants, and narcotics should be taken to relieve your symptoms of pain. Be aware that new therapies are constantly evolving for HIV and the treatment of its pain. Keep educating yourself on new discoveries and talk with your doctor about them to see if they will be beneficial in helping relieve your pain.

References

1.   Voss JG. Predictors and Correlates of Fatigue in HIV/AIDS. J Pain Symptom Manage. 2005;29(2):173-184.

2.   Robinson-Papp J, Gonzalez-Duarte A, Simpson DM, Rivera-Mindt M, Morgello S, Manhattan HIVBB. The roles of ethnicity and antiretrovirals in HIV-associated polyneuropathy: a pilot study. J Acquir Immune Defic Syndr. 2009;51(5):569-573.

3.   Sambamoorthi U, Walkup J, McSpiritt E, Warner L, Castle N, Crystal S. Racial differences in end-of-life care for patients with AIDS. AIDS Public Policy J. 2000;15(3-4):136-148.

4.   Huang MB, Ye L, Liang BY, et al. Characterizing the HIV/AIDS Epidemic in the United States and China. Int J Environ Res Public Health. 2015;13(1).

5.   Garofalo R, Gayles T, Bottone PD, Ryan D, Kuhns LM, Mustanski B. Racial/Ethnic Difference in HIV-related Knowledge among Young Men who have Sex with Men and their Association with Condom Errors. Health Educ J. 2015;74(5):518-530.

6.   Grov C, Rendina HJ, Ventuneac A, Parsons JT. Sexual Behavior Varies Between Same-Race and Different-Race Partnerships: A Daily Diary Study of Highly Sexually Active Black, Latino, and White Gay and Bisexual Men. Arch Sex Behav. 2015.

7.   Smith TK. Sexual protective strategies and condom use in middle-aged African American women: a qualitative study. J Assoc Nurses AIDS Care. 2015;26(5):526-541.

8.   Trepka MJ, Niyonsenga T, Fennie KP, McKelvey K, Lieb S, Maddox LM. Sex and Racial/Ethnic Differences in Premature Mortality Due to HIV: Florida, 2000-2009. Public Health Rep. 2015;130(5):505-513.

9.   Silverberg MJ, Jacobson LP, French AL, Witt MD, Gange SJ. Age and racial/ethnic differences in the prevalence of reported symptoms in human immunodeficiency virus-infected persons on antiretroviral therapy. J Pain Symptom Manage. 2009;38(2):197-207.

10.   Miles MS, Isler MR, Banks BB, Sengupta S, Corbie-Smith G. Silent endurance and profound loneliness: socioemotional suffering in

African Americans living with HIV in the rural south. Qual Health Res. 2011;21(4):489-501.

11.   Prentiss D, Power R, Balmas G, Tzuang G, Israelski DM. Patterns of marijuana use among patients with HIV/AIDS followed in a public health care setting. J Acquir Immune Defic Syndr. 2004;35(1):38-45.

30. Sickle Cell Pain

Sickle cell disease is a debilitating and sometimes life-threatening blood disorder. For some patients, the results are devastating, including severe pain that often requires hospitalization and can last for days. The use of preventive maintenance treatments, particularly regular blood transfusions and a drug called hydroxyurea are medically indicated. The problem is that sickle cell disease is comparatively rare. Most clinicians don't encounter it or have limited experience and expertise with respect to treatment of the associated pain.

In the United States, most people with sickle cell disease are of African ancestry or identify themselves as black. About 1 in 13 African American babies is born with sickle cell trait. About 1 in every 365 black children is born with sickle cell disease. There are also many people with this disease who come from Hispanic, southern European, Middle Eastern, or Asian Indian backgrounds. Sickle cell disease is a genetic disorder; It results in an abnormality in the oxygen-carrying hemoglobin found in red blood cells.

This leads to a rigid, sickle like shape under certain circumstances. Sickle cell disease is a severe hematologic condition that presents unique complications among affected pregnant women.[1] A 7-year-old American white boy of Greek ancestry had sickle cell anemia.[2] This is the first demonstrated example of sickle cell anemia in a white male described in the United States.

The disease causes the body to make abnormal sickle or crescent-shaped red blood cells that can block vessels, causing organ damage and pain. It is a debilitating and life-threatening illness. The recommendations urge physicians caring for sickle cell patients to use the powerful painkillers when necessary. The severity of the pain is not associated with physical findings. The drug hydroxyurea increases the production of healthy fetal hemoglobin. Patients must take hydroxyurea for three months before it becomes effective. Regular transfusions shut off the body's production of sickle cells and raise the red blood count to normal, reducing the risk of anemia. An attack can be set off by temperature changes, stress, dehydration, and high altitude. A person with a single abnormal copy does not usually have symptoms and is said to have sickle-cell trait.

Regular transfusions shut off the body's production of sickle cells and raise the red blood count to normal, which reduces the risk of anemia. Periodic episodes of pain, called crises, are a major symptom of sickle cell anemia. Pain develops when sickle-shaped red blood cells block blood flow through tiny blood vessels to your thorax, abdomen and joints. Pain can also occur in your bones. The pain may vary in intensity and can last for a few hours to a few weeks. Patients can experience a dozen or more crises a year. If a crisis is severe enough, you may need to be hospitalized. Sickle cells can damage your spleen, an organ that fights infection. This may make you more vulnerable to infections.

Some patients with sickle cell anemia experience vision problems.3 Small blood vessels that supply blood to the eyes may become plugged with sickle cells. This can permanently damage the retina. Sickle cell anemia is caused by a mutation in the gene that tells your body to make hemoglobin. Hemoglobin allows red blood cells to carry oxygen from your lungs to all parts of your body. In sickle cell anemia, the abnormal hemoglobin causes red blood cells to become rigid, sticky and misshapen. Recruits in basic training with the sickle-cell trait have a substantially increased, age-dependent risk of exercise-related sudden death.[4]

The sickle cell gene is passed from generation to generation in a pattern of inheritance called autosomal recessive inheritance. This means that both the mother and the father must pass on the defective form of the gene for a child to be affected. If only one parent passes the sickle cell gene to the child, that child will have the sickle cell trait. With one normal hemoglobin gene and one defective form of the gene, people with the sickle cell trait make both normal hemoglobin and sickle cell hemoglobin. Their blood may contain some sickle cells, but they generally don't experience symptoms. However, they are carriers of the disease, which means they can pass the defective gene on to their children. There was an association between sickle cell disease (SCD) and dental caries in African-American adults.[5]

Sickle cell anemia is caused by a mutation in the gene that tells your body to make hemoglobin. Hemoglobin allows red blood cells to carry oxygen from your lungs to all parts of your body. In sickle cell anemia, the abnormal hemoglobin causes red blood cells to become rigid, sticky and misshapen. The gene is more common in families that come from Africa, India, Mediterranean countries, Saudi Arabia, the Caribbean islands, and South and Central America. In the United States, it most commonly affects blacks.

Sickle cell anemia can lead to a host of complications. A stroke can occur if sickle cells block blood flow to an area of your brain. Signs of stroke include seizures, weakness or numbness of your arms and legs, sudden speech difficulties, and loss of consciousness. If your baby or child has any of these signs and symptoms, seek medical treatment immediately. A stroke can be fatal. Another life threatening complication of sickle cell anemia causes chest pain, fever and difficulty breathing. Acute chest syndrome can be caused by a lung infection or by sickle cells blocking blood vessels in your lungs. It may require emergency medical treatment with antibiotics and other treatments. Sickle cell anemia is also associated with significant electrocardiographic abnormalities.[6]

Patients with sickle cell anemia can also develop high blood pressure in their lungs called pulmonary hypertension. This complication usually affects adults rather than children. Shortness of breath and fatigue are common symptoms of this condition, which can be fatal. Sickle cells can block blood flow through blood vessels, immediately depriving an organ of blood and oxygen. In sickle cell anemia, blood is also chronically low on oxygen. Chronic deprivation of oxygen-rich blood can damage nerves and organs in your body, including your kidneys, liver and spleen. Organ damage can be fatal.

Sickle cell anemia can cause open sores, called ulcers, on your legs. The breakdown of red blood cells produces a substance called bilirubin. A high level of bilirubin in your body can lead to gallstones. Men with sickle cell anemia may experience painful, long-lasting erections, a condition called priapism. As occurs in other parts of the body, sickle cells can block the blood vessels in the penis. This can damage the penis and eventually lead to impotence.

The actual nature of pain experience in sickle cell disease is poorly understood and sub-optimally managed.[7,8] The experience of sickle cell disease pain is indescribable without the use of analogy, as it is unbearable, agonizing, constant, and inescapable and without limit. Difficulty describing pain creates a perception of being misunderstood or minimized by professionals.[9] Personification of pain is often employed by patients to attempt to form a relationship with their pain.

Chronic hemolytic anemia produces jaundice, gallstones, splenomegaly and poorly healing ulcers over the lower tibia. Life-threatening severe anemia can occur during hemolytic or aplastic crises, generally associated with viral or other infection or by folic acid deficiency. Acute painful episodes due to acute vaso-occlusion from clusters of sickled red cells may occur spontaneously or be provoked by infection, dehydration, or hypoxia. Common sites of acute painful episodes include the bones and the chest. These episodes last hours to days and may produce low-grade fever. Acute vasoocclusion may cause strokes.

Repeated episodes of vascular occlusion especially affect the heart, lungs, and liver. Ischemic necrosis of bone occurs, rendering the bone susceptible to osteomyelitis due to salmonellae and staphylococci. Infarction of the papillae of the renal medulla causes renal tubular concentrating defects and gross hematuria, more often encountered in sickle cell trait than in sickle cell anemia. Retinopathy similar to that noted in diabetes mellitus is often present and may lead to visual impairment. Pulmonary hypertension may develop and is associated with a poor prognosis. These patients are prone to delayed puberty. An increased incidence of infection is related to hyposplenism as well as to defects in the alternative pathway of complement.

There is a wide spectrum of severity, with some patients having no symptoms and others suffering frequent, life-changing complications. Much of this variability is unexplained, despite increasingly sophisticated genetic studies.10 Environmental factors, including climate, air quality, socio-economics, exercise and infection, are likely to be important.11 The effects of weather vary with geography, although most studies show that exposure to cold or wind increases hospital attendance with acute pain. Most of the different air pollutants correlate with increased hospital attendance, although higher concentrations of atmospheric carbon monoxide may offer some benefit for patients with sickle cell disease.

On examination, patients are often chronically ill and jaundiced. There is hepatomegaly, but the spleen is not palpable in adult life. The heart is enlarged, with a hyper-dynamic precordium and systolic murmurs. Non-healing ulcers of the lower leg and retinopathy may be present. Sickle cell anemia becomes a chronic multisystem disease, with death from organ failure. With improved supportive care, average life expectancy is now between 40 and 50 years of age. In adult patients with diabetes mellitus, spinal cord trauma, and sickle cell anemia, prophylactic cholecystectomy is generally not indicated for asymptomatic or uncomplicated gallstone disease. Right-upper-quadrant ultrasound is indicated preoperatively for those who are at high risk for developing gallstones so that cholecystectomy may be performed concomitantly if indicated however.

Patients describe experiencing unimaginable, agonizing, continuous, inescapable and limitless pain which is almost impossible to describe. Patients use analogy and personification as a way to overcome this difficulty.9 Participants spoke about a process where, ultimately, they felt obliged to accept their illness as it would never be cured; but were able to appreciate life and recognize positive life lessons as a result of living with sickle cell anemia. Painful crisis in patients with sickle cell anemia is associated with severe pain in 75% and most will require second-line therapy for adequate resolution.[12] Physicians need to provide adequate pain relief to decrease morbidity in these patients.

Diseases that can cause intrinsic tooth discoloration and dental pathology include sickle cell anemia.[13,14] Avascular necrosis of the femoral head occurs when the blood supply is disrupted. An insidious onset of pain occurs over 2-3wks and is often bilateral. The most common location of avascular necrosis is of the hip. Sickle cell anemia may be a cause of avascular necrosis. An MRI is very sensitive in detecting early stages of avascular necrosis, red marrow persistence, extramedullary hematopoiesis, changes of arthritis, infections and joint effusion.[15] Venous thromboembolism is a recognized complication of sickle cell disease.[16]

There are differences in pain management between hematologists and hospitalists. Patients cared for by hospitalists more frequently utilized home oral pain medication during admission, had shorter lengths of hospitalization, and did not have a significant increase in readmission.[17] Management of the acute painful crisis (APC) of sickle cell disease (SCD) remains unsatisfactory despite advances in the understanding and management of acute pain in other clinical settings.[18] One reason for this is an unsophisticated approach to the use of opioid analgesics for pain management. This applies to hematologists who are responsible for developing acute sickle pain management protocols for their patients, and to health care staff in the acute care setting

Stem cell transplantation can cure more than 80% of children with sickle cell anemia who have suitable HLA-matched donors. Transplantation remains investigational. Patients with sickle cell anemia should have their care coordinated with a hematologist. People with sickle cell trait may experience sudden cardiac death and rhabdomyolysis during vigorous exercise, especially at high altitudes. They may also be at increased risk for a venothromboembolism.

Sickle cell patients are often admitted for pain control of an acute pain crisis. The cause of pain is most likely due to ischemia of tissue in infarcted tissues. Acute pain crisis in sickle cell patients requires aggressive hydration and treatment of pain usually by opioids given intravenously in the initial phase. Common opioids used are hydromorphone, morphine, and oxycodone.

NSAIDs are also often used to control nociceptive pain; they're given PO as an adjunct to opioids to control the pain in sickle cell crisis. Pain from an acute crisis can be decreased by up to 50% with hydroxyurea. A low-dose ketamine infusion can be an option for pain control in sickle cell disease as well.[19] Low-dose intravenous ketamine-midazolam infusion might also be effective in reducing the patient's pain and opioid requirements in patients with sickle cell disease with severe painful crisis.[20]

Sickle cell patients may abuse pain medications as any pain patient may do. The modes of abuse of sickle cell patients ranged from obtaining analgesic prescription from multiple sources, injecting analgesics and sharing analgesics between patients in the hospital.[21] It is therefore necessary for pain physicians and to address the use of opioid in chronic sickle cell pain and provide alternatives and a suitable guideline for their use. The information provided could help propel research in sickle cell disease associated chronic pain and uncover new treatment options for clinicians.[22]

A clear directive to doctors is to take patients at their word when they say they are in pain, and to treat it promptly and aggressively.[23] Remember that the pain associated with sickle cell anemia may not be associated with physical findings. There is only a paucity of clinical trials regarding screening, management, and monitoring for individuals with sickle cell disease.

References

1.   Barfield WD, Barradas DT, Manning SE, Kotelchuck M, Shapiro-Mendoza CK. Sickle cell disease and pregnancy outcomes: women of African descent. Am J Prev Med. 2010;38(4 Suppl):S542-549.

2.   Campbell JJ, Oski FA. Sickle cell anemia in an American white boy of Greek ancestry. Am J Dis Child. 1977;131(2):186-188.

3.   Freitas LG, Isaac DL, Tannure WT, et al. [Retinal manifestations in patients with sickle cell disease referred to a University Eye Hospital]. Arq Bras Oftalmol. 2011;74(5):335-337.

4.   Kark JA, Posey DM, Schumacher HR, Ruehle CJ. Sickle-cell trait as a risk factor for sudden death in physical training. N Engl J Med. 1987;317(13):781-787.

5.   Laurence B, George D, Woods D, et al. The association between sickle cell disease and dental caries in African Americans. Spec Care Dentist. 2006;26(3):95-100.

6.   Oguanobi NI, Onwubere BJ, Ike SO, Anisiuba BC, Ejim EC, Ibegbulam OG. Electocardiographic findings in adult Nigerians with sickle cell anaemia. Afr Health Sci. 2010;10(3):235-241.

7.   Booker MJ, Blethyn KL, Wright CJ, Greenfield SM. Pain management in sickle cell disease. Chronic Illn. 2006;2(1):39-50.

8.   Taylor LE, Stotts NA, Humphreys J, Treadwell MJ, Miaskowski C. A review of the literature on the multiple dimensions of chronic pain in adults with sickle cell disease. J Pain Symptom Manage. 2010;40(3):416-435.

9.   Coleman B, Ellis-Caird H, McGowan J, Benjamin MJ. How sickle cell disease patients experience, understand and explain their pain: An Interpretative Phenomenological Analysis study. Br J Health Psychol. 2016;21(1):190-203.

10.   Tewari S, Brousse V, Piel FB, Menzel S, Rees DC. Environmental determinants of severity in sickle cell disease. Haematologica. 2015;100(9):1108-1116.

11.   Serjeant GR. Natural history and determinants of clinical severity of sickle cell disease. Curr Opin Hematol. 1995;2(2):103-108.

12.   Boyd I, Gossell-Williams M, Lee MG. The Use of Analgesic Drugs in Patients with Sickle Cell Painful Crisis. West Indian Med J. 2014;63(5):479-483.

13.   Richard PA. Pathophysiology of dental changes in sickle cell disease. J Conn State Dent Assoc. 1977;51(1):20-23.

14.   Okafor LA, Nonnoo DC, Ojehanon PI, Aikhionbare O. Oral and dental complications of sickle cell disease in Nigerians. Angiology. 1986;37(9):672-675.

15.   Sachan AA, Lakhkar BN, Lakhkar BB, Sachan S. Is MRI Necessary for Skeletal Evaluation in Sickle Cell Disease. J Clin Diagn Res. 2015;9(6):TC08-12.

16.   van Hamel Parsons V, Gardner K, Patel R, Thein SL. Venous thromboembolism in adults with sickle cell disease: experience of a single centre in the UK. Ann Hematol. 2015.

17.   Shah N, Rollins M, Landi D, Shah R, Bae J, De Castro LM. Differences in pain management between hematologists and hospitalists caring for patients with sickle cell disease hospitalized for vasoocclusive crisis. Clin J Pain. 2014;30(3):266-268.

18.   Telfer P, Bahal N, Lo A, Challands J. Management of the acute painful crisis in sickle cell disease- a re-evaluation of the use of opioids in adult patients. Br J Haematol. 2014;166(2):157-164.

19.   Tawfic QA, Faris AS, Kausalya R. The role of a low-dose ketamine-midazolam regimen in the management of severe painful crisis in patients with sickle cell disease. J Pain Symptom Manage. 2014;47(2):334-340.

20.   Uprety D, Baber A, Foy M. Ketamine infusion for sickle cell pain crisis refractory to opioids: a case report and review of literature. Ann Hematol. 2014;93(5):769-771.

21.   Kotila TR, Busari OE, Makanjuola V, Eyelade OR. Addiction or Pseudoaddiction in Sickle Cell Disease Patients: Time to Decide - a Case Series. Ann Ib Postgrad Med. 2015;13(1):44-47.

22.   Lutz B, Meiler SE, Bekker A, Tao YX. Updated Mechanisms of Sickle Cell Disease-Associated Chronic pain. Transl Perioper Pain Med. 2015;2(2):8-17.

23.   Yawn BP, Buchanan GR, Afenyi-Annan AN, et al. Management of sickle cell disease: summary of the 2014 evidence-based report by expert panel members. JAMA. 2014;312(10):1033-1048.

31. Sports Related Pain

The current trend today in the United States is physical activity. Physical exercise can help you maintain or lose your weight, maintain strength, and can be protective for your heart. However, you can develop aches and pains in your body associated with moderate physical exercise. As more individuals become more aware of the benefits of physical exercise, the incidence of exercise-related injuries is increasing. Furthermore, gender-specific differences exist as to the types of injuries that occur.

Pain essentially is your body's protective mechanism to prevent further injury to your tissues. Most pain is relatively mild and goes away relatively quickly. If your pain is severe and persists for more than seven days, however, your body is trying to tell you that something is wrong. Most significant pain should not last for more than one to three days unless you have sustained a significant injury. Your pain can be caused by muscle injury or an injury to one of your ligaments, bones or tendons.

You can also have an inflammation of one of your peripheral nerves, which are nerves outside of your brain and spinal cord. You can even have a small fracture of one of your bones. If you have an injury to a tissue in your body, this tissue is usually a muscle, tendon, or ligament. Tendons and ligaments can tear apart or tear away from their attachments. The same holds true for muscles.

Usually small fractures in bones heal quickly. The most common bone injuries are stress fractures of your small bones, such as those in your feet. These stress fractures usually take approximately eight weeks to heal. The cover of your bone called a periosteum is a wrapper around your bone that contains many small nerves. If you sustain a bruise to your periosteum, you can have significant pain for several days to several weeks.

You can develop an abnormal bone growth about the bone in your heel. This abnormal bone growth, which can be painful, is called a spur. Muscles, ligaments, and tendons are composed of fibers that run parallel to each other. These fibers are like the strings of a guitar. They are wrapped in an outer layer. If these fibers are stretched beyond their normal length, they can tear. Usually these fibers grow back together. However, sometimes scars can prevent the ends of the fibers from reattaching. As a result, scars in these areas can become painful.

Myofascial pain can occur when your muscle fibers are stretched beyond their normal elastic limits. When this happens, it is called a strain. The tender areas in your muscles are called trigger points, and these cause a myofascial pain syndrome. Usually ice or heat over the painful muscle can significantly relieve your pain. Massage therapy can also provide you with significant muscle pain relief as well. You also have cartilage in your joints. Adults who engage in strength training are less likely to experience loss of muscle mass, functional decline, and fall-related injuries than adults who do not strength train.1 Studies on strength-training interventions have indicated that inactive older adults who begin regular strength training achieve substantial strength gains within a few months.

Cartilage is a substance that exists between your bones and can be compressed. This compressive ability makes the cartilage act as a shock absorber in some of your joints. Cartilage allows your bones of your joints such as your knee joints to slide over each other. If you do not have the cartilage, one bone will slide over another bone. You would have increased friction applied to your bones in your joint, which could cause you significant pain.

You can also stretch and injure a tendon, which is called a sprain. An acute sprain is a stretch of a ligament after your injury. If you don't heal within six weeks, you are showing signs of chronic pain. If you still have pain after six months, you have chronic pain. A tendon is composed of a group of fibers that attaches your muscles to your bones. A tendon is composed of tough fibers. A tendon injury can take a long time to heal. Muscle injuries, on the other hand, can heal faster than tendon injuries. The reason for this difference is that muscles have a greater blood flow than tendons.

The flow of blood to injured tissue is necessary to bring nutrients that can heal tissue. A tendon injury can be potentially serious because if it does not heal properly you can be prone to re-injury. In other words, if your tendon does not heal properly, there can be a weak area in the nonhealed part of your tendon. If you exercise again, you may re-injure this tendon. If your tendon is partially injured or torn, you can develop inflammation in your tendon. This inflammatory process is called tendonitis. Improper healing can cause you to have scar tissue and make you prone to re-injury.

Some tendons in your body are bathed in a fluid that is surrounded by a sheath. If your tendon becomes inflamed from overuse, it may swell. When it swells, it rubs against your outer tendon sheath, which can cause you to have significant pain. This type of pain is called tenosynovitis. You need to realize that all tendons have this fluid sheath that surrounds them. Another type of tissue in your body is a tough fibrous tissue composed of fibers, as previously mentioned.

The purpose of ligaments is to hold bones together. For example, vertebrae, the bones that are stacked on top of each other in your back, are held together by ligaments. If too much stress is placed on your ligaments, the ligament may tear. As with the other tissues mentioned previously, a tear in your ligament can cause inflammation. Your ligaments can heal properly or improperly. Again like the other tissues that mentioned previously, improper healing can make you prone to re-injury. Ligaments are an example of another tissue that does not have a great blood supply. As a result of a minimal blood supply, this tissue is slow to heal.

You have probably heard the term "bursitis." Some people have bursitis of their shoulder, whereas others have a bursitis about their hip. A bursa is a sac that is filled with fluid. This fluid-filled sac is placed between either a tendon or a bone or between a ligament and a bone. A bursa allows a tendon to glide about the bone of your shoulder or hip, for example. When your tendon glides smoothly over your bone, the tendon does not become inflamed or injured. However, sometimes your bursa can become inflamed, leading to what is called bursitis. If the inflammation in your bursa progresses, the fluid can accumulate within your bursa. This expansion of the bursal sac will cause you to have pain. If this happens, you develop bursitis.

You need to be aware that scarring can form within your bursa. If a scar does form, you can have chronic irritation of your bursa. As a result, this can cause you to have chronic pain. The fascia is a tissue that covers your muscles and separates one muscle from another. The fascia is present throughout your body. This fascia enables one muscle to slide smoothly over another muscle.

Sometimes an area where your fascia and muscle come together can be separated, causing pain at this junction. This can also be an origin of what is called myofascial pain. So in a sports injury, you can have pain related to an actual tear in your muscle or pain related to an injury at the junction of your fascia and your muscle.

You usually are not aware of your elbow until you develop pain in your elbow joint. Your elbow joint is formed by one bone from your upper arm and two bones from your forearm. You can have irritation of your elbow joint or you can have a tennis player's or golfer's tendonitis.

An injury to your elbow is usually in the tendons of the muscles that attach to the bones about your elbow.

In tennis elbow, the pain runs to your outer elbow. You may also have pain about your inner elbow. This usually occurs when you play golf. Tennis elbow was named because it affected tennis players. However, anyone can develop a tennis elbow. Tennis elbow means that you have an inflamed tendon about your elbow. You can have pain on the outside of your elbow. You can develop tennis elbow if you are a weightlifter, play tennis or racquetball, or wait tables.

The problem with tennis elbow is that you can sustain a re-injury. If you have pain on the outside of your elbow, you should stop the activity that caused your pain. You should use ice over the elbow. Nonsteroidal anti-inflammatory drugs may help you control your pain. You probably have tennis elbow if the pain in your elbow is so bad that you cannot even lift a coffee cup. You usually have tenderness over a dime-sized area on the outer aspect of your elbow. X-rays of your elbow are not necessary.

A Velcro wrist splint can be helpful in controlling your pain as well. If your pain persists after four weeks, sometimes a short arm cast needs to be used. At 6 to 10 weeks, you should be feeling much better. If not, you will be referred to an orthopedic surgeon. You should gradually resume your activities. Physical therapy does play a role, but it is a minor role in the treatment of this painful entity.

You may also develop pain on your inner elbow. This inner elbow pain is called golfer's elbow. If you are scrubbing a floor vigorously, you can develop pain in your inner elbow. The pain usually starts several days after you were doing an activity. The treatment for golfer's elbow is the same as that for tennis elbow. You may also develop pain in your elbow joint. This type of pain may be due to osteoarthritis. Nonsteroidal anti-inflammatory medications will help this pain. Rarely will you need a steroid injection into the joint. You can also develop a bursitis in your elbow.

You can develop a sudden red, swollen area over your elbow. Your range of motion about your elbow will be normal. You do not need x-rays. If your pain is aggravating and persisting, your doctor may want to use a needle and syringe to remove the fluid from your bursa (a process called "aspiration") and send the fluid to a laboratory to test for crystals, bacteria, and so on. If your tests determine that you have gout, you will be treated appropriately. Injection of a steroid into your bursa can provide you with pain relief. If your pain persists, you will be referred to an orthopedic surgeon. Usually ice and nonsteroidal anti-inflammatory drugs will control this pain.

You knee, which is the largest joint in your body, may be injured if you are active in sports. Many different types of injuries can affect your knees. Jogging or running has gained popularity in the past 10 to 15 years. However, this activity has led to an increase in knee injuries. The knee is made up of your thigh bone and your shin bones. There is also a bone in front of your knee called the kneecap (patella). Your bones about your knee are held together by ligaments. There is a ligament at either side of your knee. These ligaments provide your knee with stability. Your knee also contains cartilage, which coats your bones. Your cartilage allows your bones to slide over each other with ease. If your cartilage wears out, it can cause you to have arthritis. Between your thigh bone and your shin bone is another cartilage called a meniscus. These cartilages are attached to your shin bone (tibia). You also have muscles that control your range of motion. These are called the quadriceps and hamstrings. When your quadriceps muscles contract, they make your knee straighten. When your hamstring muscles contract, these muscles make your knee and lower leg pull backward at the knee joint. To cushion your knee, you have several bursa in your knee. You can have several areas of pain within your knee.

Have you ever had pain under your kneecaps after you run? Have you ever had problems where you can't squat or kneel anymore? What is the grinding noise that I hear when I bend my knee? These symptoms are compatible with a disease called chondromalacia patellae. This disease involves a painful kneecap. You will have pain when you bend your knee and will feel areas about your knee that feel like Rice Krispies crushing. You may have swelling about your knee. If you have no swelling, you will have a normal range of motion. If your knee is arthritic, you will the symptoms of chrondromalacia patellae.

An x-ray eventually will show signs of osteoarthritis in the joint where your patella meets your femur. Injection of a local anesthetic about this area can be diagnostic of your disease. Arthroscopy, which involves inserting a scope into your knee, can identify the pathology going on with your knee. If you have pain in your knee, you should apply ice and elevate your knee. You should avoid squatting as well as kneeling. Swimming is preferred to jogging or any impact exercises. You may want to use a Velcro strap over your knee. You should take a nonsteroidal anti-inflammatory medication following your injury. If your pain persists after three months, you may benefit from an oral steroid.

After three to four months, you will need to continue daily straight-leg-raising exercises as well as doing range of motion exercises. Physical therapy is one of the main treatments for this disorder. Swelling about your knee can last for several months. You should attempt to improve your quadriceps and hamstring tone. If you do exercises to strengthen your quadriceps and hamstring muscles, you can slow down the progression of the chondromalacia to an osteoarthritis.

Occasionally, surgical procedures are done. However, injection therapy or surgery is not a substitute for increasing your muscle strength. Sometimes you can develop swelling just below your kneecap. You will feel as if you have a "fever" inside your knee. As your knee becomes swollen, you will find that you are unable to bend or straighten it.

If you have not improved after two months, an MRI of your knee may need to be done. You also may need to have an arthroscopic procedure by your orthopedic surgeon to determine what type of therapy you actually need. Physical therapy is an extremely important modality for swelling of your knee. You can have steroids injected into your knee as well. If you have rheumatoid arthritis, your surgeon can operate on your knee to improve your function and to decrease your pain. When playing sports or running, you may tear a cartilage in your knee.

Injury prevention must be emphasized to athletes. Opportunities for injury prevention might include promoting injury-prevention measures more vigorously among players of Pacific Island ethnicity, ensuring injured players are fully rehabilitated before returning to play, reducing the effects of ground hardness through ground preparation and stricter enforcement of the laws relating to foul play.[2]

The cartilage in your knee acts as shock absorbers. These shock absorbers cushion the movement between your thigh bone and your shin bone. You can have a slight tear of your cartilage or a more severe tear. With a slight tear, you may have mild to moderate pain and experience a clicking sound when you move your knee. When you have a severe cartilage tear, your knee may give way. It can also get stuck in a bent position. With a severe tear, your knee will be painful and you will notice swelling about your knee. A plain x-ray of your knee can be helpful in the diagnosis of the cause of your knee pain.

A loose body in your knee may be noted in an imaging study. An MRI image may or may not be useful. An arthroscopy can be helpful in diagnosing the cause of your pain. There is a chance that you may need surgical treatment of your torn cartilage. You should stop sports following your injury. You should not squat or kneel. You should apply ice to your knee when it swells and elevate your knee. You may need crutches so that you can avoid weight bearing.

A pull-on knee brace can provide you with relief. If you still have pain after two weeks, your doctor may want to aspirate the swelling about your knee. If you still have pain at four weeks, you will probably be referred to an orthopedic surgeon. You need to be aware that a knee injury can predispose you to premature arthritis. Physical therapy does not play an important role in the treatment of a cartilage tear. Sometimes a steroid injection into your knee will prove helpful.

You have probably suffered an ankle sprain. An ankle sprain is a partial tear of the ligaments of your ankle joint. Your ligaments can be pulled away from the location where they attach to your bones. A sprain can be classified as acute, recurrent, or chronic. If it is an acute sprain, you may have recently stepped off a high curb and come down wrong on your foot. You may have tried to turn a corner while running and your ankle suddenly gave out. I was playing basketball and jumped up and landed on the side of my foot. All of these instances are examples of an acute sprain.

Did you ever injure your ankle years ago and were recently playing basketball and re-injured your ankle? This is an example of a recurrent sprain. Did you ever injure your ankle years ago but continued to have weakness and pain in your ankle? This is an example of a chronic sprain. Usually following an acute sprain your ankle will be swollen and may be discolored on the side of the injury.

Have you had a previous ankle injury and every time you play basketball your ankle gives out? This could be the result of a chronic sprain. Your ligament may not have healed properly if you continue to have chronic pain. When this happens, you should be examined by your doctor. If you have had an ankle injury, you will have tenderness and swelling over the injured side. If you try to move your ankles sideways, you will have an aggravation of your pain.

In an acute injury, your range of motion about your ankle will be limited. With chronic pain, your range of motion will be greater. Your doctor will examine you for lack of stability of your ankle. If you have a minor ankle sprain, you will have tenderness over one of your ankle bones. These ankle bones are projections that stick out to the right and left of your ankle that is, perpendicular to your ankle. You will usually have tenderness about one of these ankle bones or both. Your acute pain can be so intense that you may have the pain while the doctor tries to examine you. You must, therefore, tell your doctor if the examination is painful. As your symptoms resolve, you may have pain with movement of your ankle. Your pain will improve gradually.

You may develop pain on the outer side of your ankle, which can be a result of a tendon injury. This tendon is called the peroneus. Sometimes the bone that forms your fifth toe could have a small fracture. When your pain has resolved, your range of motion should return to normal. After your pain subsides, you may continue to have instability of your ankle. If you rock your ankle back and forth with your hand, you may notice a knocking about your ankle. This could signify a separation of your tibia and fibula, which are the two lower bones in your leg. The lower parts of these bones form your ankle joint. If you notice this problem, consult a doctor. A chronic instability of your ankle could lead to a decreased range of motion about your ankle as well as pain with motion. As a result, you may develop arthritis of your ankle.

Following an ankle injury, you may have pain about your inner ankle or about your outer ankle. Pain just behind your inner ankle bone usually results from a tendon injury. This type of injury usually develops slowly. It can get progressively worse. If you sustain trauma to your ankle, you may injure this tendon. When this happens, your ankle may swell. This type of injury is usually caused by running or jumping sports. A lack of a proper warm-up or a lack of conditioning can contribute to this injury. This injury can be seen in soccer players or kickers in football who kick with the inner aspects of their foot. If you have an injury, stop exercising until your pain improves. Apply ice to the painful area. Also elevate your foot and ankle on a pillow. Remember that you may re-injure yourself if your injury is not properly treated.

If your pain persists for a prolonged period, your doctor may have you do physical therapy and may possibly prescribe an orthotic for you to be placed in your shoe. Remember that you should see your doctor if your acute injury does not resolve in four to seven days. Your primary care doctor may even refer you to an orthopedic surgeon. Steroid injections may provide you with relief if other modalities fail. You may need x-rays of your ankle to exclude a tear of your ligament from your bone. Upon examination of the x-ray, your doctor may notice small flecks of bone. If your pain persists beyond your normal healing time, a magnetic resonance imaging (MRI) scan may be necessary.

The overall goal of treatment is to allow your injury to heal. As previously stated, immediately after the injury you should apply ice and rest the ankle. You should also limit weight bearing. You can immobilize your ankle with an Ace wrap. You may need to temporarily use a crutch.

Usually after a week or two you can begin to do some stretching exercises. You may need to wear a Velcro ankle brace or high-top tennis shoes at this time. You should not engage in stop-and-go sports such as basketball, running, or impact aerobics. You must realize that injury healing is measured in months rather than weeks.

You need to be patient following an orthopedic injury. If you still hurt after six weeks, your doctor will probably give you an injection with a steroid as well as numbing medicine. The injection can be repeated again in two to four weeks if your pain has not significantly improved. After four weeks, you will need to increase your stretching exercises. Three to four days after your initial injury, you may notice that heat provides you with pain relief. Not only can a tendon about your outer ankle be injured, the ligament about your ankle can be injured as well.

Ligaments attach bone to bone and thus stabilize your ankle. You may experience a snap if your ligaments are injured. It takes several hours for swelling and pain to occur. Pain with this injury is similar to that when you injure your peroneal tendon. Treatment for this injury is the same as the pain associated with your peroneal tendon. You must stop activity, elevate your leg, and wrap your ankle in ice. If the pain persists, you must see a doctor. Do not attempt to bear weight on the ankle until you have a decrease in your pain. You may need physical therapy as well as injection therapy. If your pain has not improved over time and if your ligaments are totally ruptured, for example, if your arm, leg, hands, or foot does not move when you consciously try to move, you may need orthopedic surgery. If a total tear of your ligament is suspected, see an orthopedic surgeon quickly. The longer you wait the less chance that surgery will be successful.

You can also sprain your inner ankle. This happens if you have an injury where your ankle collapses inward, such as from playing football or basketball. The treatment for this injury is the same as the treatment for the outer ankle injury. Whenever you have an ankle sprain, remember that improper immobilization with improper healing can cause you to have a weak ankle, which will subject you to recurrent injury. If you need medications, usually a nonsteroidal anti-inflammatory medication will help you control your pain.

An injury to your foot and ankle is not uncommon because your feet and ankles are under a lot of stress. They support the weight of your body. You need to know that your foot has 26 joints in each foot. Furthermore, in your foot and ankles you have 15 different tendons. You also have 10 different ligaments and several bursas. With all of these anatomic structures, it is easy for you to realize that your foot and ankle can be a common source of pain if you are physically active.

Your foot and ankle act independently of each other. Examine your foot and ankle. The ankle bones are at the very ends of your lower leg bones. These two bones are connected to each other and to your foot by ligaments. Within your ankle is a joint that enables you to walk on uneven surfaces. You have a strong ligament that attaches the muscle of your calf to your heel. This tendon is called your Achilles tendon. Your foot has tendons and muscles that help pull your toes downward or pull your toes upward toward.

Another relatively common orthopedic injury is an injury about your ankle, which is an Achilles tendon injury. If you have injured your Achilles tendon, you will experience tenderness above your heel. If you try to press your foot down to the floor, you will have an aggravation of your pain. If you bring your ankle back toward your knee, you will feel pain as well. Usually your range of motion about your ankle will be normal. The tendon attaches your calf muscle to your ankle. An x-ray will not help with the diagnosis of an Achilles tendonitis. An MRI scan will help with the diagnosis.

There is scarce information on rugby league injuries in female players. It appears that females incur substantially fewer injuries than males.[3] In a post-concussion evaluation study that is of critical clinical relevance in males, African Americans and Whites did not differ significantly on baseline or post-concussion verbal memory, visual memory, reaction time, and total reported symptoms.[4] Regardless of race/ethnicity, there were significant decrements in computerized neurocognitive performance and increased symptoms following a concussion. Professional football players deficient in vitamin D levels may be at greater risk of bone fractures than White players. Black professional football players have a higher rate of vitamin D deficiency than do white players.[5] In children, more white children fracture bones than black and mixed ancestry children.[6] Female athletes sustained a higher rate of concussion and, in all sports except lacrosse, had greater time loss from concussion than male athletes.[7]

You have a bursa about your Achilles tendon. This bursa can become inflamed. If this occurs, you will have pain in the back of your heel. X-rays are not helpful in the diagnosis of a bursitis in this area. Usually the diagnosis is made if you have pain immediately above your heel. An injection of local anesthetic in this area can confirm the diagnosis. Your doctor may apply a steroid. Injection may be repeated.

You should have physical therapy. Occasionally your doctor may want to immobilize your ankle.

If you are doing repetitive exercises, you may injure one of the joints in your body. A joint is an area that exists between two bones. Your knee is an example of a joint. Your joint is surrounded by a tissue called a joint capsule. Within your joint is a fluid that is called synovial fluid. This is a viscous liquid that lubricates your joint. Your joint capsule contains many pain fibers. When this capsule becomes inflamed, you may have a painful joint. When your joint is injured, fluid increases in your joint, which can cause you pain. This increase in the fluid in your joint can decrease the range of motion of your joint.

Exercise may cause you to have shoulder pain. You may also sustain a rotator cuff tendon tear. This tendon attaches a muscle to the bone in your upper arm called the humerus. A tear in this tendon can cause weakness and pain in your shoulder. You may sustain this injury if you fall or do violent pulls on a starter cable. Excessive pushing and pulling can cause tears as well. These tears usually respond to stretch exercises as well as nonsteroidal anti-inflammatory medications. On occasion, you may need an injection with a steroid. If you do not respond to conservative care within four weeks, see an orthopedic surgeon. If you have a moderate to large rotator cuff tendon tear, you are a probable candidate for surgery.

Sports-related injuries are common and often patients do not obtain healthcare for these injuries. Among Americans with a sports-related injury, those who are Black, and those who lack insurance or a usual source of care, are at risk for not obtaining care.[8] With respect to sports injuries, you must try to avoid injury. Avoid the urge to run too much too soon. Take time off if you feel pain. Change your training routines. Get proper rest between high-intensity workouts. Stretch before and after exercise regimens. The femur, hip bone, patella (knee cap), tibia, fibula, and foot are common areas for sports-related injuries and pain as described in the sections on knee pain, ankle pain, Achilles tendon pain, and foot pain. Among Americans with a sports-related injury those who are Black, and those who lack insurance or a usual source of care, are at risk for not obtaining care for an injury.[8]

A total of 865 members of the U.S. military underwent repair of Achilles tendon ruptures at U.S. military hospitals during calendar years 1994, 1995, and 1996. Participation in the game of basketball accounted for 64.9% of all injuries in Black patients and 34.0% of all injuries in nonblack patients. Among those injured, blacks had a significantly increased risk for injury related to playing basketball than nonblack individuals.[9] There appears to be a significant relative predisposition toward lower-extremity major tendon rupture in Black U. S. service members when compared to white service members.[10] In a large sample of military recruits examined for stress fractures, it was found that stress fracture risk was elevated among recruits who were female, older, had lower body weight, had lower BMI, and/or were not of black race/ethnicity.[11] Stress fracture risk was elevated among recruits who were female, older, had lower body weight, had lower BMI, and/or were not of black race/ethnicity.[11,12]

With the increasing number of adolescent females participating in organized athletics, there has been concern over their susceptibility to injury during participation. Females were found to have a lower percentage of abnormalities of the hips, knees, and ankles than males.[13] Black males had a significantly higher rate of hip abnormalities than White males, and Black females had a higher rate of knee abnormalities than white females.

The number of injuries in male and female soccer players has decreased over the past decade.[14] A higher injury rate was seen in men but proportionally, females sustained more severe injuries. Female basketball players are more likely to tear their anterior cruciate ligament than are their male counterparts.[15] Tear rates in the Women's National Basketball Association vary by racial group, with White European American players having more than 6 times the anterior cruciate ligament tear rate of other ethnic groups combined.

There are gender-specific differences with respect to sports injuries. Women suffer certain sports injuries more than men. Women are at greater risk of injury to the anterior cruciate ligament in the knee, the kneecap, and knee joint, as well as cartilage in the knee, than are men playing the same sports. In contrast, ankle injuries show no gender-specific differences. Stress fracture in female military recruits was not correlated with bone density or calcium intake during adolescence.[16] Running had the lowest percentage of injuries and basketball had the highest percentage. Caucasians have been found to have a higher risk for stress fractures than African-American military recruits.[17]

The most frequently injured body regions were the foot and the ankle in basketball, volleyball, soccer, and running, but in wrestling, the knee. These findings suggest that injury rates are associated with the sport rather than sex of player, and the most frequently injured body regions are the lower extremities.[18] Measures of bending strengths in the forefoot are lower in females than males, and in European Americans than in African Americans, which corresponds to the respective rates of general metatarsal stress fracture in these groups.[19]

Studies are also currently being done looking at the effect of exercise on pre- and postmenopausal women. By comparing these two groups, the effects of hormones on sports injuries may be more easily studied. The question that remains to be answered is why women have a higher injury rate than men. Progesterone stimulates the injury healing process in connective tissue in women. It is imperative for the female athlete to keep her progesterone levels at the maximum level to keep ligaments and tendons strong.

You should also know that women with menstrual disturbances are at a greater risk of a sports injury. Menstrual disturbances are more prevalent in female athletes than in the general female population. Stress fractures are more frequent in female athletes with such disturbances. Lower estrogen levels may be associated with such conditions. Lower estrogen levels may have a negative effect on bone strength as well as the retention of calcium within the women's bones.

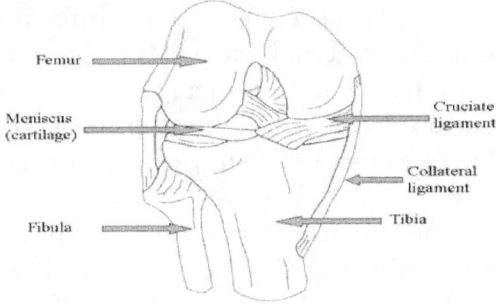

Figure 1. Knee injuries frequently occur in sports injuries.

With respect to anterior cruciate ligament injuries in women, women who are mid-cycle in their menstrual cycle are more prone to anterior cruciate ligament injuries. Hormonal differences between men and women influence a tendency toward ligament laxity in women. This ligament laxity may predispose women to sports injuries. Ligament laxity also increases during pregnancy. The anterior cruciate ligament tear rate for White European American players in the Women's National Basketball Association vary by racial group, with White European American players having more than 6 times the anterior cruciate ligament tear rate of other ethnic groups combined.[15]

High-energy intakes during the Iron Man triathlons help male athletes to accomplish faster times but have the opposite effect on females. In other words, increasing carbohydrate ingestion during the running portion of the contest may help improve performance in male athletes but not in female athletes. The reason for this finding is unknown. On the other hand, men show greater fatigue during exercise and slower recovery time than women.

Rugby is a fast sport and involves contact between players. During a club rugby season in New Zealand, it was found that the rate of injury in games decreased significantly over time in both males and females.[20] No differences were found when examined by gender, playing position, age, and ethnicity or by health and fitness types.

Women don't slow down as much as men do when they are running a marathon. This is because males may have lower fat-burning properties than females. Fat burning does provide an athlete with energy. As you can see, there are differences among studies comparing men and women athletes. The reason for this controversy appears to be hormonal. For this reason, hormonal studies with respect to athletic performance continue to be studied.

Physical therapy may help in the management of your pain and possibly prevent its reoccurrence. When you suffer the initial pain, ice, massage, and padding are indicated. Ice needs to be applied for at least 10 minutes to exert its effect. Injection therapy may also provide you with relief. Proper warm-up techniques before exercise activities and cool-down techniques after exercise activities can help prevent some sports-related injuries.

Physical therapy and stretching exercises can help relieve muscle pain from a sports-related injury. Rest, ice, compression, and elevation for strains and sprains will help decrease your pain. Over-the-counter pain medications such as ibuprofen and Tylenol can help reduce the pain and inflammation caused by your injury. Your doctor may want to prescribe muscle relaxants to help your muscles recoup from the injury.

References

1.   Centers for Disease C, Prevention. Trends in strength training--United States, 1998-2004. MMWR Morb Mortal Wkly Rep. 2006;55(28):769-772.

2.   Chalmers DJ, Samaranayaka A, Gulliver P, McNoe B. Risk factors for injury in rugby union football in New Zealand: a cohort study. Br J Sports Med. 2012;46(2):95-102.

3.   King DA, Hume PA, Milburn P, Gianotti S. Women's rugby league injury claims and costs in New Zealand. Br J Sports Med. 2010;44(14):1016-1023.

4.   Kontos AP, Elbin RJ, 3rd, Covassin T, Larson E. Exploring differences in computerized neurocognitive concussion testing between African American and White athletes. Arch Clin Neuropsychol. 2010;25(8):734-744.

5.   Maroon JC, Mathyssek CM, Bost JW, et al. Vitamin D profile in National Football League players. Am J Sports Med. 2015;43(5):1241-1245.

6.   Thandrayen K, Norris SA, Pettifor JM. Fracture rates in urban South African children of different ethnic origins: the Birth to Twenty cohort. Osteoporos Int. 2009;20(1):47-52.

7.   Covassin T, Moran R, Elbin RJ. Sex Differences in Reported Concussion Injury Rates and Time Loss From Participation: An Update of the National Collegiate Athletic Association Injury Surveillance Program From 2004-2005 Through 2008-2009. J Athl Train. 2016.

8.   Gutierrez G, Sills M, Bublitz CD, Westfall JM. Sports-related injuries in the United States: who gets care and who does not. Clin J Sport Med. 2006;16(2):136-141.

9.   Davis JJ, Mason KT, Clark DA. Achilles tendon ruptures stratified by age, race, and cause of injury among active duty U.S. Military members. Mil Med. 1999;164(12):872-873.

10.   Owens B, Mountcastle S, White D. Racial differences in tendon rupture incidence. Int J Sports Med. 2007;28(7):617-620.

11.   Knapik J, Montain SJ, McGraw S, Grier T, Ely M, Jones BH. Stress fracture risk factors in basic combat training. Int J Sports Med. 2012;33(11):940-946.

12.   Wright AA, Taylor JB, Ford KR, Siska L, Smoliga JM. Risk factors associated with lower extremity stress fractures in runners: a systematic review with meta-analysis. Br J Sports Med. 2015;49(23):1517-1523.

13.   DuRant RH, Linder CW, Sanders JM, Jr., Jay S, Brantley G, Bedgood R. Adolescent females' readiness to participate in sports. Sex and race differences in the preparticipation athletic examination. J Adolesc Health Care. 1988;9(4):310-314.

14.   Mufty S, Bollars P, Vanlommel L, Van Crombrugge K, Corten K, Bellemans J. Injuries in male versus female soccer players: epidemiology of a nationwide study. Acta Orthop Belg. 2015;81(2):289-295.

15.   Trojian TH, Collins S. The anterior cruciate ligament tear rate varies by race in professional Women's basketball. Am J Sports Med. 2006;34(6):895-898.

16.   Cline AD, Jansen GR, Melby CL. Stress fractures in female army recruits: implications of bone density, calcium intake, and exercise. J Am Coll Nutr. 1998;17(2):128-135.

17.   Nattiv A. Stress fractures and bone health in track and field athletes. J Sci Med Sport. 2000;3(3):268-279.

18.   Dane S, Can S, Gursoy R, Ezirmik N. Sport injuries: relations to sex, sport, injured body region. Percept Mot Skills. 2004;98(2):519-524.

19.   Griffin NL, Richmond BG. Cross-sectional geometry of the human forefoot. Bone. 2005;37(2):253-260.

20.   Alsop JC, Chalmers DJ, Williams SM, Quarrie KL, Marshall SW, Sharples KJ. Temporal patterns of injury during a rugby season. J Sci Med Sport. 2000;3(2):97-109.

Index